Common Clinical Dilemmas in Percutaneous Coronary Interventions

T0100695

Common Clinical Dilemmas in Percutaneous Coronary Interventions

Editors

Eulógio E Martinez MD PhD
Director, Cardiac Catheterization and
Interventional Cardiology
Heart Institute (InCor)
University of Sao Paulo Medical School.
and
Professor of Medicine
Federal University of Sao Paulo
Sao Paulo
Brazil

Pedro A Lemos MD PhD
Senior Interventional Cardiologist
Heart Institute (InCor)
University of Sao Paulo Medical School
Sao Paulo
Brazil

Andrew TL Ong MBBS FRACP
Consultant Cardiologist
Department of Cardiology
Westmead Hospital
Sydney
Australia

Patrick W Serruys MD PhD FACC FESC
Department of Interventional Cardiology
Thorax Centre
Erasmus Medical Center
Rotterdam
The Netherlands

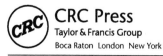

CRC Press
Taylor & Francis Group
Boca Raton London New York

CRC Press is an imprint of the
Taylor & Francis Group, an **informa** business

CRC Press
Taylor & Francis Group
6000 Broken Sound Parkway NW, Suite 300
Boca Raton, FL 33487-2742

First issued in paperback 2019

© 2007 by Taylor & Francis Group, LLC
CRC Press is an imprint of Taylor & Francis Group, an Informa business

No claim to original U.S. Government works

ISBN-13: 978-1-84184-609-5 (hbk)
ISBN-13: 978-0-367-38946-8 (pbk)

A CIP record for this book is available from the British Library.

Library of Congress Cataloging-in-Publication Data available on application

Visit the Taylor & Francis Web site at
http://www.taylorandfrancis.com

and the CRC Press Web site at
http://www.crcpress.com

Contents

Contributors

Alexander Abizaid MD PhD
*Institute Dante Pazzanese
   of Cardiology
Ibirapuera, Sao Paulo
Brazil*

John A Ambrose MD FACC
*Professor of Medicine
University of California, San Francisco
and
Chief of Cardiology
University of California, San Francisco
Fresno
and
Director of Cardiology
Community Regional Medical Center
Fresno, CA
USA*

Dominic J Angiolillo MD PhD
*Division of Cardiology
University of Florida
Jacksonville·
and
Cardiovascular Imaging Core
   Laboratories
Jacksonville, FL
USA*

David Antoniucci MD
*Division of Cardiology
Careggi Hospital
Florence
Italy*

Chourmouzios Arampatzis MD PhD
*Senior Interventional Cardiologist
Interbalkan Medical Center
Thessaloniki
Greece*

Federica Baldazzi MD
*Institute of Cardiology–University
   of Bologna
Policlinico S. Orsola–Malpighi Bologna
Italy*

Theodore Bass MD
*Division of Cardiology
University of Florida
Jacksonville, FL
USA*

Fatih Bayrak MD
*Department of Cardiology
Yeditipe University Hospital
Kozyatağı
Istanbul
Turkey*

Leonardo C Clavijo MD PhD
*Washington Hospital Center
Washington DC
USA*

Marc Cohen MD
*Division of Cardiology
Newark Beth Israel Medical Center
Newark, NJ
USA*

Antonio Colombo MD
*EMO Centro Cuore Columbus
and
San Raffaele Hospital
Milan
Italy*

John T Coppola
*Comprehensive Cardiovascular Center
Saint Vincent Catholic Medical
   Centers of New York
New York, NY
USA*

Marco A Costa MD PhD
*Division of Cardiology
University of Florida
Jacksonville
and
Cardiovascular Imaging Core Laboratories
Jacksonville, FL
USA*

Marcus N da Gama MD
Heart Institute (InCor)
University of Sao Paulo Medical School
Sao Paulo
Brazil

Muzaffer Degertekin MD PhD
Department of Cardiology
Yeditipe University Hospital
Kozyatağı
Istanbul
Turkey

Jean-Bernard Durand MD
Division of Cardiology
MD *Anderson Hospital*
Houston, TX
USA

Antonio Esteves Filho MD
Heart Institute (InCor)
University of Sao Paulo Medical School
Sao Paulo
Brazil

Pedro de Araújo Gonçalves MD
Serviço de Cardiologia
Hospital de Santa Cruz
Carnaxide
Portugal

Luis A Guzman MD
Assistant Professor of Medicine
University of Florida College of Medicine
and
Director, Peripheral Vascular Disease
   Interventional Program
The Cardiovascular Center
Jacksonville, FL
USA

Timothy D Henry MD
Director of Research
Minneapolis Heart Institute
and
Professor of Medicine
University of Minnesota
Minneapolis, MN
USA

David R Holmes Jr MD
Mayo Clinic
Rochester, MN
USA

Pedro E Horta MD
Heart Institute (InCor)
University of Sao Paulo Medical School
Sao Paulo
Brazil

Aamer H Jamali MD
Cedars-Sinai Medical Center
Los Angeles, CA
USA

Pilar Jimenez-Quevedo MD
Stem Cell Research Center
Texas Heart Institute at St Luke's
   Episcopal Hospital
Houston, TX
USA

Luiz J Kajita MD
Heart Institute (InCor)
University of Sao Paulo Medical
   School
Sao Paulo
Brazil

Giannis Kanonidis MD PhD
Professor of Cardiology
Hippokrateion Hospital
Thessaloniki
Greece

Gary E Lane MD
Director, Cardiac Catheterization
   Laboratory
Mayo Clinic
Jacksonville, FL
USA

David M Larson MD
Clinical Associate Professor
University of Minnesota
   Medical School and Emergency
   Medicine
Ridgeview Medical Center
Waconia, MN
USA

Pedro A Lemos MD PhD
Senior Interventional Cardiologist
Heart Institute (InCor)
University of Sao Paulo Medical
   School
Sao Paulo
Brazil

Raj R Makkar MD
Cedars-Sinai Medical Center
Los Angeles, CA
USA

Antonio Marzocchi MD
Head of the Catheterization Laboratory
Institute of Cardiology–University of
  Bologna
Policlinico S. Orsola–Malpighi Bologna
Italy

Eulógio E Martinez MD PhD
Director, Cardiac Catheterization
  and Interventional Cardiology
Heart Institute (InCor)
University of Sao Paulo Medical School
and
Professor of Medicine
Federal University of Sao Paulo
Sao Paulo
Brazil

Luiz Alberto Mattos MD
Institute Dante Pazzanese of Cardiology
São Paulo
Brazil

Nestor F Mercado MD PhD
Division of Cardiovascular Diseases
Scripps Clinic
La Jolla, CA
USA

Nicolai Mejevoi MD
Division of Cardiology
Newark Beth Israel Medical Center
Newark, NJ
USA

Roxana Mehran MD
Associate Professor of Medicine
Director, Outcomes Research Data
  Coordination and Analysis
Center for Interventional Vascular
  Therapies
Columbia University Medical Center,
and
Director, Data Coordinating and
  Analysis Center, Cardiovascular
  Research Foundation
New York, NY
USA

Douglass A Morrison MD PhD
The Cardiac Catheterization Laboratories
SAVAHCS
and
The Sarver Heart Center
University of Arizona College
  of Medicine
Tucson, AZ
USA

Bülent Mutlu MD
Department of Cardiology
Yeditipe University Hospital
Kozyatağı
Istanbul
Turkey

Marc C Newell MD
Chief Resident, Internal Medicine
Abbott Northwestern Hospital
Minneapolis, MN
USA

Eugenia Nikolsky MD PhD FACC
Director, Clinical Research in Invasive
  Cardiology
Rambam Medical Center
Haifa
Israel

Tugrul Okay MD
International Hospital,
  Department of Cardiology
Istanbul
Turkey

Andrew TL Ong MBBS FRACP
Consultant Cardiologist,
  Department of Cardiology
Westmead Hospital
Sydney, Australia

Emerson C Perin MD PhD
Stem Cell Research Center
Texas Heart Institute at
  St Luke's Episcopal Hospital
Houston, TX
USA

Marco A Perin MD PhD
Heart Institute (InCor)
University of Sao Paulo Medical School
Sao Paulo
Brazil

Augusto Pichard MD
Cardiac Catheterization Laboratory
Washington Hospital Center
Washington DC
USA

Pilar Jiménez Quevedo MD
Texas Heart Institute
Houston, TX
USA

Henning Rasmussen MD
Associate Professor of Medicine
University of California
San Francisco, CA
USA

Expeditio Ribeiro MD
Heart Institute (InCor)
University of Sao Paulo Medical School
Sao Paulo
Brazil

Francesco Saia MD PhD
Institute of Cardiology–University of
   Bologna
Policlinico S. Orsola–Malpighi Bologna
Italy

Ricardo Seabra-Gomes MD PhD FACC FESC
Instituto do Coração
Carnaxide
Portugal

Patrick W Serruys MD PhD FACC FASC
Department of Interventional
   Cardiology
Thorax Centre, Erasmus Medical
   Center
Rotterdam
The Netherlands

Guilherme V Silva MD
Stem Cell research Center
Texas Heart Institute at
   St Luke's Episcopal Hospital
Houston, TX
USA

Jose A Silva MD FACC FESC FSCAI
Tchefuncte Cardiovascular Associates
   and TCA Research
Covington, LA
USA

Manel Sabaté Tenas MD PhD
Unitat de Cardiologia Intervencionista
Hospital Universitari de Sant Pau
Barcelona
Spain

J Eduardo Sousa MD PhD
Instituto Dante Pazzanese de Cardiologia
São Paulo
Brazil

Goran Stankovic MD
Institute for Cardiovascular Diseases
Clinical Center of Serbia
Belgrade
Serbia

Christopher J White MD
Department of Cardiology, Ochsner Clinic
   and Alton Ochsner Medical Foundation
New Orleans, LA
USA

Philip T Zeni Jr MD
Memphis Interventional Radiology Clinic
Baptist Memorial Hospital
Memphis, TN
USA

Preface

Percutaneous coronary intervention (PCI) is rapidly becoming the first choice for myocardial revascularization in all forms of presentation of significant coronary artery disease.

In the era of drug-eluting stents the combination of high success rate and very low acute and late events prompted cardiologists and interventionalists to extend the indications of percutaneous interventions for clinical and angiographic presentations that were considered limitations to the technique just a few years ago.

Of all medical specialties, interventional cardiology is perhaps the one in which evidence-based medicine has been more extensively applied, ever since its birth when Andreas Gruntzig did the first balloon angioplasty, about 30 years ago. Strategies for the prevention of complications (stent thrombosis, restenosis, access site bleeding, acute intraprocedural ischemic episodes), or for the improvement in success rate (stents, devices for atheroablation, intracoronary ultrasound, etc) were all carefully evaluated by well-designed trials. This explains the constant changes in pharmacological adjunct therapy and in the rate of utilization of many devices in a relatively short time span. New challenges presented by treatment of total chronic coronary occlusions, the identification of plaques with increased risk of rupture and how to deal with them, treatment of bifurcation lesions, etc, are the subject of important ongoing investigations.

Although most patients referred for PCI are treated according to guidelines derived from results of multicentered randomized studies, important decisions have to be made on an individual basis, without the help of information provided by major trials, in many instances due to patient selection, as is the case in patients of very old age, and in some angiographic characteristics (ostial lesions, chronic total occlusions, very long lesions), usually excluded from randomization.

More challenging are clinical dilemmas that will probably never be addressed by major trials, due either to the relative rarity of the condition, to problems in comparing results of different treatment options, or to lack of financial support. Additionally, well-conducted major trials addressing a specific issue may yield conflicting results.

In this book many of the chapters deal with different situations in which decision making will be dependent upon clinical judgment based on individual experience and on data from less-conclusive clinical studies. Among the interventional scenarios here dealt with include the following:

- decisions regarding problems related to comorbidities, like PCI for coronary disease in patients with renal failure, in dialysis, and post-renal transplant; risks associated with interaction of iodine contrast agents and antidiabetic drugs
- choice of adjunct pharmacological therapy for patients with a past history of immunoallergic syndromes triggered by iodine contrast agents, aspirin, or IIb/IIIa inhibitors; management of patients with known aspirin and/or clopidogrel resistance
- dose adjustments for patients with prior use of oral anticoagulants, thrombolytic agents, and potent antiplatelet drugs.

- decisions regarding management and indication of percutaneous circulatory support for patients with hemodynamic complications of coronary artery disease (CAD), specifically represented by stable syndromes and very depressed left ventricular function, and acute syndromes complicated by cardiogenic shock
- options related to timing of interventions: indication for *ad hoc* angioplasty, for simultaneous treatment of culprit and non-culprit lesions in acute coronary syndromes, for staged percutaneous revascularization in multivessel disease, and for combined or staged interventions in patients with associated coronary, carotid and peripheral disease
- decisions regarding management of acute intraprocedural complications, like coronary dissection or perfuration, the no-reflow phenomenon, and distal coronary embolization
- patient selection for percutaneous intervention in massive pulmonary embolism, end-stage aortic stenosis, and hypertrophic cardiomyopathy.

To accomplish our goals, we have invited several internationally known leaders in the field of interventional cardiology.

We hope that this unique in-depth presentation of challenging patients and procedural subsets will be of great value to clinical as well as interventional cardiologists worldwide.

Eulógio E Martinez

1

Immunoallergic syndromes in interventional cardiology

Chourmouzios A Arampatzis, Giannis Kanonidis, and Patrick W Serruys

Percutaneous coronary intervention has become the dominant form of revascularization in patients with atherosclerotic disease. We have witnessed an enormous evolution in materials and equipment that has minimized the procedural risks. However, there are still complications that every physician should bear in mind.

The aim of the present chapter is to focus on issues regarding immunoallergic syndromes such as iodine contrast reactions, aspirin allergy, heparin and post-IIb/IIIa inhibitor thrombocytopenia.

The development of well-tolerated contrast agents has created conditions of maximal safety during the procedure. Currently, iodinated agents are mainly used in the interventional suites.[1] These agents have benzene rings with three bound iodine atoms, termed tri-iodinated. Ionic agents are bound to a non-radiopaque cation that results in a highly soluble, low-viscosity but high-osmolar (two particles per iodinated ring) contrast agent. On the other hand, non-ionic contrast agents are not bound with cations since they have no electrical charge, and this results in lower osmolality (one particle per ring) which improves the safety profile but increases viscosity. A large study demonstrated that the use of non-ionic agents, particularly in cardiac interventions is associated with fewer adverse events.[2] Allergic reactions to the contrast agent can be either anaphylactoid (caused by activation of the kinin system, and the activated basophils or mast cells would be directly stimulated by the contrast agent or indirectly by non-specifically activated complements), or chemotoxic (caused by the hydrophobicity and hyperosmoticity of the contrast media itself).[3] Allergic reactions range from mild inconvenience, such as itching, nausea or vomiting, to life-threatening emergencies, such as dyspnea, shock, or cardiopulmonary arrest. The overall incidence is lower with low- as compared to high-osmolality agents (Figure 1.1). However the difference is primarily due to minor reactions such as nausea, vomiting, and urticaria.

The incidence of reactions to contrast media varies between 4.6 and 8.5%. True anaphylaxis occurs in 1%, and death in 0.001–0.009% of patients who receive contrast media.[4] There are no specific diagnostic tests to track down patients susceptible to contrast media reactions. Atopy is a predisposing factor, and patients with a previous reaction have a 17–35% chance of recurrence.

When conditions such as active asthma, significant allergies, impaired cardiac function, blood–brain barrier breakdown, and marked anxiety are present, the use of a low-osmolality contrast agent is indicated, since the risk of developing contrast

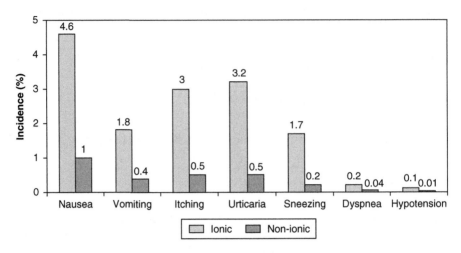

Figure 1.1   Incidence of allergic reactions.

allergy is high. The physician should be alerted when the relevant history of the patient is suspicious of allergy. Accordingly he should be able to recognize the clinical signs and symptoms of the allergic reaction. True anaphylactoid reaction may be presented with agitation, shortness of breath, stridor, wheezing, and changes in blood pressure. Dermal reactions might be present such as urticaria, pruritus, and skin flushing. A more severe reaction might present with mucosal edema, severe bronchoconstriction, and/or laryngeal edema. Generalized edema may present with edematous eyelids or perioral edema. Once the allergic reaction occurs there should be a treatment algorithm, and a subsequent protocol in order to restrain the allergy (Table 1.1).

There is no clear evidence that any regimen prevents severe reactions. Steroid pretreatment prevents mild reactions.[2] The only regimen found effective to date is methylprednisolone 32 mg orally, given 12 and 2 hours prior to intravenous (IV) contrast use.[5] Concurrent use of specific H_1, and H_2 blockers has also been recommended. In patients with allergy to iodinated contrast media, X-ray angiography with gadolinium-based contrast media is a potential alternative technique for evaluating coronary artery disease.[6]

Aspirin inhibits platelet cyclooxygenase 1 enzyme (COX 1), and prevents platelet aggregatation. Having been used for more than 100 years, it remains the cornerstone of coronary artery disease therapy. Current guidelines dictate that aspirin is indicated as a class I regimen, unless a true sensitivity reaction exists, in which case, the alternate use of thienopyridine is indicated (clopidogrel, ticlopidine). However, the long-term use of thienopyridines may be associated with severe hematological disorders. Dual antiplatelet therapy is increasingly indicated in a large portion of patients with coronary disease.[7-9]

There are three presentations of allergic reactions seen with aspirin: respiratory (exacerbated respiratory tract disease or AERD), cutaneous (urticaria), and systematic sensitivity (anaphylaxis).[10] The incidence of aspirin–respiratory disease is 10%, and for aspirin-induced urticaria it varies from 0.07 to 0.2% in the general population.[11]

Table 1.1 Treatment algorithm for allergic reactions

Symptoms and signs	Mild/minor	Moderate	Severe
Nausea, vomiting, upper respiratory congestion, limited urticaria	Monitoring vital signs, observe that symptoms do not worsen		
Symptomatic urticaria, mild bronchospasm, vasovagal reaction		Assess airway, 100% O_2, obtain vital signs, benadryl 50 mg IV, hydrocortisone 100 mg IV, albuterol (2.5 mg in 2.5 ml normal saline) inhalation nebulizer, epinephrine (1:1000 0.3 ml subcutaneous), atropine	
Laryngospasm, severe bronchospasm, cardiorespiratory collapse, generalized seizures			Secure airway, 100% O_2 epinephrine (1:10 000 3–5 ml IV or via endotracheal tube), methyl-prednisolone 125 mg or hydrocortisone 500 mg IV

Inhibition of the COX enzyme decreases the levels of prostaglandins (PGs), particularly PGE_2, thus stimulating 5-lipoxygenase-activating protein, and followed by increased secretion of leukotrienes and histamine from mast cells.[12] Leukotrienes increase vascular permeability, and mucus gland secretion, and induce bronchoconstriction (sometimes severe enough to require intubation). Patients prone to aspirin-induced respiratory tract disease usually have a history of asthma, nasal polyps, and/or rhinitis.[11] Clinical manifestations include excessive rhinorrhea, broncospasm, and even laryngospasm. This condition is usually seen in adulthood in 10–15% of asthmatics, and females have a higher prevalence.

Similar to the mechanism described just before, an individual may present with cutaneous reactions to non-steroidal anti-inflammatory drugs (NSAIDs). Indeed, the excess production of leukotrienes triggered initially by COX inhibition induces urticaria and/or angioedema reactions.[13] Atopy seems to play a significant part, since patients with history of asthma, hay fever or urticaria, are more sensitive to developing a cutaneous reaction. Moreover, the occurrence of aspirin-induced urticaria in patients with idiopathic urticaria is 20–30%.[13] Additionally, we may witness 'blended' reactions consisting of a mixed clinical picture of urticaria, angioedema, dyspnea, wheezing, cough, hoarseness, and rhinorrhea.[14]

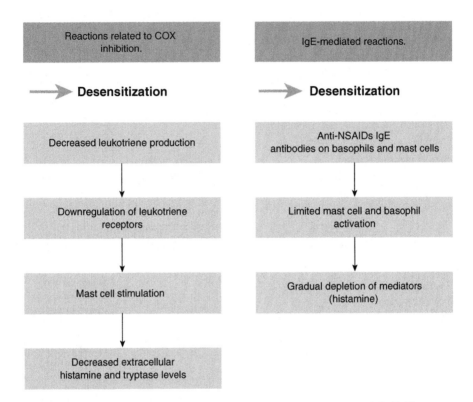

Figure 1.2   Proposed mechanisms of aspirin desensitization. IgE, immunoglobulin E.

Severe allergic reactions such as hypotension, swelling, laryngeal edema, and/or tachypnea occur minutes after aspirin consumption. Since a specific immunoglobulin E against aspirin has not been detected, these reactions are called anaphylactoid.

Aspirin desensitization is the medical process in which increasing oral doses of aspirin eradicate the pharmacological and immunological reactions of the regimen. The desensitization mechanism differs depending on the type of reaction (Figure 1.2). There are no *in vitro* tests that can identify patients with aspirin hypersensitivity, but several desensitization protocols exist.[15] Treatment protocols need the careful surveillance of an internist and an allergist. There are different protocols whether the patient has aspirin-induced respiratory or cutaneous disease (Figure 1.3).[16,17] Some patients are cross-sensitive to NSAIDs that inhibit COX enzymes. In these kinds of patients, desensitization protocols have failed, and when they undergo coronary intervention bare-metal stent implantation along with alternative adjunctive therapy such as IIb/IIIa inhibitors, direct thrombin inhibitors and thienopyridines are indicated.

Heparin-induced thrombocytopenia (HIT) is defined as a decrease in platelet count during or shortly after exposure to the drug. There are two types of HIT. The incidence of type I HIT is 10%; the mechanism is unknown, it is characterized by a mild and transient decrease in platelet count, and, importantly, it is not associated with an increased risk of thrombosis. This disorder disappears when the patient

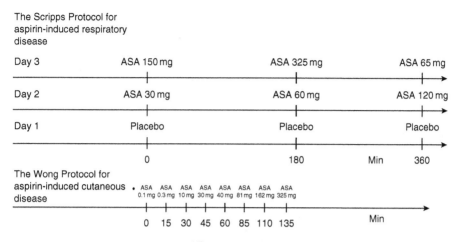

Figure 1.3 Desensitization protocols.[16,17] ASA, acetyl-salicylic acid.

becomes heparin-free.[18,19] Type II HIT is an immune-mediated disorder, and it is associated with a risk of thrombosis. The incidence that triggers this disorder is the formation of heparin-related platelet-activating antibodies that recognize platelet factor 4 bound to heparin. Consequently, platelet activation escalates thrombin generation by activating the coagulation cascade.[18] The incidence of HIT II among the heparinized patients is 1–5%, although it is established that more patients develop antibodies against heparin. HIT is more often seen in patients who receive unfractionated heparin than in those receiving low-molecular-weight heparin. The onset of the disorder might be rapid or delayed. Thrombocytopenia occurs usually between the 5th and 10th day of heparin administration, unless the patient has already been exposed to heparin. Thrombocytopenia is moderate (platelet count 50–$80 \times 10^9/l$), and sometimes is within normal values but less that 50% with respect to the preheparin value. Platelet counts starts to rise 2–3 days after heparin is discontinued, and the antibodies disappear 2–3 months afterwards. The occurrence of thrombosis is associated with a 20–30% mortality.

Warkentin has developed a clinical score for estimating the probability of HIT.[19] Thrombocytopenia, timing, thrombosis, and the absence of other explanations consist of the 4 Ts score as is delineated in Table 1.2. Preliminary evaluation suggest a low probability of developing HIT antibodies (<5%) when a low score is obtained (≤3) and high probability (>80%) when we have high score (≥6). When the clinician suspects HIT, laboratory tests for HIT antibodies must be requested. There are two types of assays for HIT: washed platelet-activating assays, and commercial platelet factor 4/polyanion enzyme immunoassays. A negative test generally rules out HIT, but it is important to interpret the test by estimating all clinical parameters.[19]

When HIT is clinically strongly suspected, in a patient requiring anticoagulation, the following should be observed: removal of the trigger (heparin cessation) is not sufficient to prevent thrombosis, so an alternative non-heparin anticoagulant is required to control thrombin formation. Currently, there are three anticoagulant regimens (danaparoid, lepirudin, and argatroban) that do not cross-react with HIT antibodies. For chronic anticoagulation, treatment is required for at least 2–3 months to prevent recurrence of thrombosis.

Table 1.2   The 'four Ts' test

Score	0	1	2
Thrombocytopenia	>50% platelet decrease to nadir >20%	30–50% platelet decrease or nadir 10–19	<30% platelet decrease or nadir <10
Timing	Days 5–10 or	>10 days or unclear timing	<day 4
Thrombosis	Proven new thrombosis, skin necrosis or acute systemic reaction after intravenous UFH heparin Progressive or recurrent thrombosis, erythematous skin lesions, suspected thrombosis	None	
Other	None evident	Possible	Definite

Several trials have demonstrated that the use of the highly effective antiplatelet drug, the glycoprotein (GP) IIb/IIIa antagonists in the setting of percutaneous coronary interventions are associated with improved clinical outcomes.[20,21] Thrombocytopenia is a complication seen in all the major published trials.[22] The incidence varies from 1.1% to 5.6% (severe thrombocytopenia with platelet count less than $20\times10^9/l$ ranges from 0.1% to 0.5%) depending on the different pharmacokinetic characteristics of the agents, the dose administered and duration of use, repetition of exposure, and the various drugs co-administered with these agents. The exact mechanism of GP IIb/IIIa-induced thrombocytopenia is not yet defined. Fistly, an immune mechanism is suggested in which the binding of the antagonist to GP IIb/IIIa receptors leads to the exposure of ligand-induced binding sites recognized by pre-existing or induced antibodies. Secondly, the receptor–drug metabolite complex itself may induce an immune response. Thrombocytopenia may occur more often with abciximab, and less often with tirofiban and eptifibatide. Patients receiving the above-mentioned drugs should be monitored for thrombocytopenia for 24 h, and for patient receiving abciximab a platelet count at 2 and 4 h after drug infusion is recommended. If the diagnosis of drug-induced thrombocytopenia is suspected, discontinuation of the agent is mandatory, and platelet transfusion considered if the thrombocytopenia is severe. Since these agents are infused mostly in patients with acute coronary syndromes and patients undergoing coronary intervention, aspirin therapy should be continued together with a thienopyridine, unless there is a high risk of major bleeding.

Immunoallergic syndromes in interventional cardiology are not frequent, but their occurrence may be associated with severe adverse events. Every interventional cardiologist should be alerted and familiar with these kinds of clinical scenarios in order to achieve optimal results for the patient.

REFERENCES

1. Kaufman J. Vascular and Interventional Radiology, the Requisites. Philadelphia, PA: Mosby; 2004.
2. Bettmann MA, Heeren T, Greenfield A, Goudey C. Adverse events with radiographic contrast agents: results of the SCVIR Contrast Agent Registry. Radiology 1997; 203: 611–20.
3. Lasser EC, Lang JH, Lyon SG, Hamblin AE. Complement and contrast material reactors. J Allergy Clin Immunol 1979; 64: 105–12.
4. Vervloet D, Durham S. Adverse reactions to drugs. BMJ 1998; 316: 1511–14.
5. Lasser EC, Berry CC, Talner LB et al. Pretreatment with corticosteroids to alleviate reactions to intravenous contrast material. N Engl J Med 1987; 317: 845–9.
6. Spinosa DJ, Kaufmann JA, Hartwell GD. Gadolinium chelates in angiography and interventional radiology: a useful alternative to iodinated contrast media for angiography. Radiology 2002; 223: 319–25; discussion 326–7.
7. Gaspoz JM, Coxson PG, Goldman PA et al. Cost effectiveness of aspirin, clopidogrel, or both for secondary prevention of coronary heart disease. N Engl J Med 2002; 346: 1800–6.
8. Morice MC, Serruys PW, Sousa JE et al. A randomized comparison of a sirolimus-eluting stent with a standard stent for coronary revascularization. N Engl J Med 2002; 346: 1773–80.
9. Moses JW, Leon MB, Popma JJ et al. Sirolimus-eluting stents versus standard stents in patients with stenosis in a native coronary artery. N Engl J Med 2003; 349: 1315–23.
10. Stevenson DD. Aspirin and NSAID sensitivity. Immunol Allergy Clin North Am 2004; 24: 491–505, vii.
11. Gollapudi RR, Teirstein PS, Stevenson DD, Simon RA. Aspirin sensitivity: implications for patients with coronary artery disease. JAMA 2004; 292: 3017–23.
12. Szczeklik A, Stevenson DD. Aspirin-induced asthma: advances in pathogenesis, diagnosis, and management. J Allergy Clin Immunol 2003; 111: 913–21; quiz 922.
13. Sanchez-Borges M, Capriles-Hulett A, Caballero-Fonseca F. Cutaneous reactions to aspirin and nonsteroidal antiinflammatory drugs. Clin Rev Allergy Immunol 2003; 24: 125–36.
14. Stevenson DD, Sanchez-Borges M, Szczeklik A. Classification of allergic and pseudoallergic reactions to drugs that inhibit cyclooxygenase enzymes. Ann Allergy Asthma Immunol 2001; 87: 177–80.
15. Ramanuja S, Breall JA, Kalaria VG. Approach to 'aspirin allergy' in cardiovascular patients. Circulation 2004; 110: e1–4.
16. Szczeklik A, Stevenson DD. Aspirin-induced asthma: advances in pathogenesis and management. J Allergy Clin Immunol 1999; 104: 5–13.
17. Wong JT, Nagy CS, Krinzman SJ, Maclean JA, Bloch KJ. Rapid oral challenge-desensitization for patients with aspirin-related urticaria-angioedema. J Allergy Clin Immunol 2000; 105: 997–1001.
18. Franchini M. Heparin-induced thrombocytopenia: an update. Thromb J 2005; 3: 14.
19. Warkentin TE. Heparin-induced thrombocytopenia: diagnosis and management. Circulation 2004; 110: e454–8.
20. Boersma E, Harrington RA, Moliterno DJ et al. Platelet glycoprotein IIb/IIIa inhibitors in acute coronary syndromes: a meta-analysis of all major randomised clinical trials. Lancet 2002; 359: 189–98.
21. Madan M, Berkowitz SD. Understanding thrombocytopenia and antigenicity with glycoprotein IIb-IIIa inhibitors. Am Heart J 1999; 138: 317–26.
22. Dasgupta H, Blankenship JC, Wood GC et al. Thrombocytopenia complicating treatment with intravenous glycoprotein IIb/IIIa receptor inhibitors: a pooled analysis. Am Heart J 2000; 140: 206–11.

2

The kidney and percutaneous coronary interventions

Eugenia Nikolsky, Alexander Abizaid,
and Roxana Mehran

Definition of chronic renal insufficiency • Impact of chronic renal insufficiency on outcomes after percutaneous coronary intervention • Hemorrhagic complications in relation to chronic renal insufficiency • Adjunctive pharmacotherapy during percutaneous coronary intervention in patients with chronic renal insufficiency • Long-term outcomes post-percutaneous coronary intervention in relation to chronic renal insufficiency • Frequency of angiographic and clinical restenosis in patients with chronic renal insufficiency • Drug-eluting stents in patients with chronic renal insufficiency • Renal function deterioration post-percutaneous coronary intervention in patients with chronic renal insufficiency: contrast-induced nephropathy • Prevention of contrast-induced nephropathy • Targeted renal therapy • Conclusion

Chronic renal insufficiency (CRI) is a prevalent condition in patients undergoing percutaneous coronary revascularization. In a pooled analysis of contemporary trials on percutaneous coronary intervention (PCI), CRI at baseline was present in approximately 25% of the patients,[1] and among patients undergoing primary PCI for acute myocardial infarction (MI), about 20% of the study population had baseline CRI.[2] Despite the high prevalence of CRI in the PCI series, no study assessed prospectively the outcomes of these patients, while the current data are available from the *post hoc* analyses from controlled randomized trials, registries, and observational studies.

DEFINITION OF CHRONIC RENAL INSUFFICIENCY

Glomerular filtration rate (GFR) equal to the sum of the filtration rates in all of the functioning nephrons is the best measure of overall kidney function.[3] The normal level of GFR varies according to age, sex, and body size. Normal GFR in young adults is approximately 120 to 130 ml/min/1.73 m^2, and declines with age. Serum creatinine solely is not a reliable indicator of renal damage, and should not be used to assess the level of kidney function.

Estimation of GFR is used to assess the degree of renal impairment, and provides a rough measure of the number of functioning nephrons.[3] By consensus, chronic renal insufficiency is defined as estimated glomerular filtration rate (eGFR) ≤ 60 ml/min (1.73 m^2), representing loss of half or more of the normal kidney function, or the presence of persistent proteinuria with an albumin/creatinine ratio >30 mg/g in the urine samples.[3] The following most widely used formulae to estimate the GFR include the Cockcroft–Gault and Modification of Diet in Renal Disease (MDRD) equations:

- The Cockcroft–Gault equation takes into account the increase in creatinine production with increasing weight, and the decline in creatinine production with age. The value obtained must be multiplied by 0.85 in women.

$$\text{Creatinine clearance (ml/min)} = \frac{(140 - \text{age}) \times \text{body weight (kg)}}{\text{Serum creatinine (mg/dL)} \times 72}$$

- The Modification of Diet in Renal Disease (MDRD) equation is based on data obtained from the MDRD study. In addition to the serum creatinine, the equation uses age, serum albumin concentration, and blood urea nitrogen value to estimate the GFR:

$$\text{eGFR (ml/min/1.73 m}^2\text{)} = 170 \times (\text{serum creatinine (mg/dl)})^{-0.999}$$
$$\times (\text{age (years)})^{-0.176} \times (\text{serum urea (mg/dl)})^{-0.170}$$
$$\times (\text{albumin (g/dl)})^{0.318} \times (0.762 \text{ if female}),$$
$$\times (1.180 \text{ if African American}).$$

- The simplified or abbreviated MDRD equation:

$$\text{eGFR (ml/min/1.73 m}^2\text{)} = 186 \times (\text{serum creatinine (mg/dl)})^{-1.154}$$
$$\times (\text{age (years)})^{-0.203} \times (0.742 \text{ if female})$$
$$\times (1.210 \text{ if African American}).$$

IMPACT OF CHRONIC RENAL INSUFFICIENCY ON OUTCOMES AFTER PERCUTANEOUS CORONARY INTERVENTION

In several large-scale PCI series, the presence of CRI is strongly associated with less favorable prognosis.[4-11] The reasons are multifactorial and include less-favorable demographic features and angiographic characteristics in patients with CRI, metabolic abnormalities, propensity to hypercoagulable state, anemia, and electrolyte disturbances, as well as impaired pharmacokinetics and pharmacodynamics of medications. In most PCI series, patients with CRI typically have higher proportion of elderly and females, and have higher prevalence of comorbidities including hypertension, diabetes mellitus, vascular disease, and congestive heart failure, as well as prior MI and coronary artery bypass grafting (CABG).[4-11] Angiographic features of patients with CRI frequently include multivessel coronary artery disease (CAD), vein graft disease, severely calcified vessels, more complex lesions, and worse left ventricular performance.[4-11] Still, the rate of angiographic success in large PCI series usually is unrelated to the renal function and exceeds 95%.[5,6]

Both in early PCI series and in contemporary PCI trials, CRI represents a powerful predictor of worse short- and long-term outcomes. In the PCI arm of the randomized Bypass Angioplasty Revascularization Investigation (BARI) trial, patients with CRI versus those without had almost 10 times higher in-hospital mortality (6.7% vs. 0.7%, respectively; $P < 0.05$).[7] Similar data were obtained in the later series on 362 patients with CRI (serum creatinine >1.5 mg/dl) compared with 2972 patients with preserved renal function (serum creatinine ≤1.5 mg/dl) (10.1% vs. 1.1%).[4] Of importance, the prognosis of patients with CRI is not necessary related to the degree of renal function impairment. In one study, in-hospital mortality was similarly high in patients with both mild and severe CRI (serum creatinine 1.6–2.0 mg/dl and >2.0 mg/dl, respectively) (11.5% vs. 9.9%).[4]

In the contemporary Randomized Evaluation in PCI Linking Bivalirudin to Reduced Clinical Events (REPLACE-2) trial of patients with stable and unstable angina and/or inducible ischemia treated with PCI, 30-day mortality was significantly higher among 886 patients with CRI compared to 4824 patients without CRI (1.6% vs. 0.1%; $P < 0.001$).[9] In the do Tirofiban and ReoPro Give Similar Efficacy Outcome (TARGET) trial, patients in the lowest quartile of creatinine clearance (< 70 ml/min) compared to those in the highest quartile (> 114 ml/min) had significantly higher rates of composite endpoint of death, MI, and urgent target vessel revascularization (TVR) (7.3% vs. 5.8%; $P = 0.005$).[10] Finally, in the largest so far randomized Controlled Abciximab and Device Investigation to Lower Late Angioplasty Complications (CADILLAC) trial of patients with acute MI treated with primary PCI, 30-day mortality was strikingly higher in patients with baseline CRI versus those without (7.5% vs. 0.8%; $P < 0.0001$), with an incremental increase in mortality for each 10 ml/min decline in baseline creatinine clearance.[2] In all of these trials, after adjusting for demographic, clinical, and procedural factors, CRI consistently represented a powerful predictor of in-hospital mortality.[4-7,9]

HEMORRHAGIC COMPLICATIONS IN RELATION TO CHRONIC RENAL INSUFFICIENCY

Patients with CRI have excess of bleeding complications. The main reasons include the alteration in the coagulation system and impaired response to medications. Several trials identified CRI as an independent predictor of hemorrhagic events irrespective of antithrombotic regimen. In the REPLACE-2 trial, patients with CRI had more than twice increased incidence of major bleeding (6.1% vs. 2.5%; $P < 0.0001$), and CRI predicted major bleeding in patients treated either with unfractionated heparin plus planned platelet glycoprotein IIb/IIIa receptor inhibitors, or with bivalirudin.[9] Similarly, when treated with tirofiban in the TARGET trial, patients in the lowest quartile of creatinine clearance compared to those in the highest quartile had significantly increased risk of major bleeding (1.6% vs. 0.3%, respectively) and red blood cell transfusions (5.3% vs. 2%).[10] Furthermore, in the CADILLAC trial, hemorrhagic complications and transfusion requirements were increased more than two-fold in patients with CRI.[11]

ADJUNCTIVE PHARMACOTHERAPY DURING PERCUTANEOUS CORONARY INTERVENTION IN PATIENTS WITH CHRONIC RENAL INSUFFICIENCY

Given that many antithrombotic medications are cleared through the renal pathway, knowledge of drug metabolism is important considering the choice of anticoagulation regimen in patients with CRI. Therapeutic doses of unfractionated heparin are cleared by a combination of a rapid, saturable mechanism, and a slower, non-saturable, dose-independent mechanism of renal clearance.[12] Close intraprocedural monitoring of anticoagulation is important in patients with CRI when heparin is used as an antithrombotic agent during PCI.

Bivalirudin (Angiomax) is cleared from plasma by a combination of renal mechanisms and proteolytic cleavage, with a half-life in patients with normal renal function of 25 min.[13] Bivalirudin clearance in patients with creatinine clearance > 60 ml/min is 3.4 ml/min/kg, and decreases to 2.7–2.8 ml/min/kg in patients with creatinine clearance of 10–60 ml/min, and 1.0 ml/min/kg in patients on dialysis. Plasma half-life of bivalirudin is approximately 25 min in patients with creatinine clearance

>60 ml/min, 34 min in patients with creatinine clearance 30–60 ml/min, nearly 1 h in patients with creatinine clearance 10–30 ml/min, and 3.5 h in hemodialysis patients. Approximately 25% of bivalirudin is removed by hemodialysis. Given the specifics of bivalirudin's pharmacodynamics and pharmacokinetics, bivalirudin dosage adjustment is required in patients with impaired renal function, and the following regimen of administration is recommended: an intravenous bolus of 0.75 mg/kg regardless of renal function, followed by an infusion of 1.75 mg/kg/h for the duration of the PCI procedure in patients with moderate renal impairment (creatinine clearance 30–59 ml/min); 1.0 mg/kg/h in patients with severe renal impairment (creatinine clearance <30 ml/min); and 0.25 mg/kg/h in patients on hemodialysis.

In the randomized REPLACE II trial, among patients with impaired renal function (creatinine clearance <60 ml/min), bivalirudin demonstrated suppression of ischemic events at 30-day follow-up to the degree provided by heparin and glycoprotein IIb/IIIa inhibition (9.7% vs. 9.4%, respectively).[9] In addition, treatment with bivalirudin was associated with a trend towards lower incidence of protocol-defined major bleeding (5.1% vs. 7.1%; $P = 0.20$), and a significant reduction in composite of major plus minor bleeding by thrombolysis in myocardial infarction (TIMI) criteria (3.2% vs. 7.1%; $P = 0.009$).[9] In a meta-analysis of three randomized trials of bivalirudin versus heparin among patients treated with PCI, there was greater absolute benefit of bivalirudin in terms of reduction of ischemic and bleeding complications in patients with worse degrees of renal impairment (2.2%, 5.8%, 7.7%, and 14.4% for patients with normal renal function, mild, moderate, and severe renal impairment, respectively).[1]

Abciximab is rapidly cleared from the circulation by the reticuloendothelial system, and increases the risk of bleeding in patients with CRI to the magnitude not exceeding that in patients without renal impairment. In the PCI series from the Mayo Clinic, there was no significant interaction between creatinine clearance and either major or minor bleeding with abciximab.[14]

In contrast to abciximab, eptifibatide and tirofiban undergo renal clearance, requiring appropriate dosing adjustments in patients with renal insufficiency. In the Enhanced Suppression of Platelet IIb/IIIa Receptor with Intregrilin Therapy (ESPRIT) trial, eptifibatide was documented to be at least as effective in patients with mild CRI as in patients with normal renal function without increasing bleeding risk.[15] In the TARGET trial, there was a trend towards greater benefit of abciximab over tirofiban with regard to 30-day ischemic complications in patients with creatinine clearance <70 ml/min (6.0% vs. 8.7%; $P = 0.07$).[10] Abciximab, compared with tirofiban, was also associated with an increased risk of minor bleeding in patients with creatinine clearance <70 ml/min (7.2% vs. 3.4%; $P = 0.004$).[10]

LONG-TERM OUTCOMES POST-PERCUTANEOUS CORONARY INTERVENTION IN RELATION TO CHRONIC RENAL INSUFFICIENCY

Long-term prognosis post-PCI is obviously affected by impaired renal function.[7,8,16,17] In the BARI trial, patients with even mild CRI experienced doubling of mortality during a 7-year period compared to patients with preserved renal function.[7] In the Mayo Clinic's PCI prospective registry on 5327 patients, 1-year mortality after successful intervention was 1.5%, 3.6%, 7.8%, and 18.3% in patients with creatinine clearance ≥70, 50–69, 30–49, and <30 ml/min, respectively. As expected, mortality rate was the highest in patients on dialysis (19.9%).[5] In the same study, by multivariate analysis, moderate or severe renal insufficiency was associated with a greater risk of death than even diabetes.[5] Furthermore, in the large-scale Prevention of Restenosis with Tranilast and its Outcomes (PRESTO) PCI trial, the risk of death at 9 months was 2.7 times higher in the lowest versus the highest creatinine clearance group (<60 ml/min vs. >89 ml/min).[8] Furthermore, in patients undergoing primary PCI for acute MI, presence of CRI was associated with a striking increase in short-term and late mortality, similar to the excess risk of anterior versus non-anterior MI location.[11]

FREQUENCY OF ANGIOGRAPHIC AND CLINICAL RESTENOSIS IN PATIENTS WITH CHRONIC RENAL INSUFFICIENCY

Patients with CRI are *not* at increased risk of restenosis after bare-metal stent implantation. Among 11 484 patients in the PRESTO trial, 83% of whom were treated with stent, patients with mild or moderate CRI (baseline serum creatinine <1.8 mg/dl) had paradoxically lower rates of restenosis post-PCI and TVR than patients with preserved renal function.[8] At 9-month angiographic follow-up in a total of 2556 patients (22% of study population), those in the lowest quartile of creatinine clearance (<60 ml/min) had 32% restenosis rate compared with 37% in patients in the highest quartile of creatinine clearance (>89 ml/min; $P = 0.02$.)[8] Similar data were obtained in the bare-metal stent arm of the randomized TAXUS IV trial, in which by multivariate analysis, an increase for each 10 ml/min in creatinine clearance was independently associated with the risk of 9-month binary restenosis (odds ratio (OR) = 1.14; $P = 0.009$).[18]

DRUG-ELUTING STENTS IN PATIENTS WITH CHRONIC RENAL INSUFFICIENCY

In the subanalysis from the TAXUS-IV pivotal randomized trial comparing outcomes after implantation of the polymer-based slow-release paclitaxel-eluting stent versus bare-metal stent in patients with stable and unstable angina and inducible ischemia, implantation of a paclitaxel-eluting stent resulted in strikingly lower rates of 9-month angiographic restenosis in patients with (2.1% vs. 20.5%; $P = 0.009$) and without (9.2% vs. 27.8%; $P < 0.0001$) baseline CRI, translating into lower rates of 1-year TLR in the TAXUS arm compared with the bare-metal stent arm, in both patients with CRI (3.3% vs. 12.2%, respectively; $P = 0.01$) and those without CRI (4.7% vs. 15.8%, respectively; $P < 0.0001$).[18] Likewise, in the Cypher Registry Experience at Washington Hospital Center with Drug-eluting Stents (C-REWARDS), patients with CRI had significantly lower rates of 6-month TLR when treated with a sirolimus-eluting stent compared with bare-metal stents (7.1% vs. 22.1%; $P = 0.02$).[19] In two studies, CRI was identified as an independent predictor of stent thrombosis after drug-eluting stent implantation,[20,21] while there were no such concerns in the TAXUS-IV trial.[18]

RENAL FUNCTION DETERIORATION POST-PERCUTANEOUS CORONARY INTERVENTION IN PATIENTS WITH CHRONIC RENAL INSUFFICIENCY: CONTRAST-INDUCED NEPHROPATHY

Chronic renal insufficiency is the most powerful predictor of renal function deterioration after the exposure to contrast media, a condition known as contrast-induced nephropathy (CIN). CIN is one of the most common sources of acute renal failure among hospitalized patients. It is associated with prolonged in-hospital stay, increased morbidity, mortality, and costs. CIN is defined as an absolute (≥ 0.5 mg/dl) or relative ($\geq 25\%$) increase in serum creatinine level after the exposure to contrast agent compared to baseline value, when alternative explanations for renal impairment have been excluded.[22,23] It occurs within 24–96 h post-exposure, and there is a return of renal function to baseline or near baseline in 1 to 3 weeks.[22,23] In 80% of cases, rise in creatinine occurs within the first 24 h, and nearly all patients who progress to serious renal failure (those requiring either nephrology consultation or dialysis) have a rise in serum creatinine within the first 24 h, with the peak of this rise commonly at 48–96 hours after contrast exposure.[22] Patients with less than an absolute rise of 0.5 mg/dl in serum creatinine at 24 h are unlikely to have any clinically significant form of CIN.[24]

Rates of CIN in patients with underlying renal disorder are extremely high, ranging from 14.8 to 55%.[22,25] Despite the use of preprocedure hydration and nonionic contrast media, CIN may occur in one-third of patients with baseline CRI.[26] The higher the baseline creatinine value, the greater is the risk of CIN. As shown in one of the studies, if baseline plasma creatinine level is ≤ 1.2 mg/dl, the risk of CIN is only 2%.[27] In patients with values of creatinine in the range of 1.4–1.9 mg/dl, the risk of CIN compared with the previous group increases five-fold (10.4%).[27] As for patients with baseline creatinine level ≥ 2.0 mg/dl, more than half of them (62%) subsequently develop CIN.[27]

A curvilinear relationship was found between estimated creatinine clearance and the risk of renal failure requiring dialysis in patients undergoing diagnostic

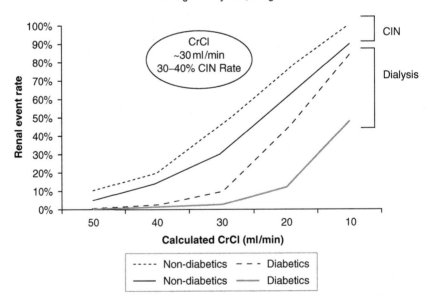

Figure 2.1 Validated risk of acute renal failure requiring dialysis after diagnostic angiography and/or angioplasty. A mean contrast dose of 250 ml and a mean age of 65 years is assumed. CrCl, creatinine clearance; CIN, contrast-induced nephropathy. Data adapted from McCullough and Sandberg.[28]

Table 2.1   Risk factors for the development of CIN

Fixed (non-modifiable) risk factors	Modifiable risk factors
Older age	Volume of contrast media
Diabetes mellitus	Hypotension
Pre-existing renal failure	Anemia
Advanced congestive heart failure	Dehydration
Low left ventricular ejection fraction	Low serum albumin level (<35 g/l)
Acute myocardial infarction	Angiotensin-converting enzyme inhibitors
Cardiogenic shock	Diuretics
Renal transplant	Non-steroid anti-inflammatory drugs
	Nephrotoxic antibiotics
	Intra-aortic balloon pump

coronary angiography with or without angioplasty (Figure 2.1).[22] Below a threshold estimated creatinine clearance of 25 ml/min, the risk of dialysis increases rapidly.[22,28]

Impaired renal function is frequent in patients with other risk factors for the development of CIN (Table 2.1). Assessment of cumulative risk is important to identify an individual patient's risk for developing CIN. A simple CIN risk score (Figure 2.2) was proposed in our institution, based on the readily available information, and is recommended for both clinical and investigational purposes.[29] The occurrence of CIN was found to be 7.5–57.3% for a low (≤ 5) and high (≥ 16) risk score, respectively, with corresponding rates of dialysis 0.04–12.6%.[29] Significant increases in rates of dialysis (Figure 2.3) and 1-year mortality were observed with increments of risk score.

Volume of contrast medium is the only modifiable risk factor of CIN, and is especially crucial in patients with CRI. In previous studies, the rates of CIN among 228 patients with normal baseline creatinine level that received high-load of contrast media (250–800 ml) were 4.3%, and much higher (11%) among 54 patients that received >400 ml of contrast agent.[30,31] In our study on diabetic population, CIN developed in approximately every fifth, fourth, and second patient who received 200–400 ml, 400–600 ml, and >600 ml of contrast, respectively.[32] In the same study, each 100 ml increment in contrast volume resulted in a 30% increase in the odds of CIN (OR 1.30, 95% confidence interval (CI) 1.16–1.46), and there was a significant ($P<0.0001$) trend towards increased covariate adjusted odds of CIN across increased amounts of contrast media.

Anemia might be one of the factors in deteriorating renal ischemia. According to our interventional cardiology database analysis, rates of CIN steadily increased as baseline hematocrit quintile decreased (from 10.3% in the highest quintile to 23.3% in the lowest quintile; $P<0.0001$).[33] Stratification by baseline eGFR and baseline hematocrit showed that the rates of CIN were the highest (28.8%) in patients who had the lowest level for both baseline eGFR and hematocrit. Patients with the lowest eGFR but relatively high baseline hematocrit values had remarkably lower rates of CIN (15.8%, 12.3%, 17.1%, and 15.4% in the second, third, fourth, and fifth quintiles of baseline hematocrit, respectively; $P<0.0001$) (Figure 2.4). The rates of CIN increased also with increment in change in hematocrit. Patients in the lowest quintile of baseline hematocrit with absolute hematocrit drop $>5.9\%$ had almost doubled

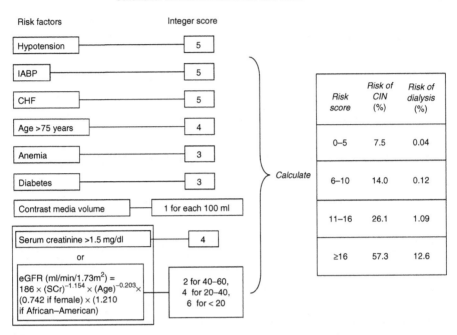

Figure 2.2 Schema to define CIN risk score. CHF, congestive heart failure class III–IV by New York Heart Association classification and/or history of pulmonary edema; eGFR, estimated glomerular filtration rate; SCr, serum creatinine; IABP, intraaortic balloon pump. Anemia: baseline hematocrit value <39% for men and <36% for women. Hypotension: systolic blood pressure <80 mmHg for at least 1 h requiring inotropic support with medications or intra-aortic balloon pump within 24 h periprocedurally.

rates of CIN compared with patients with hematocrit change <3.4% (38.1% vs. 18.8%, respectively; *P* <0.0001).[33] By multivariate analysis, lower baseline hematocrit was an independent predictor of CIN; each 3% decrease in baseline hematocrit resulted in a significant increase in the odds of CIN in patients with and without chronic kidney disease (11% and 23%, respectively). Change in hematocrit also showed a significant association with CIN.[33]

Several studies recognized advanced congestive heart failure, compromised left ventricle systolic performance, dehydration, hypotension, the use of intra-aortic balloon pump, and several drugs (angiotensin-converting enzyme (ACE) inhibitors, diuretics, and non-steroidal anti-inflammatory drugs) to be negative prognostic factors of CIN.

The role of ACE inhibitors has been controversial. In one study, patients receiving ACE inhibitors had a significant increase in serum creatinine after the procedure, compared with patients without such therapy.[34] However, prior use of ACE inhibitors predicted the occurrence of CIN only on univariate, but not on multivariate analysis.[34]

Studies from our institution highlighted the negative impact of periprocedural hypotension and the use of an intra-aortic balloon pump in the development of

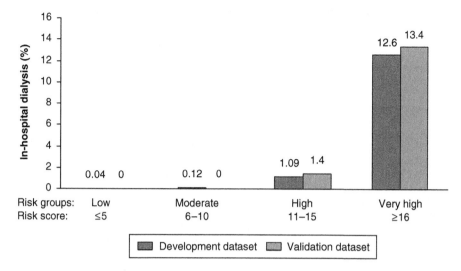

Figure 2.3 In-hospital hemodialysis can be predicted by a high or very high CIN risk score value similarly in the development and validation datasets.

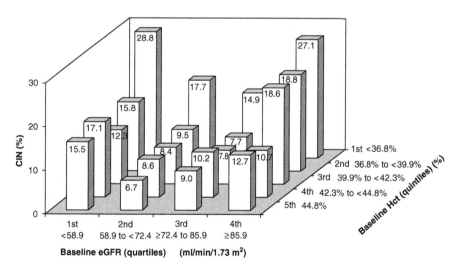

Figure 2.4 Risk of contrast-induced nephropathy in relation to baseline hematocrit (Hct) and eGFR.

CIN.[29,35] The detrimental influence of prolonged hypotension on kidney function is well known. However, even relatively short periods of hypotension may be hazardous. Intra-aortic balloon counterpulsation may signify a very high-risk population due to severe coronary atherosclerosis, and/or indicate a role of atheroembolism in the pathogenesis of CIN.

Table 2.2   Various treatment modalities assessed in randomized trials on prevention of contrast-induced nephropathy[a]

Treatment	Effect
Hydration	+
Sodium bicarbonate	+
Hemofiltration	+
Prostaglandin E_1	+
N-acetyl-L-cysteine	+/−
Dopamine	+/−
Fenoldopam	+/−
Theophylline	+/−
Calcium-channel blockers	+/−
Atrial natriuretic peptide	−
Haemodialysis	Deleterious effect

[a] + positive effect; − no effect; +/− conflicting data.

Choice of contrast agents in patients with chronic renal insufficiency undergoing percutaneous coronary intervention

Controversy exists as to whether the use of different contrast agents is of any benefit in diminishing the risk of CIN. In a study by Katholie et al, the decrease in creatinine clearance was more pronounced and lasted longer in the group that received high-osmolar contrast media compared to the arm exposed to low-osmolar contrast agent.[36] Harris et al also reported higher rates of CIN in patients that have received high-osmolar (14%) compared with low-osmolar (2%) contrast media.[37] On the contrary, Schwab et al did not show any significant differences in nephrotoxic effect between several studied contrast agents.[38] A randomized, double-blind, prospective, multicenter Nephrotoxicity in High-Risk Patients Study of Iso-Osmolar and Low-Osmolar Non-Ionic Contrast Media (NEPHRIC) trial compared the nephrotoxicity of iohexol, a non-ionic monomer, to iodixanol, a non-ionic dimer in a total of 129 subjects with diabetes mellitus and serum creatinine concentrations of 1.5–3.5 mg/dl, undergoing coronary or aortofemoral angiography.[39] Significantly more patients assigned to iohexol (26%) experienced a serum creatinine increase of 0.5 mg/dl or more, compared with patients in the iodixanol group (3%). No patient in the iodixanol group had an increase in serum creatinine of ≥ 1.0 mg/dl, compared to 10 patients (15%) in the iohexol group.[39]

In a meta-analysis of 45 trials, the greater increase in serum creatinine after administration of high- compared with low-osmolar contrast media was seen only in patients with pre-existing renal failure.[40]

Based on the available data, in current practice non-ionic low-osmolar contrast media is a preferred agent in patients with renal impairment. Further study is warranted to clarify the issue of minimizing the renal damage while using the different contrast material.

PREVENTION OF CONTRAST-INDUCED NEPHROPATHY

The unfavorable prognostic implications of CIN make its prevention of paramount importance. Multiple preventive modalities have been investigated and are summarized in Table 2.2.

Hydration

The positive effect of adequate hydration in reducing rates of CIN was established in a randomized study by Solomon et al: in patients with chronic renal insufficiency undergoing angiography, hydration with 0.45% saline provided better protection against renal function deterioration than did hydration with 0.45% saline plus mannitol or furosemide.[41] Subsequent randomized study demonstrated that in patients with mild-to-moderate renal insufficiency different modes of fluids administration (intravenous versus oral) had similar renoprotective effect.[42] Another randomized, open labeled study by Mueller et al compared two hydration regimens in a total of 1620 patients undergoing PCI, showing the superiority of isotonic versus half-isotonic saline in reducing rates of CIN (0.7% versus 2%, respectively).[43] The benefit of isotonic saline was especially prominent in women, diabetic patients, and patients receiving more than 250 ml of contrast media.[43]

In the randomized PRINCE-trial, the achievement of high urine flow rate by forced diuresis with intravenous crystalloid, mannitol, and furosemide provided, compared with control (crystalloid plus placebo), only modest benefit against CIN.[44] One prospective, single-center, randomized trial showed that preventive hydration with sodium bicarbonate before and after iopamidol administration was more effective than hydration with sodium chloride for prophylaxis of CIN.[45] In this study, among a total of 119 patients with stable serum creatinine levels of at least 1.1 mg/dl, patients that received hydration with sodium bicarbonate had significantly lower rates of CIN (1.7%) compared with patients that received a 154 mEq/l infusion of sodium chloride (13.6%).[45]

Hydration should be performed cautiously in patients with CRI and impaired left ventricle performance. In our institution, the recommended regimen of hydration in the presence of CRI is 1 ml/kg/h for 12 h pre- and post-PCI for patients with normal ejection fraction and volume replacement matching urine output, to maintain euvolemic state for 12 h pre- and post-PCI for patients with moderately or severely reduced ejection fraction.

N-acetyl-L-cysteine

The use of N-acetyl-L-cysteine, an agent with anti-oxidant properties, in the prevention of CIN, is based on the assumption that CIN is caused by reactive oxygen species, formed as a result of direct toxic effect of contrast media on tubular epithelial cells. In the first randomized placebo-controlled study of 83 patients exposed to contrast media, prophylactic oral administration of N-acetyl-L-cysteine along with hydration was superior to hydration alone in prevention of CIN in patients with elevated baseline creatinine level (2% vs. 21%).[46] The subsequent APART trial, including 54 patients and using similar design, confirmed the previous results: CIN occurred in 8% of patients in the oral N-acetyl-L-cysteine group versus 45% in the placebo group.[47]

Later on, however, the enthusiasm regarding the efficacy of N-acetyl-L-cysteine has been lessened. In the larger randomized study (183 patients), albeit lacking placebo-control, oral N-acetyl-L-cysteine plus hydration compared to hydration alone did not provide significant difference in the rates of CIN.[48] The benefit of N-acetyl-L-cysteine in this study was statistically significant only in patients that received a relatively small volume of contrast (≤ 140 ml).[48] Similarly, in the largest for today (487 patients), randomized study, intravenous N-acetyl-L-cysteine (500 mg) was ineffective in preventing CIN in patients with impaired renal function.[49] Also, no positive effect of N-acetyl-L-cysteine was obtained in several other studies.[50-53]

The results of several meta-analytic studies on the use of N-acetyl-L-cysteine are inconsistent as well: two reports supported the use of N-acetyl-L-cysteine in reducing rates of CIN,[54,55] while two others showed no evidence of N-acetyl-L-cysteine efficacy in preventing CIN.[56,57]

Dopamine

Due to a dilatory effect on the renal vasculature and the ability to increase renal blood flow (RBF), and GFR, dopamine was supposed to be useful in prevention of CIN. The results of clinical studies are conflicting. In one study, dopamine was shown to attenuate the increase in serum creatinine level after exposure to contrast medium,[58] while in other studies such effect was not documented,[59] or was present only in patients with creatinine ≥ 2.0 mg/dl.[60] Moreover, in patients with peripheral vascular disease and CIN, the effect of dopamine on renal function was found to be deleterious.[61]

Fenoldopam

Fenoldopam, a selective, dopamine D_1 receptor agonist, known to produce both systemic and renal arteriolar vasodilatation, was shown to blunt the decline in RBF and GFR after exposure to contrast media.[62] In the largest randomized radiocontrast study to date, the CONTRAST trial, 315 patients undergoing invasive cardiac procedures with a calculated creatinine clearance <60 ml/min were hydrated and then randomized to either fenoldopam (0.05 µg/kg/min, titrated up to 0.10 µg/kg/min) starting 1 h before catheterization and continuing for 12 hours after, vs. matching placebo.[63] The incidence of CIN showed a similar frequency in both groups (33.6% vs. 30.1%; $P = 0.54$). Thus, fenoldopam cannot be recommended for prophylactic use in patients at high risk for CIN.

Theophylline

Several data give evidence of adenosine involvement in renal hemodynamic response to contrast media, raising the hypothesis that theophylline, an adenosine A_1 receptor antagonist, may attenuate the decrease in RBF and GFR induced by exposure to contrast media. In a randomized, placebo-controlled study, prophylactic intravenous administration of 200 mg theophylline reduced the incidence of CIN in patients with chronic kidney disease (4% in patients treated with theophylline vs. 16% in patients treated with placebo).[64] In another randomized, placebo-controlled study, treatment with theophylline compared with placebo was accompanied by a smaller decrease in GFR, plasma erythropoietin, and renin, and a smaller increase in urinary beta$_2$ microglobulin.[65] Oral theophylline in a dose of 200 mg twice daily prescribed to diabetic patients 24 h before and 48 h after exposure to contrast, provided significantly less fall in GFR and lower creatinine values compared to placebo.[66] However, three other randomized studies did not show any benefit of theophylline compared to placebo in preventing CIN.[61,67,68]

Other treatment modalities

Atrial natriuretic peptide in three different doses failed to prevent CIN in a randomized, placebo-controlled study.[69]

Following contrast-induced alterations in calcium metabolism and the ability of calcium-channel antagonists to relieve vasoconstriction, several studies investigated the effect of calcium-channel blockers on rates of CIN. In a small (35 patients) randomized study, GFR was preserved in patients treated with nitrendipine, while it was decreased in patients that received placebo.[70] On the contrary, in three other studies, the change in creatinine level did not differ significantly between the groups.[71–73]

Based on the decreased levels of prostaglandins in patients with CIN, it was hypothesized that prophylactic administration of prostaglandin E_1 may be beneficial in reducing CIN. Double-blind, randomized, placebo-controlled study investigated the effect of intravenous administration of prostaglandin E_1 in three different doses, showing that compared with placebo patients treated with prostaglandin E_1, independently of the dose given, experienced significantly less increase in serum creatinine after exposure to contrast medium.[74]

One retrospective study analyzed the risk of CIN among 1002 patients with stable baseline serum creatinine ≥ 1.5 mg/dl undergoing cardiac catheterization. None of these patients were taking statins before admission.[75] According to results, mean serum creatinine value post-procedure, and the rates of CIN were significantly lower among 250 patients pretreated with statins before exposure to non-ionic, low-osmolality contrast, compared with 752 patients who were not pretreated with statins.[75]

Several studies examined the effect of hemodialysis, immediately after exposure to contrast media, in preventing renal function deterioration in patients with pre-existing chronic kidney disease. The results were consistent across all the studies, showing that prophylactic hemodialysis does not diminish the rates of CIN, and may even increase the risk of CIN.[76–80]

One randomized study investigated the role of hemofiltration, as compared with isotonic-saline hydration, both started 4–8 h before exposure to contrast medium, and continued for 18–24 h post-exposure, in preventing CIN in patients with chronic kidney disease (serum creatinine concentration >2 mg/dl) undergoing coronary interventions.[81] Among a total of 114 consecutive patients, CIN developed significantly less frequently in patients treated with hemofiltration (fluid replacement rate, 1000 ml/h without weight loss), compared with patients treated with isotonic-saline hydration (1 ml/kg/h) [5% vs. 50%, $P < 0.001$]. Besides, hemofiltration was associated with significantly lower rates of temporary renal-replacement therapy (3% vs. 25%, respectively), in-hospital events (9% vs. 52%), in-hospital mortality (2% vs. 14%), and cumulative one-year mortality (10% vs. 30%).

TARGETED RENAL THERAPY

Targeted renal therapy is a novel catheter-based approach aimed at delivery of renal vasodilator agents such as fenoldopam, a selective D_1 receptor agonist, and nesiritide, a B-type natriuretic peptide, directly to the kidneys via the renal arteries using Benephit Infusion System (FlowMedica, Inc., Fremont, CA, USA) to maximize the beneficial kidney effects of drugs while minimizing systemic side-effects (Figure 2.5). Ongoing trials are addressing the issue of whether local drug delivery will allow the reduction of CIN rates in patients undergoing contrast medium exposure.[82]

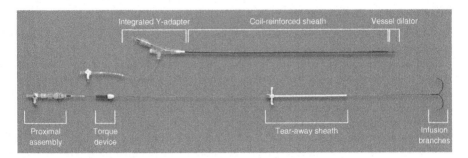

Figure 2.5 Benephit Infusion System (FlowMedica, Inc., Fremont, CA).

CONCLUSION

Chronic renal insufficiency is a frequent comorbidity in patients undergoing PCI. Renal impairment, even mild, in patients undergoing PCI confers a clinically significant risk for excess mortality and morbidity. Patients with impaired renal function are at increased risk of CIN, known to worsen further the prognosis of patients with CRI. Although rare in the general population, CIN has high incidence in patients with underlying renal dysfunction. The use of a risk score may identify patients predisposed to developing CIN. So far, the best way to prevent CIN is to identify the patients at risk and to provide adequate periprocedural hydration, accounting for the left ventricle performance. Temporary periprocedural discontinuation of nephrotoxic agents is essential. Non-ionic contrast agents provide lower rates of CIN and are, therefore, preferred in patients with impaired renal function. The amount of contrast should be minimized, and repeated use of contrast media within a short period of time should be avoided. The role of various drugs in prevention of CIN is still controversial and warrants future studies.

REFERENCES

1. Chew DP, Bhatt DL, Kimball W et al. Bivalirudin provides increasing benefit with decreasing renal function: a meta-analysis of randomized trials. Am J Cardiol. 2003; 92: 919–23.
2. Stone GW, Grines CL, Cox DA et al. Comparison of angioplasty with stenting, with or without abciximab, in acute myocardial infarction. The Controlled Abciximab and Device Investigation to Lower Late Angioplasty Complications (CADILLAC) Investigators. N Engl J Med 2002; 346: 957–66.
3. Levey AS, Coresh J, Balk E et al; National Kidney Foundation. National Kidney Foundation practice guidelines for chronic kidney disease: evaluation, classification, and stratification. Ann Intern Med. 2003; 139: 137–47.
4. Rubenstein MH, Harrell LC, Sheynberg BV et al. Are patients with renal failure good candidates for percutaneous coronary revascularization in the new device era? Circulation. 2000; 102: 2966–72.
5. Best PJ, Lennon R, Ting HH et al. The impact of renal insufficiency on clinical outcomes in patients undergoing percutaneous coronary interventions. J Am Coll Cardiol 2002; 39: 1113–19.
6. Gruberg L, Dangas G, Mehran R et al. Clinical outcome following percutaneous coronary interventions in patients with chronic renal failure. Catheter Cardiovasc Interv 2002; 55: 66–72.

7. Szczech LA, Best PJ, Crowley E et al; Bypass Angioplasty Revascularization Investigation (BARI) Investigators. Outcomes of patients with chronic renal insufficiency in the bypass angioplasty revascularization investigation. Circulation 2002; 105: 2253–8.
8. Best PJ, Berger PB, Davis BR et al; PRESTO Investigators. Impact of mild or moderate chronic kidney disease on the frequency of restenosis: results from the PRESTO trial. J Am Coll Cardiol. 2004; 44: 1786–91.
9. Chew DP, Lincoff AM, Gurm H et al; REPLACE-2 Investigators. Bivalirudin versus heparin and glycoprotein IIb/IIIa inhibition among patients with renal impairment undergoing percutaneous coronary intervention (a subanalysis of the REPLACE-2 trial). Am J Cardiol 2005; 95: 581–5.
10. Berger PB, Best PJ, Topol EJ et al. The relation of renal function to ischemic and bleeding outcomes with 2 different glycoprotein IIb/IIIa inhibitors: the do Tirofiban and ReoPro Give Similar Efficacy Outcome (TARGET) trial. Am Heart J 2005; 149: 869–75.
11. Sadeghi HM, Stone GW, Grines CL et al. Impact of renal insufficiency in patients undergoing primary angioplasty for acute myocardial infarction. Circulation 2003; 108: 2769–75.
12. Hirsh J, Anand SS, Halperin JL, Fuster V; American Heart Association. Guide to anticoagulant therapy: Heparin: a statement for healthcare professionals from the American Heart Association. Circulation 2001; 103: 2994–3018.
13. Robson R. The use of bivalirudin in patients with renal impairment. J Invasive Cardiol 2000; 12(Suppl F): 33F-6.
14. Best PJ, Lennon R, Gersh BJ et al. Safety of abciximab in patients with chronic renal insufficiency who are undergoing percutaneous coronary interventions. Am Heart J 2003; 146: 345–50.
15. Reddan DN, O'Shea JC, Sarembock IJ et al. Treatment effects of eptifibatide in planned coronary stent implantation in patients with chronic kidney disease (ESPRIT Trial). Am J Cardiol 2003; 91: 17–21.
16. Nikolsky E, Mehran R, Turcot D et al. Impact of chronic kidney disease on prognosis of patients with diabetes mellitus treated with percutaneous coronary intervention. Am J Cardiol 2004; 94: 300–5.
17. Rinehart AL, Herzog CA, Collins AJ et al. A comparison of coronary angioplasty and coronary artery bypass grafting outcomes in chronic dialysis patients. Am J Kidney Dis 1995; 25: 281–90.
18. Halkin A, Mehran R, Casey CW et al. Impact of moderate renal insufficiency on restenosis and adverse clinical events after paclitaxel-eluting and bare metal stent implantation: results from the TAXUS-IV Trial. Am Heart J 2005; 150: 1163–70.
19. Kuchulakanti PK, Torguson R, Chu WW et al. Impact of chronic renal insufficiency on clinical outcomes in patients undergoing percutaneous coronary intervention with sirolimus-eluting stents versus bare metal stents. Am J Cardiol 2006; 97:792–7.
20. Iakovou I, Schmidt T, Bonizzoni E et al. Incidence, predictors, and outcome of thrombosis after successful implantation of drug-eluting stents. JAMA 2005; 293: 2126–30.
21. Kuchulakanti PK, Chu WW, Torguson R et al. Correlates and long-term outcomes of angiographically proven stent thrombosis with sirolimus- and paclitaxel-eluting stents. Circulation 2006; 113: 1108–13.
22. McCullough PA, Wolyn R, Rocher LL, Levin RN, O'Neill WW. Acute renal failure after coronary intervention: incidence, risk factors, and relationship to mortality. Am J Med 1997; 103: 368–75.
23. Mehran R, Nikolsky E. Contrast-induced nephropathy: definition, epidemiology, and patients at risk. Kidney Int Suppl 2006; 100: S11–15.
24. Guitterez NV, Diaz A, Timmis GC et al. Determinants of serum creatinine trajectory in acute contrast nephropathy. J Interv Cardiol 2002; 15: 349–54.
25. Rihal CS, Textor SC, Grill DE et al. Incidence and prognostic importance of acute renal failure after percutaneous coronary intervention. Circulation 2002; 105: 2259–64.
26. Gruberg L, Mehran R, Dangas G et al. Acute renal failure requiring dialysis after percutaneous coronary interventions. Catheter Cardiovasc Interv 2001; 52: 409–16.

27. Hall KA, Wong RW, Hunter GC et al. Contrast-induced nephrotoxicity: the effects of vasodilator therapy. J Surg Res 1992; 53: 317–20.
28. McCullough PA, Sandberg KR. Epidemiology of contrast-induced nephropathy. Rev Cardiovasc Med 2003; 4(Suppl 5): S3–9.
29. Mehran R, Aymong ED, Nikolsky E et al. A simple risk score for prediction of contrast-induced nephropathy after percutaneous coronary intervention: development and initial validation. J Am Coll Cardiol 2004; 44: 1393–9.
30. Rosovsky MA, Rusinek H, Berenstein A et al. High-dose administration of nonionic contrast media: a retrospective review. Radiology 1996; 200: 119–22.
31. Kahn JK, Rutherford BD, McConahay DR et al. High-dose contrast agent administration during complex coronary angioplasty. Am Heart J 1990; 120: 533–6.
32. Nikolsky E, Mehran R, Turcot D et al. Impact of chronic kidney disease on prognosis of patients with diabetes mellitus treated with percutaneous coronary intervention. Am J Cardiol 2004; 94: 300–5.
33. Nikolsky E, Mehran R, Lasic Z et al. Low hematocrit predicts contrast-induced nephropathy after percutaneous coronary interventions. Kidney Int 2005; 67: 706–13.
34. Kini AS, Mitre CA, Kim M et al. A protocol for prevention of radiographic contrast nephropathy during percutaneous coronary intervention: effect of selective dopamine receptor agonist fenoldopam. Catheter Cardiovasc Interv 2002; 55: 169–73.
35. Dangas GD, Iakovou I, Nikolsky E et al. Contrast induced nephropathy after percutaneous coronary interventions in relation to chronic kidney disease: importance of periprocedural hemodynamic variables. Am J Cardiol 2005; 95: 13–19.
36. Katholi RE, Taylor GJ, Woods WT et al. Nephrotoxicity of nonionic low-osmolarity versus ionic high-osmolarity contrast media: a prospective double-blind randomized comparison in human beings. Radiology 1993; 186: 183–7.
37. Harris KG, Smith TP, Cragg AH, Lemke JH. Nephrotoxicity from contrast material in renal insufficiency: ionic versus nonionic agents. Radiology 1991; 179: 849–52.
38. Schwab SJ, Hlatky MA, Pieper KS et al. Contrast nephrotoxicity: a randomized controlled trial of a nonionic and an ionic radiographic contrast agent. N Engl J Med 1989; 320: 149–53.
39. Aspelin P, Aubry P, Fransson SG et al. Nephrotoxicity in High-risk Patients Study of Iso-Osmolar and Low-Osmolar Non-Ionic Contrast Media Study Investigators. Nephrotoxic effects in high-risk patients undergoing angiography. N Engl J Med 2003; 348: 491–9.
40. Barrett BJ, Carlisle EJ. Metaanalysis of the relative nephrotoxicity of high- and low-osmolarity iodinated contrast media. Radiology 1993; 188: 171–8.
41. Solomon R, Werner C, Mann D, D'Elia J, Silva P. Effects of saline, mannitol, and furosemide to prevent acute decreases in renal function induced by radiocontrast agents. N Engl J Med 1994; 331: 1416–20.
42. Taylor AJ, Hotchkiss D, Morse RW, McCabe J. PREPARED: Preparation for Angiography in Renal Dysfunction: a randomized trial of inpatient vs outpatient hydration protocols for cardiac catheterization in mild-to-moderate renal dysfunction. Chest 1998; 114: 1570–4.
43. Mueller C, Buerkle G, Buettner HJ et al. Prevention of contrast media-associated nephropathy: randomized comparison of 2 hydration regimens in 1620 patients undergoing coronary angioplasty. Arch Intern Med 2002; 162: 329–36.
44. Stevens MA, McCullough PA, Tobin KJ et al. A prospective randomized trial of prevention measures in patients at high risk for contrast nephropathy: results of the PRINCE study. Prevention of Radiocontrast Induced Nephropathy Clinical Evaluation. J Am Coll Cardiol 1999; 33: 403–11.
45. Merten GJ, Burgess WP, Gray LV et al. Prevention of contrast-induced nephropathy with sodium bicarbonate: a randomized controlled trial. JAMA 2004; 291: 2328–34.
46. Tepel M, van der Giet M, Schwarzfeld C et al. Prevention of radiographic-contrast-agent-induced reductions in renal function by acetylcysteine. N Engl J Med 2000; 343: 180–4.
47. Shyu KG, Cheng JJ, Kuan P. Acetylcysteine protects against acute renal damage in patients with abnormal renal function undergoing a coronary procedure. J Am Coll Cardiol 2002; 40: 1383–8.

48. Briguori C, Manganelli F, Scarpato P et al. Acetylcysteine and contrast agent-associated nephrotoxicity. J Am Coll Cardiol 2002; 40: 298–303.
49. Webb JG, Pate GE, Humphries KH et al. A randomized controlled trial of intravenous N-acetylcysteine for the prevention of contrast-induced nephropathy after cardiac catheterization: lack of effect. Am Heart J 2004; 148: 422–9.
50. Durham JD, Caputo C, Dokko J et al. A randomized controlled trial of N-acetylcysteine to prevent contrast nephropathy in cardiac angiography. Kidney Int 2002; 62: 2202–7.
51. Vallero A, Cesano G, Pozzato M et al. [Contrast nephropathy in cardiac procedures: no advantages with prophylactic use of N-acetylcysteine (NAC)] [Article in Italian] G Ital Nefrol 2002; 19: 529–33.
52. Allaqaband S, Tumuluri R, Malik AM et al. Prospective randomized study of N-acetylcysteine, fenoldopam, and saline for prevention of radiocontrast-induced nephropathy. Catheter Cardiovasc Interv 2002; 57: 279–83.
53. Goldenberg I, Shechter M, Matetzky S et al. Oral acetylcysteine as an adjunct to saline hydration for the prevention of contrast-induced nephropathy following coronary angiography. A randomized controlled trial and review of the current literature. Eur Heart J 2004; 25: 212–18.
54. Misra D, Leibowitz K, Gowda RM, Shapiro M, Khan IA. Role of N-acetylcysteine in prevention of contrast-induced nephropathy after cardiovascular procedures: a meta-analysis. Clin Cardiol 2004; 27: 607–10.
55. Alonso A, Lau J, Jaber BL, Weintraub A, Sarnak MJ. Prevention of radiocontrast nephropathy with N-acetylcysteine in patients with chronic kidney disease: a meta-analysis of randomized, controlled trials. Am J Kidney Dis 2004; 43: 1–9.
56. Bagshaw SM, Ghali WA. Acetylcysteine for prevention of contrast-induced nephropathy after intravascular angiography: a systematic review and meta-analysis. BMC Med 2004; 2: 38.
57. Kshirsagar AV, Poole C, Mottl A et al. N-acetylcysteine for the prevention of radiocontrast induced nephropathy: a meta-analysis of prospective controlled trials. J Am Soc Nephrol 2004; 15: 761–9.
58. Kapoor A, Sinha N, Sharma RK et al. Use of dopamine in prevention of contrast induced acute renal failure – a randomised study. Int J Cardiol 1996; 53: 233–6.
59. Gare M, Haviv YS, Ben-Yehuda A et al. The renal effect of low-dose dopamine in high-risk patients undergoing coronary angiography. J Am Coll Cardiol 1999; 34: 1682–8.
60. Hans SS, Hans BA, Dhillon R, Dmuchowski C, Glover J. Effect of dopamine on renal function after arteriography in patients with pre-existing renal insufficiency. Am Surg 1998; 64: 432–6.
61. Abizaid AS, Clark CE, Mintz GS et al. Effects of dopamine and aminophylline on contrast-induced acute renal failure after coronary angioplasty in patients with pre-existing renal insufficiency. Am J Cardiol 1999; 83: 260–3, A5.
62. Tumlin JA, Wang A, Murray PT, Mathur VS. Fenoldopam mesylate blocks reductions in renal plasma flow after radiocontrast dye infusion: a pilot trial in the prevention of contrast nephropathy. Am Heart J 2002; 143: 894–903.
63. Stone GW, McCullough PA, Tumlin JA et al; CONTRAST Investigators. Fenoldopam mesylate for the prevention of contrast-induced nephropathy: a randomized controlled trial. JAMA 2003; 290: 2284–91.
64. Huber W, Ilgmann K, Page M et al. Effect of theophylline on contrast material-nephropathy in patients with chronic renal insufficiency: controlled, randomized, double-blinded study. Radiology 2002; 223: 772–9.
65. Kolonko A, Wiecek A, Kokot F. The nonselective adenosine antagonist theophylline does prevent renal dysfunction induced by radiographic contrast agents. J Nephrol 1998; 11: 151–6.
66. Kapoor A, Kumar S, Gulati S et al. The role of theophylline in contrast-induced nephropathy: a case-control study. Nephrol Dial Transplant 2002; 17: 1936–41.
67. Shammas NW, Kapalis MJ, Harris M, McKinney D, Coyne EP. Aminophylline does not protect against radiocontrast nephropathy in patients undergoing percutaneous angiographic procedures. J Invasive Cardiol 2001; 13: 738–40.

68. Erley CM, Duda SH, Rehfuss D et al. Prevention of radiocontrast-media-induced nephropathy in patients with pre-existing renal insufficiency by hydration in combination with the adenosine antagonist theophylline. Nephrol Dial Transplant 1999; 14: 1146–9.
69. Kurnik BR, Allgren RL, Genter FC et al. Prospective study of atrial natriuretic peptide for the prevention of radiocontrast-induced nephropathy. Am J Kidney Dis 1998; 31: 674–80.
70. Neumayer HH, Junge W, Kufner A, Wenning A. Prevention of radiocontrast-media-induced nephrotoxicity by the calcium channel blocker nitrendipine: a prospective randomised clinical trial. Nephrol Dial Transplant 1989; 4: 1030–6.
71. Carraro M, Mancini W, Artero M et al. Dose effect of nitrendipine on urinary enzymes and microproteins following non-ionic radiocontrast administration. Nephrol Dial Transplant 1996; 11: 444–8.
72. Khoury Z, Schlicht JR, Como J et al. The effect of prophylactic nifedipine on renal function in patients administered contrast media. Pharmacotherapy 1995; 15: 59–65.
73. Spangberg-Viklund B, Berglund J et al. Does prophylactic treatment with felodipine, a calcium antagonist, prevent low-osmolar contrast-induced renal dysfunction in hydrated diabetic and nondiabetic patients with normal or moderately reduced renal function? Scand J Urol Nephrol 1996; 30: 63–8.
74. Sketch MH Jr, Whelton A, Schollmayer E et al. Prostaglandin E1 Study Group. Prevention of contrast media-induced renal dysfunction with prostaglandin E1: a randomized, double-blind, placebo-controlled study. Am J Ther 2001; 8: 155–62.
75. Attallah N, Yassine L, Musial J, Yee J, Fisher K. The potential role of statins in contrast nephropathy. Clin Nephrol 2004; 62: 273–8.
76. Vogt B, Ferrari P, Schonholzer C et al. Prophylactic hemodialysis after radiocontrast media in patients with renal insufficiency is potentially harmful. Am J Med 2001; 111: 692–8.
77. Lehnert T, Keller E, Gondolf K et al. Effect of haemodialysis after contrast medium administration in patients with renal insufficiency. Nephrol Dial Transplant 1998; 13: 358–62.
78. Huber W, Jeschke B, Kreymann B et al. Haemodialysis for the prevention of contrast-induced nephropathy: outcome of 31 patients with severely impaired renal function, comparison with patients at similar risk and review. Invest Radiol 2002; 37: 471–81.
79. Sterner G, Frennby B, Kurkus J, Nyman U. Does post-angiographic hemodialysis reduce the risk of contrast-medium nephropathy? Scand J Urol Nephrol 2000; 34: 323–6.
80. Berger ED, Bader BD, Bosker J, Risler T, Erley CM. Contrast media-induced kidney failure cannot be prevented by hemodialysis. Dtsch Med Wochenschr 2001; 126: 162–6.
81. Marenzi G, Marana I, Lauri G et al. The prevention of radiocontrast-agent-induced nephropathy by hemofiltration. N Engl J Med 2003; 349: 1333–40.
82. Ng MK, Tremmel J, Fitzgerald PJ, Fearon WF. Selective renal arterial infusion of fenoldopam for the prevention of contrast-induced nephropathy. J Interv Cardiol 2006; 19: 75–9.

3

Treatment of coronary artery disease in diabetic patients

Pilar Jiménez Quevedo and Manel Sabaté Tenas

Introduction • Coronary angioplasty in diabetic patients • Coronary bypass grafting in diabetic patients • Complications of revascularization procedures in diabetic patients • Adjunctive medical treatment in diabetic patients undergoing coronary revascularization • Summary

INTRODUCTION

It has been estimated that more than 50% of diabetic patients have significant coronary atherosclerotic lesions. This prevalence is 10-fold higher than that in the general population. A significant proportion of diabetic patients with coronary artery disease (CAD) are candidates for revascularization. Nearly 1.5 million revascularization procedures are performed each year in the United States, and approximately 15–25% of those occur in diabetic patients.[1]

Diabetes mellitus has been shown to be a predictor of poor outcomes in all modes of coronary revascularization. CAD of diabetic patients exhibits distinctive characteristics that infer an increased risk. Likewise, CAD in diabetics is characterized by being diffuse, affecting more often the left main and also the distal coronary tree, and presenting a more rapid progression as compared with non-diabetic patients (Figure 3.1).[2,3] Moreover, myocardial ischemia typically occurs without symptoms. As a result, diabetic patients have more incidence of multivessel atherosclerosis at the time of the diagnosis.[4]

In this chapter we will focus on the different modalities for the treatment of CAD in diabetic patients, and we will discuss their potential complications and also the adjunctive medical therapy.

CORONARY ANGIOPLASTY IN DIABETIC PATIENTS

Several attempts have been made to improve the acute and long-term outcomes of diabetic patients who need coronary revascularization. Traditionally, percutaneous balloon angioplasty in diabetic patients presented poorer outcomes as compared to the non-diabetic population.[5] With the advent of the stent, a significant reduction of both restenosis and clinical events were observed in diabetic patients,[6] however, long-term outcome remains poorer than in non-diabetic individuals, especially in the subgroup of insulin-dependent diabetics.[7] The prevailing mechanism of restenosis after stenting is accelerated intimal hyperplasia, which is exaggerated in diabetic patients.[8] Therefore, in recent years, attempts to reduce the restenosis after stent implantation have been focused on the creation of site-specific delivery of agents

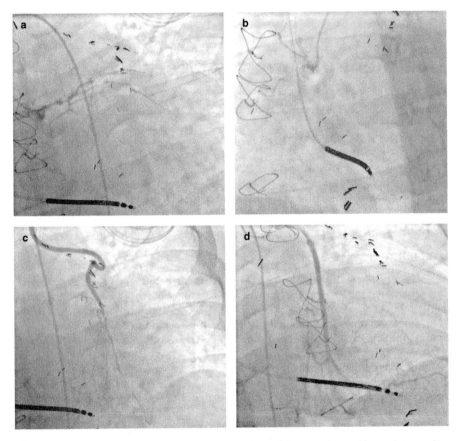

Figure 3.1 Coronary anatomy of an insulin-dependent diabetic patient with previous cardiac surgery. (a) Left coronary tree with a severe lesion in the distal part of the left main followed by the left anterior descending (LAD) and the circumflex artery occluded. (b) Occlusion of the proximal segment of the right coronary artery. (c) Patent left internal mammary artery to the LAD with the distal part of the native LAD severely and diffusely diseased. (d) Patent saphenous graft to the circumflex but once again the distal part has a small size and is diffusely diseased.

capable of interrupting cellular replication. In this regard, two drugs, sirolimus and paclitaxel, delivered from stent platforms, have been shown to be effective in randomized trials.

Sirolimus (rapamycin) is a macrocyclic lactone agent that interacts with cell cycle-regulating proteins, and inhibits cell division between phases G1 and S1. Following promising results from the first clinical studies with this stent, including very favourable lesions (the FIM [First in Man] and RAVEL [RAndomized study with the sirolimus-eluting Bx VELocity balloon-expandable stent] trials),[9,10] a randomized, large-scale trial designed to assess the safety and efficacy of sirolimus-eluting stent (SES) implantation in complex lesions was performed. Thus, the SIRIUS [SIRolImUS-coated Bx Velocity balloon-expandable stent in the treatment of patients with de novo coronary artery lesions] trial involved 1058 patients who were randomized to receive SES or bare-metal stent (BMS) implantation in *de novo* lesions.[11] The primary endpoint was the rate of target vessel failure (cardiac death, myocardial infarction, and repeat percutaneous or surgical revascularization of the target vessel) within 270 days. At follow-up, there was a significant reduction in the primary endpoint in the SES group (16.6% vs. 4.1%; P <0.001), as well as in restenosis (35.4% vs. 3.2%; P <0.001), and in target lesion revascularization rates (16.6% vs. 4.1%; P <0.001). These results were also confirmed in the Canadian and the European arms of the SIRIUS trials series (C- SIRIUS and E-SIRIUS).[12,13] The diabetic subgroup analyses of the SIRIUS trial demonstrated that in diabetic patients (n=279: 131 received SES and 148 BMS), the restenosis rates were significantly reduced in the SES group as compared with the BMS group (in-lesion: 50.5% vs. 17.6%; P <0.001; in-stent: 48.5% vs. 8.3%; P<0.001).[14] Major adverse cardiac events were also reduced in diabetic patients (25% in BMS vs. 9.2% in SES; P <0.001). However, when the effect of SES was analyzed according to diabetes status, the subgroup of diabetics treated with insulin presented a higher in-lesion restenosis rate as compared with those treated with oral agents (35% vs. 12.3%), and this was mainly due to restenosis at stent edges.[14] These results must be interpreted with caution because of the nature of a subgroup analysis with a relatively small sample size, especially in insulin-dependent diabetic patients (n=82).

The DIABETES (DIABETes and drug-Eluting Stent) trial was the only randomized study comparing SES and BMS implantation in diabetics.[15] This study was a multicenter, randomized, and placebo-controlled trial. One-hundred and sixty diabetic patients were included, 80 patients randomized to BMS, and 80 to SES. This trial was stratified according to diabetes treatment status. The primary endpoint of the study was late lumen loss as assessed by quantitative coronary angiography (QCA) at a 9-month follow-up. Both in-segment late lumen loss and restenosis rate were reduced in the SES group as compared to the BMS group (0.47 ± 0.5 mm vs. 0.06 ± 0.4 mm; P <0.001, and 33.7% vs. 7.8%; P <0.001, respectively). Of interest, this benefit was independent of diabetes status. Likewise, insulin-dependent diabetic patients showed a significant reduction in restenosis rate compared with BMS group (6.7% vs. 46.8%; P=0.001). This positive effect of SES in the subgroup of insulin-dependent diabetics is one of the main important contributions of this study, in contrast to the above-mentioned observations in the SIRIUS trial.

Furthermore, the paclitaxel eluting-stent (PES) has also proven to be effective in the prevention of restenosis. Paclitaxel is a lipophilic molecule derived from the Pacific yew tree, *Taxus brevifolia*, which is capable of inhibiting cellular division, motility, cellular activation, the secretory process, and signal transduction. The use of this stent appears to be efficacious in the reduction of restenosis after treatment of short, focal coronary lesions as demonstrated in TAXUS I and II trials.[16,17] The TAXUS IV trial was the first prospective, randomized and large-scale study performed to assess the safety and efficacy of the slow release PES.[18] In this trial 1326 patients were randomized to the implantation of a PES (n=667) or BMS (n=659). Overall, the PES group had a significant reduction in restenosis rate (26.6% vs. 7.9%, P <0.0001). Diabetes mellitus was identified in 28% of the entire cohort of patients included in the study. In diabetic patients, the use of PES reduced the risk of binary restenosis by 77% within the stent, and by 70% in the analysis segment. This reduction was also observed in the cohort of insulin-dependent diabetic patients (42.9% vs. 7.7%, P=0.007). Relative risk reduction of target lesion revascularization with the use of drug-eluting stent in the subgroup analyses of SIRIUS y TAXUS IV trial is shown in Table 3.1.[19]

Table 3.1 Relative risk reduction of target lesion revascularization with the use of drug-eluting stent in the subgroup analyses of SIRIUS y TAXUS IV trial

	Relative risk reduction SIRIUS trial (%)[11]	Relative risk reduction TAXUS IV trial (%)[18]
Overall population	75	73%
Non-diabetic group	79	76%
Diabetic group	68%	ID: 68
		NID: 67
Vessel size	71 (<2.75 mm)	76 (≤2.5 mm)
	83 (≤2.75 mm)	71 (>2.5–3.0 mm)
		68 (>3.0 mm)
Lesion length	73 (>13.5 mm)	77 (>20 mm)
	79 (≤13.5 mm)	70 (10–20 mm)
		73 (<10 mm)
Left anterior descending artery	74	69
Non-left anterior descending artery	77	76

ID; insulin-dependent; NID, non-insulin-dependent.

Adapted with permission from Sabaté M. Insulinodependencia, ¿Rapamicina resistencia? Rev Esp Cardiol 2006; 59: 91–3.[19]

The ISAR (Intracoronary Stenting and Antithrombotic Regimen)-DIABETES was a randomized trial designed to compare the safety and efficacy of the two drug-eluting stent (SES and PES) in diabetic patients.[20] In this study the late lumen loss and restenosis rate were significantly lower in the SES group as compared with the PES group (0.43 ± 0.45 mm vs. 0.67 ± 0.62 mm; $P=0.002$, and 6.9% vs. 16.5%; $P=0.03$, respectively). However, this study was underpowered to demonstrate differences in clinical restenosis.

In summary, the rates of angiographic restenosis and need for repeat target lesion revascularization have substantially decreased with the use of drug-eluting stents. However, these remain higher in diabetic as compared to non-diabetic patients.

CORONARY BYPASS GRAFTING IN DIABETIC PATIENTS

The incidence of diabetes in the population undergoing coronary bypass grafting (CABG) ranges from 12% to 38%.[21] Diabetes has been associated with increased morbidity and mortality after CABG, and is a strong predictor of death.[21] Several early studies comparing CABG surgery with balloon angioplasty in patients with multivessel disease showed an increase in mortality in the subgroup of diabetic patients treated with percutaneous coronary intervention.[22,23] However, in the stent era the randomized trials comparing both revascularization techniques did not show any significant differences in terms of mortality. The Arterial Revascularization Therapy Study (ARTS) was a prospective, randomized trial designed to compare coronary stenting versus CABG for the treatment of multivessel disease.[24] The subgroup analyses of diabetic patients ($n=208$) showed comparable survival rates free from stroke or myocardial infarction between both strategies at 1- and 3-year follow-up.[25,26] However, patients who underwent stent implantation more often required repeat revascularization procedures (1-year follow-up: 21.2% stent arm vs. 3.8% CABG arm; $P<0.001$, and 3-year follow-up: 26.7% stent arm vs. 6.6% CABG arm; $P<0.001$, respectively). The greater need for CABG following angioplasty was attributed to a less complete revascularization rate obtained in the stent arm (70.5% versus 84.1%; $P<0.001$).

After the introduction of drug-eluting stents in clinical practice, a significant decrease of clinical and angiographic restenosis has been demonstrated.[11] The potential impact of this reduction in restenosis after drug-eluting stent implantation compared with CABG in multivessel disease has been evaluated in the ARTS II trial.[27] The ARTS II trial compared the 1-year outcome of patients with multivessel disease treated with SES with the historical cohorts of patients (PCI and CABG arms) included in the ARTS I trial. In this study a lower incidence of MACE (death, stroke, or myocardial infarction) was evidenced in the SES group. However, the need for repeat revascularization was still higher than that of the historical CABG arm of the ARTS I trial. In the subgroup of diabetic patients ($n=267$) (Macaya C et al, personal communication), the overall MACE-free survival of patients treated with SES was similar to the ARTS I-CABG arm (84.3% versus 85.4%; $P=0.86$). However, as observed in the entire population, diabetic patients treated with SES presented a higher rate of repeat revascularization as compared with the historical CABG arm (12.6% versus 4.2%; $P=0.027$).

Considering the above-mentioned data, Flaherty et al proposed an algorithm to guide the type of coronary revascularization in diabetic patients (Figure 3.2).[28] Two ongoing randomized trials will compare the drug-eluting stent implantation versus surgery in diabetic patients with multivessel disease: the ongoing FREEDOM (Future Revascularization Evaluation in Patients With Diabetes Mellitus: Optimal Management of Multivessel Disease) and the CARDIA (Coronary Artery Revascularization in Diabetes) trials. These trials, which include the use of new technology (off-pump and complete arterial revascularization for surgical strategy and adjunctive platelet glycoprotein IIb/IIIa inhibitors in percutaneous intervention strategy), will shed light on this issue in future years.

COMPLICATIONS OF THE REVASCULARIZATION PROCEDURES IN DIABETIC PATIENTS

Complications after percutaneous coronary interventions in diabetic patients

Diabetes is a significant independent predictor of *death* and *myocardial infarction* after percutaneous coronary intervention.[29] One of the main complications after coronary angiography in diabetic patients is the development of contrast-induced nephropathy. *Contrast-induced nephropathy* is a severe complication that has been associated with an adverse prognostic impact. It is defined as a fixed (0.5 mg/dl) or proportionate (25%) rise in serum creatinine levels after the use of contrast agents. The major determinant of deterioration in renal function after angiography is previous renal insufficiency. However, in the absence of renal disease, diabetic patients have an increased risk compared with non-diabetic patients. As a result, according to the PCI guidelines, patients with renal dysfunction and diabetes should be monitored for

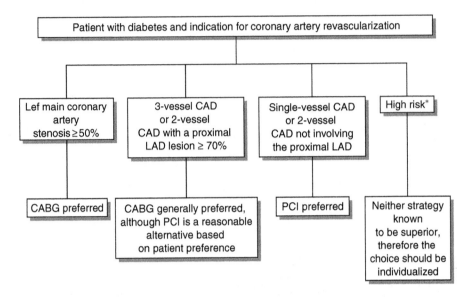

Figure 3.2 Coronary revascularization in diabetic patients. CAD, coronary artery disease; CABG, coronary artery bypass graft surgery; LAD, left anterior descending artery; PCI, percutaneous coronary intervention. *Based on AWESOME (Angina With Extremely Serious Operative Mortality Evaluation trial) criteria. Adapted from Flaherty JD, Davidson CJ. Diabetes and coronary revascularization. JAMA 2005; 293: 1501–8[28] with permission from the American Medical Association.

contrast-induced nephropathy.[30] Whenever possible, nephrotoxic drugs (certain antibiotics, non-steroidal anti-inflammatory agents, ciclosporin and metformin), especially in those with pre-existing renal dysfunction, should be withheld for 24–48 h prior to PCI and for 48 h afterwards.[31] The administration of fluids is generally recommended to reduce the risk of nephropathy following contrast administration; however, further data are needed to recommend N-acetylcysteine or intravenous sodium bicarbonate administration for the prevention of contrast-medium-induced nephropathy (Table 3.2).[32]

The development of *metformin-induced lactic acidosis* following intravascular use of contrast media is controversial. No conclusive evidence has been found to indicate that the intravascular use of contrast media precipitated the development of metformin-induced lactic acidosis in patients with normal S-creatinine ($<130 \, \mu mol/l$). The complication was almost always observed in non-insulin-dependent diabetic patients with decreased renal function before injection of contrast media.[32] Thus, it is recommended that in those patients taking metformin with evidence of renal impairment, metformin should be stopped and diabetic control obtained using alternative therapy before proceeding with angiography. On the other hand, patients with normal renal function taking metformin are not at risk of lactic acidosis following the use of iodinated contrast agents for angiography.[33]

Stroke is an uncommon (0.07–0.3%) but one of the most serious complications of PCI due to a high mortality and important morbidity. Diabetes has been reported as a predictor of stroke in patients with non-ST elevation acute coronary syndrome.[34] However, in diabetic patients undergoing PCI, an increased risk of stroke or vascular complication has not been reported.[35,36]

Table 3.2 Recommendations for reducing the risk of contrast-induced nephropathy[32]

Drug	Doses	Level of recommendation
Low osmolality contrast medium	Lowest required to complete the procedure	Recommended
Intravenous saline therapy	0.9% saline at 1 ml/kg/h for 24 h, beginning 2–12 h before administration of contrast agent	Generally recommended
Intravenous sodium bicarbonate	1. Before administration of contrast medium: sodium bicarbonate 154 mmol/l at 3 ml/kg/h	Not generally recommended. Further trials are needed
	2. After administration of contrast medium: 1 ml/kg/h for 6 h	
N-acetylcysteine	600 mg orally every 12 h, four doses beginning before administration of contrast medium	Not generally recommended. Further trials are needed

Coronary artery bypass grafting

Diabetic patients who undergo CABG have an increased morbidity and mortality. They suffer more frequently from *graft occlusion, cerebral events, and sternal wound problems* such as *mediastinitis* than the non-diabetic population.

Bilateral mammary artery grafting has been demonstrated to increase the long-term outcome compared to the implantation of only a single arterial graft. However, one of the main concerns for using bilateral internal mammary artery (IMA), especially in diabetics, has been the potential increased risk of mediastinitis. In this regard, recent studies have shown that if the IMA is harvested in a skeletonized fashion, the incidence of sternal wound problems is reduced. Calafiore et al compared single versus bilateral internal mammary artery in diabetic patients.[37] Five-hundred and fifty-eight diabetic patients were enrolled in this study. At 8-years' follow-up the group treated with bilateral mammary artery showed a significant increase in survival free from cardiac death, or myocardial infarction in the grafted area compared with those treated with a single left mammary artery.

ADJUNCTIVE MEDICAL TREATMENT IN DIABETIC PATIENTS UNDERGOING CORONARY REVASCULARIZATION

Two studies have demonstrated the relationship between glycemic control and outcome after PCI. In this setting, poor glycemic control was identified as a predictor of angiographic and clinical restenosis, as well as of progression of the atherosclerotic disease.[38–40] Conversely, in diabetic patients who underwent PCI, an optimal glycemic control (glycohaemoglobin $HbA_{1c} \leq 7\%$) is associated with a significant reduction in both rehospitalization for cardiac reasons, and recurrent angina.[39]

Table 3.3   Treatment effect of IIb/IIIa inhibitors in diabetic patients

Trial	Number[o] of diabetic patients	Death/MI (%) (IIb/IIIa vs. placebo)	Follow-up (days)	P value
EPILOG[42]	391	4.1 vs 14.8	180	<0.05
EPISTENT[41]	335	6.2 vs 12.7	180	0.040
PRISM-PLUS	362	11.2 vs 19.2	180	0.003
METANALYSIS[43,a]	1462	2.5 vs 4.5[c]	365	0.031
METANALYSIS[44,b]	6458	4.6 vs 6.2[c]	30	0.007

In all of these trials abciximab was administered, with the exception of PRISM-PLUS, which used tirofiban.

MI, myocardial infarction.

[a]This meta-analysis included the EPIC, EPILOG, and EPISTENT trials.

[b]This meta-analysis included the PRISM, PRISM-PLUS, PARAGON A, PARAGON B, PURSUIT, and GUSTO-IV trials.

[c]Death only.

EPIC: Evaluation of c7E3 for the Prevention of Ischemic Complications trial. EPILOG: Evaluation in PTCA to Improve Long-term Outcome with abciximab GP IIb/IIIa blockade trial. EPISTENT: Evaluation of Platelet IIb/IIIa Inhibitor for Stenting trial. PRISM: Platelet Receptor Inhibition in Ischemic Syndrome Management trial. PRISM-PLUS: Platelet Receptor Inhibition in Ischemic Syndrome Management in Patients Limited by Unstable Signs and Symptoms trial. PARAGON A: Platelet IIb/IIIa Antagonism for the Reduction of Acute coronary syndrome events in a Global Organization Network A trial. PARAGON B: Platelet IIb/IIIa Antagonism for the Reduction of Acute coronary syndrome events in a Global Organization Network B trial. PURSUIT: Platelet Glycoprotein IIb/IIIa in Unstable Angina: Receptor Suppression Using Integrilin Therapy trial. GUSTO-IV: Global Use of Strategies to Open Occluded Coronary Arteries IV trial.

Diabetic patients exhibit a hypercoagulable state, which is translated into an increased risk of thrombotic events and in laboratory abnormalities. Post hoc analyses from randomized trials have demonstrated that abciximab improves long-term outcome in diabetic patients after PCI (Table 3.3).[41,42] In a meta-analysis[43] of all studies evaluating the efficacy of abciximab in diabetic patients ($n=1462$), the association of abciximab and stent implantation reduced the 1-year mortality in diabetic patients from 4.5% to 2.5% ($P=0.03$).[43] Roffi et al performed a meta-analysis of diabetic patients enrolled in six large-scale platelet glycoprotein IIb/IIIa inhibitor trials.[44] More than 6000 diabetic patients were included, and IIb/IIIa inhibition therapy was associated with a significant reduction in mortality at 30 days (6.2% to 4.6%; $P=0.007$).[44] Among 1279 diabetic patients undergoing PCI, the use of these agents was associated with a mortality reduction at 30 days from 4.0% to 1.2% ($P=0.002$). Recently, a randomized trial has been performed in diabetic patients undergoing PCI: the ISAR-REACT 2 (Intracoronary Stenting and Antithrombotic Regimen: Rapid Early Action for Coronary Treatment) trial.[45] Seven-hundred and one patients were included, who received 600 mg of clopidogrel before PCI, and were randomly assigned to abciximab or placebo. At one year there were no significant differences in the incidence of death or myocardial infarction between groups. However, a significant decrease in restenosis rate was observed in the abciximab group. Data on the impact of abciximab and the incidence of restenosis in diabetic patients are inconsistent. The EPISTENT (Evaluation of Platelet IIb/IIIa Inhibitors for STENTING) trial showed a reduction of target lesion revascularization in diabetic patients treated with abciximab.[41] However, two randomized trials (the DANTE [Diabetes Abciximab steNT Evaluation] and ASIAD [Abciximab in Stenting Inhibits restenosis Among Diabetics] trials), did not demonstrate that the use of abciximab compared with placebo reduced neointimal hyperplasia or restenosis rate in this population.[46,47]

Platelet dysfunction, among other mechanisms, contributes to the increased risk of atherothrombotic complications in the diabetic population.[48] Platelets from diabetic subjects are less sensitive to antiplatelet drugs, which have been associated with an increased risk of ischemic events.[49,50] Aspirin treatment represents a gold standard for secondary prevention in patients with cardiovascular disease, as it reduces the incidence of clinical events.[51] Thienopyridine derivatives (ticlopidine and clopidogrel) have an additive effect in platelet aggregation, and could be particularly efficacious in preventing ischemic events in diabetic patients.[52] Clopidogrel therapy in addition to aspirin as primary prevention has not demonstrated any significant clinical benefit but has shown an increase in moderate bleeding in high-risk patients (the CHARISMA [Clopidogrel for High Atherothrombotic Risk, Ischemic Stabilization, Management, and Avoidance] trial).[53] However, in the setting of an acute myocardial infarction, dual antiplatelet therapy with aspirin and clopidogrel (COMMIT [ClOpidogrel and Metoprolol in Myocardial Infarction Trial] trial) showed a clear reduction in mortality.[54] Besides, during coronary stenting the combination of clopidogrel and aspirin results in a significant reduction in clinical events. In this regard, recent studies (CREDO [Clopidogrel for Reduction of Events During Observation] and PCI-CURE [Percutaneous Coronary Intervention – The Clopidogrel in Unstable Angina to Prevent Recurrent Events Trial]) have shown a significant reduction in the incidence of death, myocardial infarction or stroke with long-term (9–12 months') treatment with clopidogrel in patients undergoing elective percutaneous coronary interventions.[55,56] However, this reduction did not reach statistical significance in the diabetic subgroup, probably due to an underpowered sample size. Following the results of these studies, the 7th ACCP (American College of Chest Physicians) Conference on Antithrombotic and Thrombolytic Therapy increased the recommended duration of double antiaggregation after stent placement up to 9–12 months.[57]

SUMMARY

Diabetes mellitus, as a vascular disease, increases the risk for CAD and is identified as an independent predictor of poor outcomes after coronary revascularization. The recent development of drug-eluting stents has decreased the need for repeat revascularization after percutaneous coronary interventions. However, this is still higher than that of coronary artery bypass graft. In this regard, the ongoing FREEDOM and CARDIA trials may answer the issue of the preferred technique in diabetic patients with multivessel disease. Finally, accurate glycemic control and proper antiplatelet therapy are mandatory during and after percutaneous coronary interventions to ensure better immediate and long-term outcomes.

REFERENCES

1. Kip KE, Faxon DP, Detre KM et al. Coronary angioplasty in diabetic patients. The National Heart, Lung, and Blood Institute Percutaneous Transluminal Coronary Angioplasty Registry. Circulation 1996; 94: 1818–25.
2. Waller BF, Palumbo PJ, Lie JT, Roberts WC. Status of the coronary arteries at necropsy in diabetes mellitus with onset after 30 years: analysis of 229 diabetic patients with and without clinical evidence of coronary heart disease and comparison. Am J Med 1980; 69: 498–506.
3. Rozenman Y, Sapoznikov D, Mosseri M et al. Long-term angiographic follow-up of coronary balloon angioplasty in patients with diabetes mellitus a clue to the explanation of the results of the BARI study. J Am Coll Cardiol 1997; 30: 1420–5.
4. Wingard DL, Barrett-Connor EL, Scheidt-Nave C, McPhillips JB. Prevalence of cardiovascular and renal complication in older adults with normal or impaired glucose tolerance or NIDDM: a population-based study. Diabetes Care 1993; 16: 1022–5.
5. Stein B, Weintraub WS, Gebhart SP et al. Influence of diabetes mellitus on early and late outcome after percutaneous transluminal coronary angioplasty. Circulation 1995; 91: 979–89.
6. Van Belle E, Perie M, Braune D et al. Effects of coronary stenting on vessel patency and long-term clinical outcome after percutaneous coronary revascularization in diabetic patients. J Am Coll Cardiol 2002; 40: 410–17.
7. Abizaid A, Kornowski R, Mintz GS et al. The influence of diabetes mellitus on acute and late clinical outcomes following coronary stent implantation. J Am Coll Cardiol 1998; 32: 584–9.
8. Kornoswki R, Mintz GS, Kent KM et al. Increase restenosis in diabetes mellitus after coronary interventions is due to exaggerated intimal hyperplasia: a serial intravascular study. Circulation 1997; 95: 1366–9.
9. Sousa JE, Costa MA, Abizaid A et al. Four-year angiographic and intravascular ultrasound follow-up of patients treated with sirolimus-eluting stents. Circulation 2005; 111: 2326–9.
10. Morice MC, Serruys PW, Sousa JE et al. A randomized comparison of a sirolimus-eluting stent with a standard stent for coronary revascularization. N Engl J Med 2002; 346: 1773–80.
11. JW Moses, MB Leon and JJ Popma et al. Sirolimus-eluting stents versus standard stents in patients with stenosis in a native coronary artery, N Engl J Med 2003; 349: 1315–23.
12. Schampaert E, Cohen EA, Schluter M et al. The Canadian study of the sirolimus-eluting stent in the treatment of patients with long de novo lesions in small native coronary arteries (C-SIRIUS). J Am Coll Cardiol 2004; 43: 1110–15.
13. Schoefer J, Schluter M, Gershlick AH et al. Sirolimus- eluting stents for treatment of patients with long atherosclerotic lesions in small coronary arteries: double-blind, randomised controlled trial (E-SIRIUS). Lancet 2003; 362: 1093–9.
14. Moussa I, Leon MB, Baim DS et al. Impact of sirolimus-eluting stents on outcome in diabetic patients: a SIRIUS (SIRolImUS-coated Bx Velocity balloon-expandable stent in the treatment of patients with de novo coronary artery lesions) substudy. Circulation 2004; 109: 2273–8.
15. Sabate M, Jimenez-Quevedo P, Angiolillo DJ et al; DIABETES Investigators. Randomized comparison of sirolimus-eluting stent versus standard stent for percutaneous coronary revascularization in diabetic patients: the diabetes and sirolimus-eluting stent (DIABETES) trial. Circulation 2005; 112: 2175–83.
16. Grube E, Silber S, Hauptmann KE, et al. TAXUS I: six- and twelve-month results from a randomized, double-blind trial on a slow-release paclitaxel-eluting stent for de novo coronary lesions. Circulation 2003; 107: 38–42.
17. Colombo A, Drzewiecki J, Banning A et al. Randomized study to assess the effectiveness of slow- and moderate-release polymer-based paclitaxel-eluting stents for coronary artery lesions. Circulation 2003; 108: 788–94.
18. Stone GW, Ellis SG, Cox DA et al. A polymer-based paclitaxel-eluting stent in patients with coronary artery disease. N Engl J Med 2004; 350: 221–31.
19. Sabaté M. Insulinodependencia, ¿Rapamicina resistencia? Rev Esp Cardiol 2006; 59: 91–3.

20. Dibra A, Kastrati A, Mehilli J et al; ISAR-DIABETES Study Investigators. Paclitaxel-eluting or sirolimus-eluting stents to prevent restenosis in diabetic patients. N Engl J Med 2005; 353: 663–70.
21. Leavitt BJ, Sheppard L, Maloney C et al; Northern New England Cardiovascular Disease Study Group. Effect of diabetes and associated conditions on long-term survival after coronary artery bypass graft surgery. Circulation 2004; 110(Suppl 1): II41–4.
22. BARI Investigators. Influence of diabetes on 5-year mortality and morbidity in a randomized trial comparing CABG and PTCA in patients with multivessel disease. Circulation 1997; 96: 1761–9.
23. Niles N, McGrath PD, Malenka D et al. Survival of patients with diabetes and multivessel coronary artery disease after surgical or percutaneous coronary revascularization: results of a large regional prospective study. J Am Coll Cardiol 2001; 31: 1008–15.
24. Serruys PW, Unger F, Sousa JE et al for The Arterial Revascularization Therapies Study Group. Comparison of coronary-artery bypass surgery and stenting for the treatment of multivessel disease. N Engl J Med 2001; 344: 1117–24.
25. van den Brand MJ, Rensing BJ, Morel MA et al. The effect of completeness of revascularization on vent-free survival at one year in the ARTS trial. J Am Coll Cardiol 2002; 39: 559–64.
26. Legrand VMG, Serruys PW, Unger F, of the Arterial Revascularization Therapy Study (ARTS) Investigators. Three-year outcome after coronary stenting versus bypass surgery for the treatment of multivessel disease. Circulation 2004; 109: 1114–20.
27. Serruys PW, Ong ATL, Morice AC et al; on behalf of the ARTS II investigators. Arterial revascularization therapies study part II – sirolimus-eluting stent for the treatment of patients with multivessel de novo coronary artery lesions. EuroInterv 2005; 1: 147–56.
28. Flaherty JD, Davidson CJ. Diabetes and coronary revascularization. JAMA 2005; 293: 1501–8.
29. Mathew V, Gersh BJ, Williams BA et al. Outcomes in patients with diabetes mellitus undergoing percutaneous coronary intervention in the current era: a report from the Prevention of REStenosis with Tranilast and its Outcomes (PRESTO) trial. Circulation 2004; 109: 476–80.
30. Smith SC Jr, Dove JT, Jacobs AK et al; American College of Cardiology/American Heart Association Task Force on Practice Guidelines (Committee to revise the 1993 guidelines for percutaneous transluminal coronary angioplasty); Society for Cardiac Angiography and Interventions. ACC/AHA Guidelines for Percutaneous Coronary Intervention (revision of the 1993 PTCA guidelines) – executive summary: a report of the American College of Cardiology/American Heart Association task force on practice guidelines (Committee to revise the 1993 guidelines for percutaneous transluminal coronary angioplasty) endorsed by the Society for Cardiac Angiography and Interventions. Circulation 2001; 103: 3019–41.
31. Barrett BJ, Parfrey PS. Clinical practice. Preventing nephropathy induced by contrast medium. N Engl J Med 2006; 354: 379–86.
32. Thomsen HS, Morcos SK. Contrast media and metformin: guidelines to diminish the risk of lactic acidosis in non-insulin-dependent diabetics after administration of contrast media. ESUR Contrast Media Safety Committee. Eur Radiol 1999; 9: 738–40.
33. Nawaz S, Cleveland T, Gaines PA, Chan P. Clinical risk associated with contrast angiography in metformin treated patients: a clinical review. Clin Radiol 1998; 53: 342–4.
34. Cronin L, Mehta SR, Zhao F et al. Stroke in relation to cardiac procedures in patients with non-ST-elevation acute coronary syndrome: a study involving > 18 000 patients. Circulation 2001; 104: 269–74.
35. Fuchs S, Stabile E, Kinnaird TD et al. Stroke complicating percutaneous coronary interventions: incidence, predictors, and prognostic implications. Circulation 2002; 106: 86–91.
36. Berry C, Kelly J, Cobbe SM, Eteiba H. Comparison of femoral bleeding complications after coronary angiography versus percutaneous coronary intervention. Am J Cardiol 2004; 94: 361–3.
37. Calafiore AM, Di Mauro M, Di Giammarco G et al. Single versus bilateral internal mammary artery for isolated first myocardial revascularization in multivessel disease: long-term clinical results in medically treated diabetic patients. Ann Thorac Surg 2005; 80: 888–95.

38. Mazeika P, Prasad N, Bui S, Seidelin PH. Predictors of angiographic restenosis after coronary intervention in patients with diabetes mellitus. Am Heart J 2003; 145: 1013–21.
39. Corpus RA, George PB, House JA et al. Optimal glycemic control is associated with a lower rate of target vessel revascularization in treated type II diabetics patients undergoing elective percutaneous coronary intervention. J Am Coll Cardiol 2004; 43: 8–14.
40. Nathan DM, Lachin J, Cleary P et al. Intensive diabetes therapy and carotid intima-media thickness in type 1 diabetes mellitus. N Engl J Med 2003; 348: 2294–303.
41. Marso SP, Lincoff M, Ellis S et al.. Optimizing the percutaneous interventional outcomes for patients with diabetes mellitus Results of the EPISTENT (evaluation of platelet IIb/IIIa inhibitors for stenting trial) Diabetics substudy. Circulation 1999; 100: 2477–84.
42. Kleiman NS, Lincoff AM, Kereiakes D et al.. Diabetes mellitus, glycoprotein IIb/IIIa blockade, and heparin. Circulation 1998; 97: 1912–20.
43. Bhatt DL, Marso SP, Lincoff AM et al. Abciximab reduces mortality in diabetics following percutaneous coronary intervention. J Am Coll Cardiol 2000; 35: 922–8.
44. Roffi M, Chew DP, Mukherjee D et al. Platelet glycoprotein IIb/IIIa inhibitors reduce mortality in diabetics with non ST segment-elevation acute coronary syndromes. Circulation 2001; 104: 2767–71.
45. Kastrati A, Mehilli J, Neumann FJ et al. Abciximab in patients with acute coronary syndromes undergoing percutaneous coronary intervention after clopidogrel pretreatment: The ISAR-REACT 2 Randomized Trial. JAMA 2006; 295: 1531–8.
46. Chaves AJ, Sousa AG, Mattos LA et al. Volumetric analysis of in-stent intimal hyperplasia in diabetic patients treated with or without abciximab: results of the Diabetes Abciximab steNT Evaluation (DANTE) randomized trial. Circulation 2004; 109: 861–6.
47. Chen WH, Kaul U, Leung SK et al. A randomized, double-blind, placebo-controlled trial of abciximab for prevention of in-stent restenosis in diabetic patients after coronary stenting: results of the ASIAD (Abciximab in Stenting Inhibits restenosis Among Diabetics) Trial. J Invasive Cardiol 2005; 17: 534–8.
48. Vinik AI, Erbas T, Park TS, Nolan R, Pittenger GL. Platelet dysfunction in type 2 diabetes. Diabetes Care 2001; 24: 1476 –85.
49. Angiolillo DJ, Fernandez-Ortiz A, Bernardo E et al. Platelet function profiles in patients with type 2 diabetes and coronary artery disease on combined aspirin and clopidogrel treatment. Diabetes 2005; 54: 2430–5.
50. Eikelboom JW, Hirsh J, Weitz JI et al. Aspirin-resistant thromboxane biosynthesis and the risk of myocardial infarction, stroke, or cardiovascular death in patients at high risk for cardiovascular events. Circulation 2002; 105: 1650–5.
51. Collaborative overview of randomised trials of antiplatelet therapy-I: prevention of death, myocardial infarction, and stroke by prolonged antiplatelet therapy in various categories of patients. Antiplatelet Trialists' Collaboration. BMJ 1994; 308: 81–106.
52. Bhatt DL, Marso SP, Hirsch AT, Ringleb PA, Hacke W. Amplified benefit of clopidogrel versus aspirin in patients with diabetes mellitus. Am J Cardiol 2002; 90: 625–8.
53. Bhatt DL, Fox KA, Hacke W et al. Clopidogrel and aspirin versus aspirin alone for the prevention of atherothrombotic events. N Engl J Med 2006; 3504: 1706–17.
54. Chen ZM, Jiang LX, Chen YP et al; COMMIT (ClOpidogrel and Metoprolol in Myocardial Infarction Trial) collaborative group. Addition of clopidogrel to aspirin in 45 852 patients with acute myocardial infarction: randomised placebo-controlled trial. Lancet 2005; 366: 1607–21.
55. Yusuf S, Zhao F, Mehta SR et al. Effects of clopidogrel in addition to aspirin in patients with acute coronary syndromes without ST-segment elevation. The clopidogrel in unstable angina to prevent recurrent events trial investigators. N Engl J Med 2001; 345: 494–502.
56. Mehta SR, Yusuf S, Peters RJ, Bertrand ME, Lewis BS. Effects of pretreatment with clopidogrel and aspirin followed by long-term therapy in patients undergoing percutaneous coronary intervention: the PCI-CURE study. Lancet 2001; 358: 527–33.
57. Popma JJ, Berger P, Ohman EM, Harrington RA, Grines C. Antithrombotic therapy during percutaneous coronary intervention: the Seventh ACCP Conference on Antithrombotic and Thrombolytic Therapy. Chest 2004; 126(3 Suppl): 576S–599S.

4

Ad hoc percutaneous coronary intervention

Francesco Saia, Federica Baldazzi,
and Antonio Marzocchi

Introduction • *Ad hoc* angioplasty versus deferred procedure • Safety and efficacy of *ad hoc* angioplasty • Patient selection for *ad hoc* percutaneous coronary intervention • Economic considerations • Transradial approach • Summary

INTRODUCTION

Ad hoc angioplasty is defined as a percutanous coronary intervention (PCI) performed at the same time as diagnostic cardiac catheterization.

At the beginning of the angioplasty era, PCI procedures were generally deferred to a later time with respect to the coronary angiography, mainly for safety reasons. Remarkable technical improvements of the materials and devices for angiography and percutaneous interventions, together with clear advancement of peri-procedural medications and operators' skills, led to progressively increasing rates of *ad hoc* PCI. In the last several years PCI has increasingly been performed immediately after the diagnostic coronary angiographic procedure, with reported incidence ranging from 52% to 83%.[1-3] Reduction of hospitalization length of stay, and potential cost reduction were the major determinants of this strategy's modification.[4]

General guidelines for *ad hoc* angioplasty were issued by the American College of Cardiology/Society for Cardiovascular Angiography and Interventions (ACC/SCAI), in order to reduce the risk of invasive cardiology procedures when performed in settings without full-support services.[5] In the recent SCAI statement about *ad hoc* versus separate performance of diagnostic cardiac catheterization and coronary intervention, it is declared that '*ad hoc* intervention is reasonable for many, but not appropriate for all patients and should not be considered standard therapy'.[6] These guidelines suggest that a planned PCI procedure would be preferred for higher-risk patients with severe clinical condition.[5,6]

This chapter describes briefly pros and cons of *ad hoc* PCI, with the aim of helping the interventional cardiologist in the choice of the correct approach for each individual patient, and to provide useful suggestions for laboratories in which *ad hoc* PCI is performed.

AD HOC ANGIOPLASTY VERSUS DEFERRED PROCEDURE

Several conditions can determine and influence the feasibility and safety of *ad hoc* coronary angioplasty as compared to a deferred, planned procedure. For this reason, it is not possible to affirm *tout court* the superiority of an interventional approach over the other. A randomized study comparing the safety and efficiency of separate

Table 4.1   Theoretical differences between *'ad hoc'* and 'planned' PCI

Ad hoc PCI	Planned PCI
Advantages	
Reduces length of hospitalization	Allows scrupulous procedural planning
Reduces healthcare costs	Allows consultation with colleagues and cardiothoracic surgeons
Reduces patient's total X-ray exposure	Guarantees appropriate patient information about the risk/benefit ratio, and informed consent collection
	(Increases hospital reimbursement)
Reduces the likelihood of vascular complication	
Is generally preferred by patients	Decreases hemodynamic and renal effects of contrast loading
Disadvantages	
Difficult to plan the procedure and prepare the appropriate materials beforehand	Prolongs hospitalization
Increases the acute contrast loading	Increases healthcare costs
Does not always allow adequate pharmacological pretreatment	Increases total X-ray exposure
Informed consensus more "aleatory"	Increases the likelihood of access site complications
Lack of collegial and interdisciplinary discussion	Is generally less appreciated by patients

PCI, Percutaneous coronary intervention.

versus *ad hoc* procedures has never been performed. However, there are some specific characteristics that might suggest the shrewd choice of one or the other of the two strategies in different situations.

Ad hoc PCI offers several theoretical advantages over deferred, planned angioplasty (Table 4.1):

- reduction of hospitalization length
- reduction of healthcare costs
- reduction of patient's total X-ray exposure
- reduction of vascular complication (one access and one invasive procedure with its relative associated risks and well-known morbidity).

In addition, this procedure is more comfortable and generally preferred by patients.

However, *ad hoc* PCI carries a number of possible disadvantages that should be carefully evaluated on a case-by-case basis. Combining diagnostic and interventional procedures is obviously associated with prolonged procedural time. Longer procedures are directly associated with increased acute contrast loading, higher acute X-ray exposure,[7] and greater operators' fatigue. Pharmacological pretreatment might not be adequate for the patient's condition, especially in terms of antiplatelet agents.[8–10]

A planned, elective PCI procedure allows careful evaluation of the angiography, and stimulates ample discussion and meeting with colleagues and cardiac surgeons to decide the best strategy for revascularization for the patient. In addition, planned PCI permits preparation of material and devices necessary to accomplish the procedure, and allows availability of all possible instrumentation and devices that might be useful in the event of a complicated procedure (e.g. intra-aortic balloon pump or other left ventricular assist devices, temporary pacemakers etc). Adoption of an *ad hoc* PCI strategy makes it more difficult to inform the patient and the family about the risks and benefits of the procedure, and about alternative treatments, and may raise doubts about the correct obtaining of informed consent.

SAFETY AND EFFICACY OF *AD HOC* ANGIOPLASTY

In the pre-stent era, studies that compared outcomes of separate PCI to outcomes of *ad hoc* PCI found no significant differences in angiographic success rates or complications.[6] However, in two studies, *ad hoc* procedures were associated with an increased risk of complications in patients with unstable angina or other high-risk features.[3,11]

More recently, Shubrooks et al reported the outcome of 4136 PCIs performed in seven centers in 1997.[12] Overall, 42% were performed *ad hoc* (range 7–77% among centers). Stents were used in 72% of the *ad hoc* group and in 60% of those having separate procedures. Adjusted rates of clinical success were not different between *ad hoc* and non-*ad hoc* procedures (93.7% vs. 93.6%); there was no difference in the incidence of death (0.6% vs. 0.5%), emergency (0.9% vs. 0.8%), or any (1.4% vs. 0.8%) coronary artery bypass surgery, or myocardial infarction (2.6% vs. 2.0%). Vascular complications were lower in patients undergoing an *ad hoc* PCI procedure (0.6% versus 1.5%; $P = 0.006$).[12]

Goldstein et al evaluated data from the New York State Department of Health angioplasty database from 1995 to 1998, which included information from 33 centers using *ad hoc* PCI in 7–86% of procedures.[13] The cohort included 38 411 patients undergoing *ad hoc* PCI, and 23 462 patients undergoing separate procedures during the same hospitalization. Patients with staged interventions occurring in hospitals or admissions different from those of the initial cardiac catheterization ($n = 32 620$) were excluded. Stents were used in 63% of patients. Univariate and logistic regression analyses showed that *ad hoc* versus separate performance of PCI was not a predictor of mortality. The *ad hoc* strategy was associated with an increased risk of mortality in those with congestive heart failure during the same admission (odds ratio (OR) = 1.6; $P = 0.04$), and Canadian Cardiovascular Society class IV status (OR = 1.6; $P = 0.04$). The investigators concluded that overall mortality rates were similar for *ad hoc* and separate procedures, but that *ad hoc* PCI was associated with an increase in mortality for some high-risk subgroups.[13]

Another multicenter study showed that the risk of major complication (myocardial infarction, emergency coronary artery bypass graft (CABG) or death) was more frequent for an *ad hoc* strategy than for a staged procedure (2% vs. 1.6%).[11] In this study, multivariate analysis identified several subgroups of patients who had an increased risk for *ad hoc* procedures: patients with multivessel disease (OR 1.64, 95% confidence interval (CI) 1.13 to 2.39); female sex (OR 1.64, 95% CI 1.05 to 2.55); age >65 years (OR 1.40, 5% CI 1.02 to 1.93); and patients undergoing multilesion PTCA (OR 1.53, 95% CI 1.06 to 2.21).[11]

Vascular complications (bleeding from the site of puncture, hematoma, pseudoaneurysm, etc) represent an important issue for interventional procedures, and they are directly related to length of hospitalization and costs. Vascular complication can be related to the number of accesses used to perform the procedure (one or more for a staged strategy), and to the different accesses used (transradial vs. transbrachial vs. transfemoral). Some closure devices do not allow early repuncture of the access site where they are positioned, and in any case a double puncture of the same vessel may be more problematic. Change of the site of arterial puncture in some cases may force the operator to use a less familiar approach to accomplish the intervention. Furthermore, a double procedure is intuitively related to an increased risk of vascular complications, since it exposes twice to the same risks. As previously mentioned, this was confirmed in the study by the Northern New England Cardiovascular Disease Study Group.[12]

Ad hoc PCI requires utilization of higher amounts of contrast medium in a single procedure. Contrast loading may be a serious problem, especially for patients with hemodynamic instability (volume loading) and renal failure. Contrast-induced acute renal failure after PCI is a very serious complication associated with significant in-hospital and long-term morbidity and mortality.[14,15] Independent predictors of this untoward event are baseline creatinine clearance, diabetes mellitus, acute myocardial infarction, shock, and contrast dose.[14-16] Some data suggest that a second contrast load should be delayed for at least 72 h to minimize the risk of contrast-induced nephropathy.[17] Preventive strategies to minimize contrast-induced nephropathy are needed, and they include pretreatment with vigorous hydration and acetylcysteine, and venovenous hemofiltration, that must be co-ordinated and sometimes initiated before the PCI.[18,19] Clearly these measures may be more easily undertaken in elective, planned procedures. However, in many cases they could, and should, be considered also for diagnostic catheterization, thus opening up the way to *ad hoc* angioplasty with appropriate pretreatment, at least for interventions with expected low additional amounts of dye.

PATIENT SELECTION FOR *AD HOC* PERCUTANEOUS CORONARY INTERVENTION

In the absence of randomized trials to guide selection of patients for *ad hoc* PCI, published guidelines have been based on observational series and the opinions of experts. *Ad hoc* PCI is generally considered safe and feasible, but it is important to detect a population of patients at high risk of major complication, for whom a deferred PCI strategy would be preferable. A summary of these recommendations, mainly based on the results of relatively old studies, is given in Table 4.2.

Shaw et al analyzed the American College of Cardiology National Cardiovascular Data Registry and identified a population at high risk of major complications and death following PCI.[20] This population included patients older than 50 years, left ventricular ejection less than 30%, complex lesion morphology, and renal failure. Goldstein et al identified congestive heart failure (NYHA [New York Heart Association] III e IV) and angina CCS (Canadian Cardiovascular Society) class IV as other high-risk features for *ad hoc* PCI.[13] However, the concept of high-risk procedure has gradually changed over the years. Liberal utilization of stents (> 90% of the procedures) and the reduction of periprocedural events in high-risk PCI linked to glyco-protein IIb/IIIa utilization, provide a strong rationale for a more widespread

Table 4.2 Clinical and angiographic parameters that may indicate preference for one interventional strategy over the other according to current guidelines

Ad hoc PCI preferred	Planned PCI preferred
Clinical factors	
Acute myocardial infarction	Congestive heart failure (NYHA III/IV)[a]
Previous PCI	Age greater than 75 years[a]
Refractory unstable angina in need of urgent revascularization	Renal failure[a]
High risk of vascular complication	Very low LVEF[a]
Angiographic parameters	
Low-risk patients with simple lesion morphology	Severe multivessel disease[a]
Restenotic lesions	Very complex lesions[a]
Intermediate lesions when immediate invasive physiological evaluation is available	Borderline or controversial indication for PCI (e.g. unprotected left main procedures) Intermediate lesions when invasive physiological evaluation is not possible

LVEF, left ventricular ejection fraction; PCI, percutaneous coronary intervention.

[a]The Authors suggest that these parameters should be considered in combination. Sometimes, this may paradoxically lead to consider *ad hoc* PCI more appropriate than a deferred PCI (e.g. severe multivessel disease in very old patients and patients with renal failure, in whom it might be wiser to treat one or two vessels immediately, and defer the completion of treatment to a second session; see text).

utilization of an *ad hoc* PCI strategy.[21] Accordingly, for example, more recent data suggest that rapid triage of unstable patients to the catheterization laboratory, with aggressive antithrombotic therapy followed by *ad hoc* PCI results in superior 30-day outcomes compared to prolonged antithrombotic treatment for 3–5 days before angiography.[22]

A recently issued ACC/AHA/SCAI 2005 guideline update for PCI state that '*ad hoc* percutaneous revascularization should not be routinely performed in patients in whom the angiographic findings are unanticipated or the indication, suitability, or preferences for percutaneous revascularization is unclear'.[1] On the other hand, an *ad hoc* strategy is particularly suitable for patients with high suspicion of restenosis (angina within 6–12 months after the initial procedure), acute myocardial infarction, refractory unstable angina in need of urgent revascularization, single-vessel disease, in the absence of morphological features predictive of an adverse outcome.[1,23,24]

The SCAI recommend that patient safety should be the paramount consideration when contemplating *ad hoc* intervention, and that *ad hoc* PCI must be individualized and not be a standard or required strategy for all patients.[6] Obviously, we fully agree with the necessity of taking patient's safety into maximal consideration, and we are profoundly convinced about the opportunity of scrupulous individualized selection of the strategy for PCI. However, based on the experience of many centers that are routinely performing *ad hoc* PCI,[25] we suggest that this strategy could be safely accomplished in most cases. In our opinion, the factors listed in Table 4.2 which would favor a deferred PCI strategy, should be appropriately considered as general warnings to seriously consider before proceeding to PCI, but they cannot individually favor one approach over the other. Advanced age, for example, should not *per se* prevent *ad hoc* PCI. The same holds true for patients with mild and moderate renal failure, provided the procedure can be completed without excessive contrast loading. Paradoxically, in very old patients, in patients with heart failure, and in patients with renal failure, *ad hoc* PCI could be strongly preferred for very complex and multivessel PCI. In these cases, PCI can be more appropriately initiated in the first procedure and completed later on (staged procedure), to reduce the risks and the discomfort of a single, very long, session. Another issue that deserves some attention for *ad hoc* PCI is the the potentially problematic effect of the *oculo-stenotic reflex* on decision making for lesions of intermediate severity. Several practical approaches for the application of coronary physiological measurements in the catheterization laboratory have been identified, refined, simplified, and validated. In patients with intermediate lesions and no objective evidence of ischemia, *ad hoc* intervention should be undertaken only if equipment to invasively identify hemodynamically important lesions is available in the catheterization laboratory.[6]

ECONOMIC CONSIDERATIONS

One of the underlying assumptions of pursuing an *ad hoc* strategy is that a more rapid and definitive resolution of the ischemic coronary problem will yield significant cost savings through a shortened length of hospital stay and improved patient convenience. However, this theoretical intuitive conviction has been the subject of controversy. In the past, several studies have been performed to demonstrate this correlation between *ad hoc* procedures and reduced healthcare costs. O'Keefe et al reported in 1991 on charges associated with *ad hoc* versus separate PCI, and found significantly lower charges with *ad hoc* procedures.[26] However, their evaluation was done in a pre-stent era, and data were derived from hospital charges and not from direct cost accounting, so they may not accurately represent actual costs.

Adele et al performed a cost analysis study, to evaluate the cost advantage for a strategy of same-sitting diagnostic catheterization and PCI in comparison with staged PCI.[27] Almost half of the patients received a stent. Patients were stratified into three groups according the clinical indication: stable angina, unstable angina, and recent myocardial infarction. The use of various interventional technologies did not differ between the *ad hoc* and staged PCI groups. Surprisingly, the length of hospital stay was not significantly different between the *ad hoc* and staged groups in any of the clinical strata. There was a cost saving of borderline significance with an *ad hoc* strategy in patients with stable angina. Patients with unstable angina or post-myocardial infarction patients who were treated in an *ad hoc* fashion tended to incur a greater frequency of complications, although this trend was not statistically significant. Nevertheless, complications were a major driver of hospital costs, and lack of difference could have been influenced by this factor. Interestingly, for patients who received stents, in all cases an *ad hoc* strategy had significantly lower overall costs as compared with the staged strategy.

A single-centre retrospective study of a 10-year PCI experience (1990–2000), confirmed the safety and efficacy of *ad hoc* PCI in the stent era.[28] Length of hospital stay, throughout all years decreased for both the staged strategy and for an *ad hoc* procedure, but patients who underwent the combined procedure had a consistently

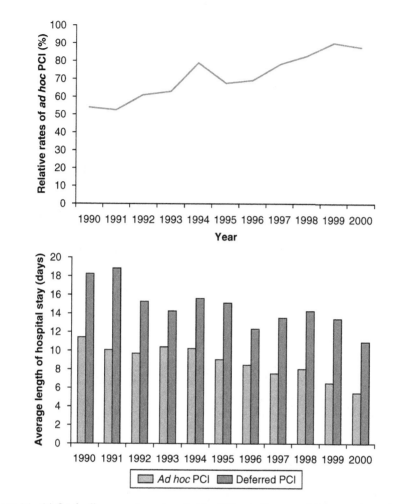

Figure 4.1   (a) Gradually increasing rates of *ad hoc* PCI over the years. (b) Progressive reduction of length of hospital stay in both *ad hoc* and deferred PCI strategies. *Ad hoc* PCI is consistently associated with lower average length of hospital stay compared to the deferred PCI group.[28]

shorter hospital stay (on average by 45%; Figure 4.1). This was true for patients with both stable and unstable angina. After adjusting for clinical and angiographic differences between the two groups and the use of stents, *ad hoc* PCI was an independent predictive factor of the length of hospital stay. The hospitalization cost was 40% lower in the combined strategy; for patients with stable angina the saving was 49%, and for unstable angina it was 29%.[28]

TRANSRADIAL APPROACH

The transradial artery approach is a good alternative to transfemoral access both for diagnostic catheterization and for PCI. This relatively new approach is characterized by reduction of vascular complication, duration of hospitalization and resultant over-all procedural costs, and the degree of the patient's discomfort.[29]

The feasibility of routine *ad hoc* angioplasty performed with the transradial approach has been recently evaluated.[30] The intention to perform *ad hoc* procedures via radial approach failed in 1.7% of the patients because of important subclavian tortuosity and/or severe radial artery spasm. Procedural results were similar between an *ad hoc* radial PCI group and a control matched group of deferred femoral PCI. No differences in fluoroscopy time, contrast volume, or catheters per case were found. Access site bleeding complications were significantly reduced in the radial group ($P < 0.01$). The total length of hospital (including the time for diagnostic and interventional procedures in the planned group) was slightly longer in the femoral-staged group, although this difference was not statistically significant (mean 2.9 days (range 2–6 days) compared to 1.9 days (range 1–5 days) in the combined group). The total hospital charge showed a cost saving of 7800 euros per patient with respect to a staged femoral strategy.[30]

The major advantages of transradial access are probably the reduction of costs as a consequence of a reduced incidence of site-related complications (bleeding from access site etc).[30]

SUMMARY

Ad hoc percutaneous coronary intervention (performing diagnostic angiography and coronary intervention within the same session) has gradually become more common, largely because of its convenience for patients and efficiency for physicians. This strategy is associated with lower vascular complications rates, a reduction of length of hospital stay, and decreased healthcare costs.

Ad hoc PCI is feasible and safe for most of the patients, but for some high-risk sub-groups of patients a deferred planned procedure would be preferable, to prevent serious complications. Clinical judgment for each individual patient is very impor-tant in deciding to proceed directly with PCI as opposed to a separate intervention. Informed consent may be a delicate issue, therefore detailed and complete information must be given to the patient before proceeding to PCI.

REFERENCES

1. Smith SC Jr, Feldman TE, Hirshfeld JW et al. ACC/AHA/SCAI 2005 guideline update for percutaneous coronary intervention. A report of the American College of Cardiology/American Heart Association Task Force on Practice Guidelines (ACC/AHA/SCAI Writing Committee to Update the 2001 Guidelines for Percutaneous Coronary Intervention). J Am Coll Cardiol 2006; 47: e1–121.
2. Rozenman Y, Gilon D, Zelingher J et al. One-stage coronary angiography and angioplasty. Am J Cardiol 1995; 75: 30–3.
3. Breisblatt WM, Ruffner RJ, Uretsky BF et al. Same-day angioplasty and diagnostic catheter-ization: safe and effective but riskier in unstable angina. Angiology 1991; 42: 607–13.
4. Clark VL, Dolce J. Unplanned admissions after outpatient cardiac catheterization. Clin Cardiol 1993; 16: 823–6.
5. Bashore TM, Bates ER, Kern MJ et al. American College of Cardiology/Society for Cardiac Angiography and Interventions clinical expert consensus document on cardiac catheteriza-tion laboratory standards: summary of a report of the American College of Cardiology Task Force on clinical expert consensus documents. Catheter Cardiovasc Interv 2001; 53: 281–6.

6. Blankenship JC, Klein LW, Laskey WK et al. SCAI statement on ad hoc versus the separate performance of diagnostic cardiac catheterization and coronary intervention. Catheter Cardiovasc Interv 2004; 63: 444–51.
7. Betsou S, Efstathopoulos EP, Katritsis D et al. Patient radiation doses during cardiac catheterization procedures. Br J Radiol 1998; 71: 634–9.
8. Steinhubl SR, Ellis SG, Wolski K et al. Ticlopidine pretreatment before coronary stenting is associated with sustained decrease in adverse cardiac events: data from the Evaluation of Platelet IIb/IIIa Inhibitor for Stenting (EPISTENT) Trial. Circulation 2001; 103: 1403–9.
9. Steinhubl SR, Berger PB, Mann JT 3rd et al. Early and sustained dual oral antiplatelet therapy following percutaneous coronary intervention: a randomized controlled trial. JAMA 2002; 288: 2411–20.
10. Mehta SR, Yusuf S, Peters RJ et al. Effects of pretreatment with clopidogrel and aspirin followed by long-term therapy in patients undergoing percutaneous coronary intervention: the PCI-CURE study. Lancet 2001; 358: 527–33.
11. Kimmel SE, Berlin JA, Hennessy S et al. Risk of major complications from coronary angioplasty performed immediately after diagnostic coronary angiography: results from the Registry of the Society for Cardiac Angiography and Interventions. J Am Coll Cardiol 1997; 30: 193–200.
12. Shubrooks SJ Jr, Malenka DJ, Piper WD et al. Safety and efficacy of percutaneous coronary interventions performed immediately after diagnostic catheterization in northern New England and comparison with similar procedures performed later. Am J Cardiol 2000; 86: 41–5.
13. Goldstein CL, Racz M, Hannan EL. Impact of cardiac catheterization-percutaneous coronary intervention timing on inhospital mortality. Am Heart J 2002; 144: 561–7.
14. McCullough PA, Wolyn R, Rocher LL et al. Acute renal failure after coronary intervention: incidence, risk factors, and relationship to mortality. Am J Med 1997; 103: 368–75.
15. Rihal CS, Textor SC, Grill DE et al. Incidence and prognostic importance of acute renal failure after percutaneous coronary intervention. Circulation 2002; 105: 2259–64.
16. Mehran R, Aymong ED, Nikolsky E et al. A simple risk score for prediction of contrast-induced nephropathy after percutaneous coronary intervention: development and initial validation. J Am Coll Cardiol 2004; 44: 1393–9.
17. Tommaso CL. Contrast-induced nephrotoxicity in patients undergoing cardiac catheterization. Cathet Cardiovasc Diagn 1994; 31: 316–21.
18. Birck R, Krzossok S, Markowetz F et al. Acetylcysteine for prevention of contrast nephropathy: meta-analysis. Lancet 2003; 362: 598–603.
19. Marenzi G, Marana I, Lauri G et al. The prevention of radiocontrast-agent-induced nephropathy by hemofiltration. N Engl J Med 2003; 349: 1333–40.
20. Shaw RE, Anderson HV, Brindis RG et al. Updated risk adjustment mortality model using the complete 1.1 dataset from the American College of Cardiology National Cardiovascular Data Registry (ACC-NCDR). J Invasive Cardiol 2003; 15: 578–80.
21. Lincoff AM, Califf RM, Topol EJ. Platelet glycoprotein IIb/IIIa receptor blockade in coronary artery disease. J Am Coll Cardiol 2000; 35: 1103–15.
22. Neumann FJ, Kastrati A, Pogatsa-Murray G et al. Evaluation of prolonged antithrombotic pretreatment ('cooling-off' strategy) before intervention in patients with unstable coronary syndromes: a randomized controlled trial. JAMA 2003; 290: 1593–9.
23. Alfonso F, Macaya C, Iniguez A et al. Repeat coronary angioplasty during the same angiographic diagnosis of coronary restenosis. Am Heart J 1990; 119: 237–41.
24. Myler RK, Stertzer SH, Clark DA et al. Coronary angioplasty at the time of initial cardiac catheterization: 'ad hoc' angioplasty possibilities and challenges. Cathet Cardiovasc Diagn 1986; 12: 213–14.
25. Varani E, Balducelli M, Lucchi GR et al. [Ad-hoc coronary angioplasty: organizational model, clinical results and costs]. Ital Heart J Suppl 2002; 3: 630–7.
26. O'Keefe JH Jr, Gernon C, McCallister BD et al. Safety and cost effectiveness of combined coronary angiography and angioplasty. Am Heart J 1991; 122: 50–4.

27. Adele C, Vaitkus PT, Wells SK et al. Cost advantages of an ad hoc angioplasty strategy. J Am Coll Cardiol 1998; 31: 321–5.
28. Le Feuvre C, Helft G, Beygui F et al. Safety, efficacy, and cost advantages of combined coronary angiography and angioplasty. J Interv Cardiol 2003; 16: 195–9.
29. Kiemeneij F, Laarman GJ, Odekerken D et al. A randomized comparison of percutaneous transluminal coronary angioplasty by the radial, brachial and femoral approaches: the access study. J Am Coll Cardiol 1997; 29: 1269–75.
30. Galli M, Di Tano G, Mameli S et al. Ad hoc transradial coronary angioplasty strategy: experience and results in a single centre. Int J Cardiol 2003; 92: 275–80.

5

Dilemmas in non-ST elevation acute coronary syndromes

John A Ambrose, John T Coppola,
and Henning Rasmussen

Pathophysiology • Patient selection and risk stratification • The role of an invasive strategy in non-ST elevation acute coronary syndromes • Drug-eluting stents and acute coronary syndromes • Long-term follow-up after the invasive strategy • The role of adjunctive pharmacotherapy • Reduced bleeding during invasive studies in acute coronary syndromes • Short- and long-term implications • Conclusions

Non-ST elevation acute coronary syndromes (NSTACS) comprised of unstable angina (UA) and non-ST segment elevation infarction account for about 1.7 million discharges from US hospitals each year.[1] Over the last 15 years, multiple randomized clinical trials have considered such questions as the optimal acute medical and antithrombotic management, the role and timing of an invasive approach and the best long-term strategies.

As clinicians, the questions we are required to answer in dealing with sick patients can be summarized in four words: *who, what, when* and *why*. *Why* is the simplest question to answer, as we strive to make our patients feel better or live longer. *Who* (which patient) is often the hardest and requires the most judgment. Next, who benefits from *what* (therapy)? Finally, once it is known who will benefit and from what, it must be then decided *when* it should be administered. In NSTACS, much work has gone into determining who will benefit by development of risk scores for predicting adverse outcomes.[2] The large studies of the last decade have investigated the what of early revascularization versus ischemia-driven revascularization,[3,4] and the use of adjunctive pharmacotherapy,[5–7] along with the *when* of therapy (for an invasive strategy, the options are acutely versus after a cooling off period versus only with recurrent ischemia).[8]

PATHOPHYSIOLOGY

Anything that acutely alters the supply/demand ratio can precipitate a bout of NSTACS. In most cases, this is caused by a plaque rupture or erosion leading to platelet deposition and intraluminal thrombus formation. If the thrombus results in complete coronary occlusion and there are no or few collaterals, ST segment elevation usually results. In non-ST segment elevation infarction and unstable angina, complete occlusion is less common, and one or sometimes more than one new and severe culprit lesion is responsible for the clinical presentation. When complete occlusion on angiography is present in NSTACS, collaterals have usually acutely formed to limit the amount of necrosis.[9]

While thrombus generally represents the final insult in NSTACS, inflammation contributes to several aspects of its pathophysiology, leading to progression of the atherosclerotic process and facilitating thrombus formation.[10] Plaque formation is initiated after mononuclear leukocytes adhere to the endothelial surface and enter the intima and accumulate lipid. A large lipid pool covered by a fibrous cap may ultimately form.[11] Initially, the vessel will expand outwardly (positive remodeling) to allow the plaque to expand without luminal narrowing.[12] The border between the normal vessel and plaque is often the point of rupture.[13] Macrophages and other inflammatory cells play a key role in plaque rupture by secretion of substances that degrade the fibrous cap. The initial thrombus formed is platelet rich. Extension of the thrombus into the lumen represents the fibrin, red cell component.

Once plaque rupture occurs, or if the underlying pathology is plaque erosion in which case a lipid-rich plaque with a thin fibrous cap may not be responsible, the resultant thrombus formed represents the balance between prothrombotic/ antithrombotic forces, fibrinolytic/antifibrinolytic activity of the vessel wall and blood as well as hemodynamic factors. If the milieu is prothrombotic or antifibrinolytic, the intraluminal thrombus formation may grow and result in a NSTACS or ST elevation myocardial infarction (MI). Otherwise; the plaque event could remain quiescent and not produce clinical sequelae. Embolization of thrombotic material to the distal vascular bed at or after the time of initial thrombus deposition may contribute to the clinical presentation of the patient and be primarily responsible for increases in biomarkers such as troponin. With the plaque rupture or erosion and thrombus formation, the patient will present with ischemic discomfort at rest or on minimal exertion. If biomarkers of necrosis are present, then a diagnosis of non-ST segment MI is made. Without necrosis, the clinical diagnosis is unstable angina.

PATIENT SELECTION AND RISK STRATIFICATION

Who will benefit from what therapy when symptoms of ischemia at rest lead a patient to seek medical attention can often be determined by looking at easily obtainable clinical data. In the mid 1980s, the Diltiazem Reinfarction Study showed an increased post-hospital risk for patients with non-ST elevation MI.[14] Long-term mortality rates of 5.5% for patients with no ST depression to 10% for those with ST depression on admission and 22% for patients with ST depression persistent through hospitalization were reported. Nicod et al found a 1-year mortality rate of 13.7% for non-ST elevation MI.[15] The strongest predictors of death after discharge were persistent ST depression, in-hospital reinfarction, congestive heart failure (CHF), advancing age, and diabetes.

The Thrombolysis in Myocardial Infarction (TIMI) Risk Score for UA/non-ST elevation MI was designed to provide clinical assessment of the chance of an unfavorable outcome using baseline clinical variables.[16] The TIMI risk score was developed using the 1957 patients in TIMI 11B randomized to unfractionated heparin therapy.[17] A list of 12 patient characteristics that could be identified at presentation and previously reported to be important in predicting outcome were tested. A multivariate regression model identified seven independent, statistically significant predictors of the composite endpoint at 14 days of death, MI, or severe recurrent ischemia prompting urgent revascularization (Table 5.1). The model was validated using

Table 5.1 TIMI risk score

Historical

- Age ≥ 65 years
- ≥ 3 risk factors for coronary artery disease
- Known lesion ≥ 50 [**units?**]; stenosis
- Aspirin use within the last 7 days.

Presentation

- Severe angina: two or more episodes in the last 24 h
- ST segment depression ≥ 0.5 m
- Increased cardiac markers of necrosis

If present 1 point

Table 5.2 Event rate for death, MI, ischemia requiring urgent revascularization at 14 days

TIMI risk score	Event rate (%)
0	0
1	4.7
2	8.3
3	13.2
4	19.2
5	26.2
6–7	40.9

three separate patient groups from three different trials.[18] The score was also tested retrospectively in the Platelet Receptor Inhibition in Ischemic Syndrome Management in Patients Limited by Unstable signs and Symptoms (PRISM-PLUS),[19] and prospectively in the Treat Angina with Aggrastat and Determine Cost of Therapy with and Invasive or Conservative Strategy (TACTICS – TIMI 18),[5] and the pattern of TIMI risk scores followed a normal distribution with a statistically significant increase of risk with increasing score. Event rates were as follows: 0% with a score of 0; 4.7% with a score of 1; 8.3% for a score of 2; 13.2% with a score of 3; 19.2% with a score of 4; 26.2% with a score of 5, and 40.9% with a score of 6–7) (Table 5.2)

The TIMI risk score serves as a simple bedside tool for predicting acute events, death and ischemic events after discharge. The risk score can also be used to guide therapy with adjunctive pharmacotherapy such as low-molecular-weight heparin and glycoprotein IIb/IIIa inhibitor agents. In TIMI 11B, and the Efficacy and Safety of Subcutaneous Enoxaparin in Unstable Angina and Non Q-Wave MI (ESSENCE) study, treatment with the low-molecular-weight heparin, enoxaparin, had a similar efficacy to unfractionated heparin with a risk score of 0–2.[17,18] Enoxaparin conferred a 17% relative risk reduction with a score of 3–4, and a 25% relative risk reduction with a score of 5–7. In PRISM-PLUS,[19] tirofiban had little benefit over heparin in

Table 5.3   High-risk factors

- Patients presenting with ischemia and pulmonary edema
- Ongoing episodes at rest pain > 20 min
- Angina associated with:
- CHF
- S_3
- New murmur of mitral regurgitation
- Hypotension
- Dynamic > 1 mm ST depression

patients with risk score < 4, but showed a 34% relative risk reduction in patients with a risk score ≥ 4.[19]

In addition to the TIMI Risk Score, the American College of Cardiology (ACC)/ American Heart Association (AHA) recognize as high risk patients who present with pulmonary edema, ongoing rest pain greater than 20 min in duration, angina associated with findings of CHF; S_3 gallop rhythm, new or worsening mitral regurgitation, hypotension or dynamic ST changes of greater than 1 mm. The physical examination can also identify precipitating causes of myocardial ischemia and evaluate comorbid conditions. Special attention to the hemodynamic effects of ischemia, blood pressure, heart rate, presence of signs of left ventricular (LV) dysfunction or mitral insufficiency increases the likelihood of a poor outcome (Table 5.3).

Profound hemodynamic instability is also not that uncommon in NSTACS. In the Global Use of Strategies to Open Occluded Coronary Arteries (GUSTO II), and the Platelet Glycoprotein IIb/IIIa in Unstable Angina Receptor Suppression Using Integrilin Therapy (PURSUIT) trials, 5% of patients with non-ST elevation MI had cardiogenic shock with a 60% in-hospital mortality.[20,21]

Troponins are sensitive and accurate in identifying myocardial necrosis. In general, the higher the troponin, the worse is the prognosis. With increasing troponin levels, the Fragmin During Instability in Coronary Artery Disease, FRISC, trial showed increasing risk of death or non-fatal MI over 40 days.[22] The GUSTO IV trial data showed a 30 day risk of mortality of 5.5% in those with a troponin T level of > 0.1 µg/l versus a 1.1% risk in patients who were troponin T negative.[23] However, not all necrosis is secondary to atherothrombossis. Fleming et al reported a 3.1% incidence of false-positive troponin, reinforcing the need for integration of all clinical data with the troponin value.[24] There is no substitute for good clinical judgment and common sense in clinical practice when dealing with NSTACS patients.

THE ROLE OF AN INVASIVE STRATEGY IN NSTACS

Currently, patients presenting with NSTACS who appear to benefit from an early invasive strategy include the following (Table 5.4): those with either recurrent ischemia at rest or with low activity on medical therapy, elevated troponin levels or new ST segment depression on electrocardiogram (ECG), ischemia with signs of CHF, depressed LV systolic function (ejection fraction (EF) < 40%), hemodynamic instability, sustained ventricular tachycardia, percutaneous coronary intervention (PCI) within 6 months, and prior coronary artery bypass graft (CABG). Patients with

Table 5.4   Invasive strategy indicated

- Recurrent ischemia at rest or low-level activity
- Elevated tropin levels
- New ST depression
- CHF
- Depressed ejection < 40%
- Hemodynamic instability
- Sustain ventricular tachycardia
- PCI within the last 6 months
- Prior CABG
- TIMI risk score ≥3 or 4

a prior PCI in the last 6 months and recurrent angina may have developed restenosis which can be effectively treated with repeat PCI. Prior CABG patients have a complex interplay between progression of native disease and graft disease, making non-invasive data difficult to interpret. Typical angiographic profiles of patients undergoing an invasive evaluation include the possibility of no epicardial disease in 10–20%, single vessel disease in 30–35%, multivessel disease in 10–50%, and in 4–10% left main stenosis.

The above indications for an invasive approach are based on clinical trial data as well as clinical judgment. Several randomized trials (Table 5.5) have assessed the role of acute angiography and intervention in the acute management of patients with NSTACS. Early trials such as TIMI-3B and the Veterans Affairs Non-Qwave Infarction Strategies in Hospital (VANQUISH), showed no benefit or even a hazard for the invasive strategy.[3,4] However, these trials were done before the widespread use of glycoprotein IIb/IIIa inhibitors, coronary stents, and clopidogrel.

Later trials showed greater benefit for the invasive strategy over the conservative approach. The Fragmin and Fast Revascularization during Instability in Coronary Artery Disease (FRISC II) trial found a significant event reduction at 6 months in the invasive cohort of patients with unstable angina or non-ST segment elevated infarction.[25] The invasive group underwent angiography within 7 days of hospitalization and treatment with low-molecular-weight heparin. At 6 months, the rate of death, MI or both was 9.4% for invasive versus 12.1% in the conservative group ($P=0.031$). The benefit of an early invasive strategy, however, was not seen in troponin-negative patients, or in patients with no demonstrable ST-T wave changes.

TACTICS-TIMI 18 randomized 2200 patients with ACS to catheterization and revascularization within 4–48 h versus a conservative, ischemia-driven strategy.[26] At 6 months, death MI, and rehospitalization occurred in 15.9% of the invasive strategy group and 19.4% of the conservative group ($P<0.025$). The rate of death and non-fatal myocardial infarction was also lower in the invasive group 7.3% versus 9.5% ($P<0.05$) Again, subgroup analysis revealed the benefit to be greatest in the troponin-positive patients. In troponin-positive patients, the endpoint was reached in 14.3% of the invasive versus 24.2% of the conservative group ($P<0.001$). Furthermore, patients with an intermediate to high TIMI score also benefited from an invasive approach.

The Randomized Intervention Trial of Unstable Angina, (RITA 3) compared optimal anti-anginal, antiplatelet, and antithrombic therapy with enoxaparin to an early

Table 5.5 Invasive strategy versus ischemic driven

	Invasive better	Ischemic driven better	Comments
TIMI III		+	Prior to stents and II$_b$ III$_a$ inhibitors
VANQUISH		+	High surgical mortality; prior to stents and II$_b$ III$_a$
TACTICS TIMI 18	+		
FRISC III	+		
RITA	+		High revascularization rate in the conservative arm
ICTUS		+	

invasive strategy.[6] There was a significant reduction in the endpoint of death, MI, or refractory angina at 4 months in the invasive group of 9.6% versus 14.5% ($P = 0.001$). The difference was mainly attributed to a reduction in refractory angina. Subgroup analysis found a reduction of death and MI in men, but not in women.

These last three trials all agreed on the benefits of an early invasive strategy over a conservative (ischemia-driven) strategy in reducing adverse events, particularly rehospitalization for recurrent angina. This benefit of the invasive strategy was also confirmed in a recent meta analysis.[27]

However, not all the recent data are positive. In the Invasive versus Conservative Treatment in Unstable Coronary Syndromes (ICTUS) trial reported in 2005, no benefit could be demonstrated for the early invasive strategy over the selective invasive approach.[7] Does this now change the paradigm of invasive management in NSTACS? While this trial assessed similar endpoints to the other trials, the lack of a significant difference between strategies could be related to the high rate of revascularization in the conservative strategy (54% at 1 year) which was higher than that seen in the other trial data favoring the invasive strategy. Also, it appears that the hospital stays in ICTUS were inordinately long in the conservative arm, as the median time to PCI during initial hospitalization was 283 h. This is not how most treat an ACS, at least not in the USA!

In spite of the findings of the ICTUS trial, we still believe that in high-risk and most moderate-risk patients with an ACS an early invasive strategy remains preferable. Not only might it reduce adverse events, an early catheterization can shorten the length of stay and it identifies those patients presenting with an ACS but without significant CAD. With advancements in PCI, more patients will probably undergo percutaneous intervention for multivessel disease. As studies now show, the safety of drug-eluting stents in ACS maintains the long-term durability of the initial percutaneous treatment.[28,29] However, interventional therapy targeted at a focal lesion in a disease known to have diffuse involvement necessitates a complementary role for medical therapy as well.[30]

Early catheterization in the invasive group does not always require intervention, since at least 10–15% of patients will have normal or non-obstructive epicardial arteries allowing for rapid discharge of the patient. Another finding at angiography that requires consideration is the less than critical lesion (<70% diameter stenosis) in the patient who presents with a possible ACS episode. Thus, a common dilemma is equating symptoms with anatomy. This cannot be answered by a large clinical trial. It is well known that angiography underestimates the amount of atherosclerosis, but typical rest angina is not normally caused by moderate lesions, particularly if the vessel has been visualized properly in orthogonal views, without foreshortening etc. Unless this lesion is associated with intracoronary thrombus or is very hazy and/or demonstrates hemodynamic significance (pressure wire or Doppler flow wire), this is not the cause of symptoms and the lesion should not undergo intervention. Again, there is no substitute for judgment and taking a good history on your patient! Is the history typical or are the symptoms unlikely to be caused by coronary artery disease? The only other exception for the intervening on a less than severe lesion might be in a patient with documented coronary spasm refractory to therapy which at least in the USA is an uncommon occurrence. With the introduction of 64-slice computed tomography (CT) scanning, some ACS patients may be evaluated by non-invasive scanning and, based on anatomy, referred for revascularization.

Another dilemma relates to the timing of intervention in the hospital. If a patient is in the high- or moderate-risk category, is it necessary to 'cool off' the patient with medical therapy prior to invasive therapy? The recent evaluation of prolonged antithrombotic pretreatment before intervention in patients with unstable Coronary Syndrome (ISAR Cool) allocated patients to pretreatment for 3–5 days prior to angiography/intervention with unfractionated heparin, aspirin and oral clopidogrel (with a 600 mg loading dose followed by 75 mg twice a day) and intravenous tirofiban versus angiography/intervention within 6 h.[8] The two groups were matched with respect to baseline risk. The endpoint death and infarction was reached in 5.9% of the early treatment versus 11.6% of the 'cooling off' strategy ($P=0.04$). Unfortunately, this study does not answer the common dilemma of a shorter delay of 12–24 h before invasive studies are performed. Is this shorter time period safe? Ronner et al used PURSUIT data to stratify patients by the time of PCI.[31] The occurrence of MI or death was influenced by the timing of PCI in patients treated with eptifibatide, with early treatment (within 24 h of treatment) having a lower 30-day event rate. Early intervention with glycoprotein IIb/IIIa inhibitors led to a lower risk of MI or death, but these patients also had a higher restenosis rate. The use of drug-eluting stents would probably modify this risk. It is our opinion that unless there is ongoing ischemia and continued pain, most patients can usually be stabilized for a short period of time (<24 h) if needed with beta-blockers, intravenous nitroglycerin and appropriate antithrombotic therapy until invasive evaluation.

DRUG-ELUTING STENTS AND ACUTE CORONARY SYNDROMES

The use of drug-eluting stents in ACS has been assessed with both paclitaxel- and sirolimus-eluting stents. Lemos et al reported a single-center experience with sirolimus-eluting stents in patients with acute coronary syndrome, using historic controls of bare-metal stents.[28] The drug-eluting stent group had more primary angioplasty, bifurcating lesions and less glycoprotein IIb/IIIa utilization, all factors associated with a high risk of subacute thrombosis. Despite the differences, the 30 major acute coronary events (MACE) rates were similar between both groups, with no difference in stent thrombosis. In the TAXUS-IV study 34% of patients enrolled had ACS. The control group was treated with bare-metal stents, and the 30-day outcome was similar in both groups. At one year, the drug-eluting stent group had lower target lesion revascularization rates, 3.9% versus 16% ($P<0.0001$). By multivariate analysis, ACS was an independent predictor of restenosis in bare-metal stents but not in paclitaxal-eluting stents.[29] Thus, it appears from current data that the use of drug-eluting stents in ACS does not increase the risk of stent thrombosis, and offers a reduction in target lesion revascularization when compared to bare-metal stents

LONG-TERM FOLLOW-UP AFTER THE INVASIVE STRATEGY

Fox et al reported 5-year follow-up from the RITA 3 trial.[32] The early results showed a halving of refractory angina at 4 months, but no significant difference in mortality or non-fatal infarction at 1 year. The 5-year outcome data have shown increasing benefit over time, favoring interventional therapy. The majority of benefit was seen in the high-risk patient, (older, diabetic, smoker prior MI). The longer follow-up neutralized some of the early mortality due to CABG, and the increased infarction due to periprocedure enzyme increase. Of course, all patients must be treated long term with a regimen to reduce cholesterol, control blood pressure, etc.

THE ROLE OF ADJUNCTIVE PHARMACOTHERAPY

The pharmacological therapy of ACS is designed to decrease recurrent ischemia and prevent MI (reMI) or death. In patients with an acute coronary syndrome, the use of beta-blockers and nitrates to control symptoms is warranted. Recent studies have suggested not only a long-term benefit to statin therapy but some acute benefits as well.[33,34]

Guidelines recommend initiation of aspirin and, based on the results of Clopidogrel in Unstable angina to prevent Recurrent Events (CURE) trial, clopidogrel for at least 9 months after an ACS.[35,36] Currently, many cardiologists will withhold clopidogrel loading in patients with NSTACS prior to catheterization, for fear of increased rates of bleeding if bypass surgery is required. As the percentage of patients requiring bypass is acutely low and there actually may be benefit to clopidogrel use prior to CABG, pre-catheterization use may become the rule rather than the exception.

Increasing the loading dose of clopidogrel from 300 mg to 600 mg shortens the time to peak effect, with the peak effect of 300 mg at 12 h, compared to 2 h for 600 mg. The higher loading dose also decreases the incidence of clopidogrel non-responsiveness to 25% of the rate seen with a 300 mg loading dose.[37] The European Society of Cardiology recommends this higher loading dose of clopidogrel for PCI.[38]

A randomized trial of 600 mg versus a 300 mg loading dose of clopidogrel prior to PCI in stable patients showed a reduction in periprocedure MI with the higher loading dose.[39] In the Intracoronary Stenting and Antithrombotic Regimen: Rapid Early Action for Coronary Treatment (ISAR React-2) trial, high-risk ACS patients were all given 600 mg clopidogrel at least 2 h prior to PCI and randomized to procedural abciximab versus placebo. There was a significant decrease in ischemic complications in those treated with abciximab without a significant increase in bleeding. The benefit was limited to those with an elevated troponin.[40]

Antithrombin agents

Unfractionated heparin had for many years been the standard anticoagulant used in ACS patients. In the last 10 years, multiple randomized trials have compared it to low-molecular-weight heparins. Low-molecular-weight heparins have the advantage of greater bioavailability, resistance to inhibition by activated platelets, higher anti-factor X_a/II_a ratios, and more predictable anticoagulant effects.

An overview of six trials with over 21 000 patients comparing enoxaparin to unfractionated heparin in patients with ACS found a 9% reduction in death and non-fatal MI at 30 days, favoring enoxaparin.[41] There was no difference in the incidence of major bleeding. To achieve adequate levels of anti-X_a it appears that if no intra-venous (IV) bolus is given the patient must have reviewed at least two doses of low-molecular-weight heparin within 12 h.[42] Due to the more reliable anticoagulation, lack of the need to monitor routinely and simple weight-adjusted dosing, enoxaparin should be preferred over unfractionated heparin, particularly if the patient is not immediately going to the catheterization laboratory. On the other hand, we believe that a patient immediately undergoing an invasive strategy (< 6–12 h) can be bolused with unfractionated heparin and placed on a drip until the procedure. While the Superior Yield of the New strategy of Enoxaparin Revascularization and GLYcoprotein IIb/IIIa inhibitors (SYNERGY) trial suggested a worse outcome for patients in whom heparin therapy was switched from one form to another,[43] a common scenario in many catheterization labs is to give a dose or two of enoxaparin and on the following morning withhold the next dose and switch to unfractionated heparin at the time of PCI. Experienced interventionalists should be able to minimize bleeding complications in these situations with careful attention to catheter size, site of intervention, closure devices etc.

The value of a direct thrombin inhibitor, bivalirudin in elective angioplasty was demonstrated in the Randomized Evaluation in PCI Linking Angiomax to Reduced Clinical Events (REPLACE) 2 trial.[44] At the ACC meeting in 2006, the preliminary results of the Acute Catheterization and Urgent Intervention Triage strategY (ACU-ITY) trial were presented by G. Stone. This trial showed that bivalirudin alone in comparison to either type of heparin plus a glycoprotein IIb/IIIa inhibitor had similar efficacy (no increase in ischemic events) but a significant reduction in bleeding in moderate- to high-risk ACS patients. Thus, the preliminary results of this trial sug-gest that patients with NSTACS who are triaged to an early invasive strategy can be safely managed with bivalirudin alone.

Glycoprotein IIb/IIIa inhibitors

The ACC/AHA Guidelines recommend the use of these agents in high-risk patients prior to catheterization based on the results of several randomized clinical trials.[45] Kong et al, in a review of 16 randomized trials of glycoprotein IIb/IIIa inhibitors could find no benefit in reducing mortality at 48–96 h, 30 days or 6 months in the patients with ACS.[46] However, the combined endpoint of death or non-fatal MI was reduced early and at 30 days.

One would think that with longer follow-up time, the early reduction in infarction before and during revascularization will translate into better survival. In diabetics, however, glycoprotein IIb/IIIa inhibitors appear to reduce mortality, and the best data are with the use of abciximab.[47] However, in general, these agents are not routinely being used in ACS. The National Registry of Myocardial Infarction reported only 25% of eligible patients received early glycoprotein IIb/IIIa inhibitors. The eld-erly patient, females and minority patients received these agents less often.[48,49]

In a substudy of the ACUITY trial presented at ACC 2006 by G. Stone,[50] patients who were to undergo an invasive strategy underwent a second randomization to upstream glycoprotein IIb/IIIa blockade, with either eptifibitide or tirofiban versus procedural glycoprotein IIb/IIIa inhibition, only with either eptifibitide or abciximab. There was a slight increase in ischemic complications with procedural use only, but also a significant reduction in bleeding. Further analysis of this trial may sort out which glycoprotein IIb/IIIa strategy is preferable in specific circumstances. Bolognese et al recently compared upstream use of tirofiban to selective use of either high-dose tirofiban or abcixmab in the catheterization lab only, and found that upstream use was superior in reducing peri-PCI troponin release.[51]

REDUCING BLEEDING DURING INVASIVE STUDIES IN ACUTE CORONARY SYNDROMES

The early invasive strategy in ACS requires the utilization of powerful antithrombin in combination with antiplatelet therapy, increasing the risk of access site bleeding. There are several possible 'tricks of the trade' to reduce bleeding during angiography. These include: (1) checking the site of femoral artery entry radiographically before puncture, to ensure one is below the inguinal ligament; (2) the use of micropuncture of the femoral artery to minimize the consequences of puncturing the back wall of the artery; (3) small sheaths (5 and 6 French) for intervention; (4) closure devices; and (5) the radial approach to angiography and intervention.

Several laboratories have now switched to the radial approach almost exclusively, with great success in both stable and ACS patients. However, as this approach is still relatively uncommon in certain regions, a short history is warranted. Kiemeneij initially used the transradial approach for stenting when anticoagulation with warfarin was standard care for patients having elective Palmaz–Schatz stent implantations.[52] He showed that with an international normalized ratio (INR) of 2.5, stenting through the radial approach could be safely performed with no access-site complications.[52] Mann et al in 1998 reported a randomized trial in ACS between radial and femoral intervention.[53] All patients received aspirin, and heparin with a goal of an activated clotting time (ACT) of 300 or greater, and abciximab was used as clinically indicated. The radial group had a slightly higher percentage of abciximab use. Primary success rates were not statistically different. Bleeding complications only occurred in the femoral group, with three large hematomas, which prolonged hospitalization. Saito et al randomized 149 patients with acute MI to transfemoral versus transradial intervention and showed similar success rates and procedure times.[54] The transfemoral group had a 3% incidence of major bleeding, the investigators did not use glycoprotein IIb/IIIa agents. The radial group did not have any access site bleeding.

Philippe et al, in a study comparing femoral to radial intervention using abciximab in primary angioplasty, had a 3% risk of major access site bleeding in the femoral cohort and no access site bleeding with the radial approach.[55] Louvard and Ludwig reported results from two large European centers.[56] In these experienced centers, success and procedure times were similar with femoral versus radial procedures, but bleeding at the access site only occurred in the femoral-treated patients. One of the centers routinely used a closure device and had a 2% bleeding complication. The other site did not use a closure device, but had a 7% rate of severe bleeding. Thus, with more aggressive antiplatelet and antithrombin use in ACS, the radial approach may offer an alternative to offset the increased risk of bleeding seen with the femoral approach.

SHORT- AND LONG-TERM IMPLICATIONS

The role of coronary bypass grafting versus multivessel intervention

When evaluating a patient with ACS and multivessel disease, the interventionist must be able to determine the likelihood of complete revascularization with a percutaneous procedure versus bypass grafting. In this evaluation the long-term durability and risk of the procedure must be factored into any decision. Patients seen in clinical practice often do not fit into randomized trials, and extrapolation to everyday practice can be misleading. Malenka et al used data from the northern New England registries of coronary revascularization.[57] The group of patients undergoing bypass was older, had worse LV function and more comorbidities. The adjusted long-term survival showed bypass surgery in patients with three-vessel disease to be better in spite of high stent use.[58] Mercado et al performed a meta-analysis on data from four recent randomized trials comparing multiple stents to coronary bypass, and at 1 year both provided a similar degree or protection from death, MI or stroke.[58] The only difference was the higher rate of repeat revascularization in the PCI group. Nevertheless, in diabetic patients with multivessel disease and NSTACS, until the results of randomized studies using drug-eluting stents and glycoprotein IIb/IIIa inhibitors are complete, it would seem that in most patients, bypass would be the best approach particularly with three-vessel disease and LV dysfunction, or when a percutaneous procedure will result in incomplete revascularization.[59]

Another related question for consideration concerns the wisdom of a percutaneous interventional approach for a systemic disease with focal manifestations in multiple vessels. Klein recently suggested that with multivessel disease, more potential plaque burden is present and can advance over time.[60] Focal therapy with stents may be inferior to CABG, which can bypass not only the hemodynamically significant but also the vulnerable plaques that might develop into culprit lesions at a later date. This may explain the long-term benefit in some studies of CABG over PCI in patients with multivessel disease. However, this suggestion does not take into account the fact that focal multivessel disease can often be managed effectively with PCI followed by the use of appropriate systemic therapies to reduce and, in the future, even reverse the progression of atherosclerosis.

Complete versus incomplete percutaneous revascularization

Another dilemma in the catheterization laboratory relates to the preferred interventional strategy in NSTACS patients. Ijsselmuiden et al randomly assigned 52 patients with ACS and multivessel disease with an identifiable culprit lesion to complete revascularization or stenting of only the culprit lesion.[61] The 1-year endpoint of death, MI, or the need for further revascularization was evaluated. Both strategies had similar rates of death and MI, but the culprit lesion group required more revascularization over the year of follow-up. What then should the interventionalist do with the ACS patient with multivessel disease destined for the catheterization laboratory? Is it appropriate to intervene on the culprit alone and bring him/her back for the other lesion or lesions, or to attempt initially complete revascularization? The treatment of the culprit lesion followed by intervention on other arteries with critical stenosis must be based on the benefit of reduced admissions and/or procedures for intervention versus the risk of a large one-time dose of contrast, prolonged procedure times, and the likelihood of success. Unfortunately, the interventionalist's decision may sometimes be driven by other factors such as hospital economics. Multiple drug-eluting stents, the norm in the USA, are not reimbursed during the same procedure, necessitating, in many instances, more than one procedure in multivessel patients amenable to complete revascularization with PCI.

Plaque stabilization and future coronary events

The concept of plaque stabilization may help extend the long-term benefits of interventional therapy in patients with an ACS by reducing the conversion of other vulnerable plaques into new culprit lesions. This can be most easily demonstrated with lipid-lowering agents, and recent trial data support the concept that the lower the low-density lipoprotein (LDL) in secondary prevention, the better. In TIMI 22, intensive lipid-lowering therapy (LDL in the range of 70 mg/dl with therapy) led to a reduction in early events that was sustained throughout the study.[33] The A–Z trial also showed a trend to event reduction in patients started on early intensive statin therapy when followed over 24 months.[34] As suggested by Ambrose and D'Agate, drugs with biological plausibility and clinical evidence (a significant reduction in non-fatal and fatal MI) such as statins, beta-blockers, angiotensin-converting enzyme inhibitors, and aspirin should be considered part of the interventional therapy for ACS, as they are potentially plaque stabilizing and may reduce conversion of vulnerable plaques into symptomatic thrombosed plaques.[62]

CONCLUSIONS

The dilemmas surrounding NSTACS relating to who, what, and when in general revolve around the appropriateness, timing and antithrombotic approaches of an invasive strategy. While the vast majority of patients presenting to the emergency department with a primary complaint of chest pain do not have obstructive coronary artery disease as the cause of symptoms, there is no substitute for taking a good history and utilizing good 'old fashioned' clinical judgment in decision making. It is our opinion that if there is a high index of suspicion for significant obstructive coronary artery disease, and particularly when the risk is high by conventional scores, that anatomic visualization of the coronary arteries is appropriate as an early (in-hospital) strategy in most cases. However, as the main goal of therapy is to benefit the patient, it is imperative that the risks/benefits are acceptable. Otherwise, the initial approach should be stress testing or nuclear imaging. If an invasive strategy is utilized, complications must be minimized.

Non-invasive definition of the coronary arteries with multislice CT scans will continue to evolve and probably replace diagnostic angiography in the future management of a large percentage of stable coronary disease patients. However, either the need for immediate intervention or the inappropriateness of multiple contrast procedures in NSTACS patients should limit its use, particularly in moderate- and high-risk patients. For the foreseeable future, we will probably utilize invasive techniques solely in the majority of these patients.

REFERENCES

1. Giugliano RP, Braunwald E. The year in non-ST-segment elevation acute coronary syndromes. J Am Coll Cardiol 2005; 46: 906–19.

2. Antman EM, Cohen M, Bernink PJ et al. The TIMI risk score for unstable angina/non-ST elevation MI: a method for prognostication and therapeutic decision making. JAMA 2000; 284: 835–42.
3. Effects of tissue plasminogen activator and a comparison of early invasive and conservative strategies in unstable angina and non-Q-wave myocardial infarction. Results of the TIMI IIIB Trial. Thrombolysis in Myocardial Ischemia. Circulation 1994; 89: 1545–56.
4. Boden WE, O'Rourke RA, Crawford MH et al. Outcomes in patients with acute non-Q-wave myocardial infarction randomly assigned to an invasive as compared with a conservative management strategy. Veterans Affairs Non-Q-Wave Infarction Strategies in Hospital (VANQWISH) Trial Investigators. N Engl J Med 1998; 338: 1785–92.
5. Cannon CP, Weintraub WS, Demopoulos LA et al. Comparison of early invasive and conservative strategies in patients with unstable coronary syndromes treated with the glycoprotein IIb/IIIa inhibitor tirofiban. N Engl J Med 2001; 344: 1879–87.
6. Fox KA, Poole-Wilson PA, Henderson RA et al. Interventional versus conservative treatment for patients with unstable angina or non-ST elevation myocardial infarction: the British Heart Foundation RITA 3 randomized trial. Randomized Intervention Trial of unstable Angina. Lancet 2002; 360: 743–51.
7. de Winter RJ, Windhausen F, Cornel JH et al. Early invasive versus selectively invasive management for acute coronary syndromes. N Engl J Med 2005; 353: 1095–104.
8. Neumann FJ, Kastrati A, Pogatsa-Murray G et al. Evaluation of prolonged antithrombotic pretreatment ('cooling-off' strategy) before intervention in patients with unstable coronary syndromes: a randomized controlled trial. JAMA 2003; 290: 1593–9.
9. Ambrose JA. Plaque disruption and the acute coronary syndromes of unstable angina and myocardial infarction: if the substrate is similar, why is the clinical presentation different? J Am Coll Cardiol 1992; 19: 1653–8.
10. Falk E, Shah PK, Fuster V. Coronary plaque disruption. Circulation 1995; 92: 657–71.
11. Libby P. Current concepts of the pathogenesis of the acute coronary syndromes. Circulation 2001; 104: 365–72.
12. Schoenhagen P, Ziada KM, Kapadia SR et al. Extent and direction of arterial remodeling in stable versus unstable coronary syndromes: an intravascular ultrasound study. Circulation 2000; 101: 598–603.
13. Pasterkamp G, Schoneveld AH, van der Wal AC et al. Relation of arterial geometry to luminal narrowing and histologic markers for plaque vulnerability: the remodeling paradox. J Am Coll Cardiol 1998; 32: 655–62.
14. Schechtman KB, Capone RJ, Kleiger RE et al. Risk stratification of patients with non-Q wave myocardial infarction. The critical role of ST segment depression. The Diltiazem Reinfarction Study Research Group. Circulation. 1989; 80: 1148–58.
15. Nicod P, Gilpin E, Dittrich H et al. Short- and long-term clinical outcome after Q wave and non-Q wave myocardial infarction in a large patient population. Circulation 1989; 79: 528–36.
16. Sabatine MS, Antman EM. The thrombolysis in myocardial infarction risk score in unstable angina/non-ST-segment elevation myocardial infarction. J Am Coll Cardiol 2003; 41: 89S–95S.
17. Antman EM, McCabe CH, Gurfinkel EP et al. Enoxaparin prevents death and cardiac ischemic events in unstable angina/non-Q-wave myocardial infarction. Results of the thrombolysis in myocardial infarction (TIMI) 11B trial. Circulation 1999; 100: 1593–601.
18. Goodman SG, Barr A, Sobtchouk A et al. Low molecular weight heparin decreases rebound ischemia in unstable angina or non-Q-wave myocardial infarction: the Canadian ESSENCE ST segment monitoring substudy. J Am Coll Cardiol 2000; 36: 1507–13.
19. Theroux P, Alexander J Jr, Pharand C et al. Glycoprotein IIb/IIIa receptor blockade improves outcomes in diabetic patients presenting with unstable angina/non-ST elevation myocardial infarction: results from the Platelet Receptor Inhibition in Ischemic Syndrome Management in Patients Limited by Unstable Signs and Symptoms (PRISM-PLUS) study. Circulation 2000; 102: 2466–72.

20. Armstrong P,Yuling F,Wei-Ching C et al for the GustoII Investigators. Acute Coronary syndrome in GustoIIb Trial. Circulation 1998; 98: 1860–8.
21. The Pursuit Trial Investigators. Inhibitor of platelet glycoprotein IIb/IIIa with eptifibatide in patients with acute coronory syndromes. N Engl J Med 1998; 339: 436–43.
22. Lagergvist B, Diderhom E, Lindahl B et al. FRISC score for selction of patients for an early invasive treatment strategy in unstable cornary artery disease. Heart 2005; 91: 1047–52.
23. James S, Armstrong P, Califf R et al. Troponin T levels and risk of 30-day outcomes in patients with the acute coronary syndrome: prospective verfication in the Gusto-IV trial. Am J Med 2003; 115: 17–84.
24. Fleming SM, O'Byrne L, Finn J, Grimes H, Daly KM. False-positive cardiac troponin I in a routine clinical population. Am J Cardiol 2002; 89: 1212–15.
25. FRISC II Investigators. Invasive compared with non-invasive treatment in unstable coro-nary-artery disease: FRISC II prospective randomized multicare study. Lancet 1999; 354: 708–15.
26. Mehta SR, Cannon CP, Fox KA, Wallentin L, Boden WE, Spacek R, Widimsky P, McCullough PA, Hunt D, Braunwald E, Yusuf S. Routine vs selective invasive strategies in patients with acute coronary syndromes: a collaborative meta-analysis of randomized trials. JAMA. 2005;293:2908–17.
27. Bavry AA, Kumbhani DJ, Quiroz R et al. Invasive therapy along with glycoprotein IIb/IIIa inhibitors and intracoronary stents improves survival in non-ST-segment elevation acute coronary syndromes: a meta-analysis and review of the literature. Am J Cardiol 2004; 93: 830–5.
28. Lemos PA, Lee CH, Degertekin M et al. Early outcome after sirolimus-eluting stent implan-tation in patients with acute coronary syndromes: insights from the Rapamycin-Eluting Stent Evaluated At Rotterdam Cardiology Hospital (RESEARCH) registry. J Am Coll Cardiol 2003; 41: 2093–9.
29. Moses JW, Mehran R, Nikolsky E et al. Outcomes with the paclitaxel-eluting stent in patients with acute coronary syndromes: analysis from the TAXUS-IV trial. J Am Coll Cardiol 2005; 45: 1165–71.
30. Nissen SE. Pathobiology, not angiography, should guide management in acute coronary syndrome/non-ST-segment elevation myocardial infarction: the non-interventionist's per-spective. J Am Coll Cardiol 2003; 41: 103S–112S.
31. Ronner E, Boersma E, Laarman G et al. Early angioplasty in acute coronary syndromes without persistent ST segment elevation improves outcome but increases the need for 6 month repeat revascularization. An analysis of pursuit trial. J Am Coll Cardiol 2002; 39: 1924–9.
32. Fox KA, Poole-Wilson P, Clayton TC et al. 5-year outcome of an interventional strategy in non-ST elevation acute coronary syndrome: the British Heart Foundation RITA 3 ran-domised trial. Lancet 2005; 366: 914–20.
33. Cannon CP, Braunwald E, McCabe CH et al. Intensive versus moderate lipid lowering with statins after acute coronary syndromes. N Engl J Med 2004; 350: 1495–504.
34. de Lemos JA, Blazing MA, Wiviott SD et al. Early intensive vs a delayed conservative sim-vastatin strategy in patients with acute coronary syndromes: phase Z of the A to Z trial. JAMA 2004; 292: 1307–16.
35. Yusuf S, Zhao F, Mehta SR, Chrolavicius S, Tognoni G, Fox KK. Effects of clopidogrel in addition to aspirin in patients with acute coronary syndromes without ST-segment elevation. N Engl J Med 2001; 345: 494–502.
36. Mehta SR, Yusuf S. Short- and long-term oral antiplatelet therapy in acute coronary syn-dromes and percutaneous coronary intervention. J Am Coll Cardiol 2003; 41: 79S–88S.
37. Williams DO. Clopidogrel pretreatment for percutaneous coronary intervention: double, double, dose in trouble? Circulation 2005; 111: 2019–21.
38. The Task Force for Percutaneous Coronary Interventions of the European Society of Cardiology. Guidelines for Percutaneous Coronary Interventions. European Heart Journal 2005; 26: 804–47.

39. Patti G, Colonna G, Pasceri V et al. Randomized trial of high loading dose of clopidogrel for reduction of periprocedural myocardial infarction in patients undergoing coronary intervention: results from the ARMYDA-2 (Antiplatelet therapy for Reduction of MYocardial Damage during Angioplasty) study. Circulation 2005; 111: 2099–106.
40. Kastrati A, Mehilli J, Neumann FJ et al. Abciximab in patients with acute coronary syndromes undergoing percutaneous coronary interventions after clopidogrel pretreatment: the ISAR-REACT 2 randomized trial. JAMA 2006; 295: 1531–38.
41. Petersen JL, Mahaffey KW, Hasselblad V et al. Efficacy and bleeding complications among patients randomized to enoxaparin or unfractionated heparin for antithrombin therapy in non-ST-segment elevation acute coronary syndromes: a systematic overview. JAMA 2004; 292: 89–96.
42. Cohen M. The role of low-molecular-weight heparin in the management of acute coronary syndromes. J Am Coll Cardiol 2003; 41: 55S–61S.
43. The SYNERGY Trial Investigators. Enoxaprin vs. unfractionated heparin in high-risk patients with non-ST-segment elevation acute coronary syndromes managed with an intended early invasive strategy. JAMA 2004; 299: 45–54.
44. Lincoff AM, Kleiman NS, Kereiakes DJ et al. Long-term efficacy of bivalirudin and provisional glycoprotein IIb/IIIa blockade vs heparin and planned glycoprotein IIb/IIIa blockade during percutaneous coronary revascularization: REPLACE-2 randomized trial. JAMA 2004; 292: 696–703.
45. Braunwald E, Antman EM, Beasley JW et al. AHA/ACC 2002 update for the management of patients with unstable angina and non-ST elevation myocardial infarction – summary article: a report of the task force on practice guidelines. J Am Coll Cardiol 2002; 40: 1366–74.
46. Kong DF, Califf RM, Miller DP et al. Clinical outcomes of therapeutic agents that block the platelet glycoprotein IIb/IIIa integrin in ischemic heart disease. Circulation 1998; 98: 2829–35.
47. Moliterno DJ, Chan AW. Glycoprotein IIb/IIIa inhibition in early intent-to-stent treatment of acute coronary syndromes: EPISTENT, ADMIRAL, CADILLAC, and TARGET. J Am Coll Cardiol 2003; 41: 49S–54S.
48. Anand SS, Xie CC, Mehta S et al. Differences in the management and prognosis of women and men who suffer from acute coronary syndromes. J Am Coll Cardiol 2005; 46: 1845–51.
49. Bhatt DL, Roe MT, Peterson ED et al. Utilization of early invasive management strategies for high-risk patients with non-ST-segment elevation acute coronary syndromes: results from the CRUSADE Quality Improvement Initiative. JAMA 2004; 292: 2096–104.
50. Ambrose JA. ACC 2006 Annual Session Highlights – myocardial ischemia and infarction. J Am Coll Cardiol 2006; 47: D13–D17.
51. Bolognese L, Falsini G, Liistro F et al. Randomized comparison of upstream tirofiban versus downstream high bolus dose of tirofiban or abciximab on tissue level perfusion and troponin release in high risk acute coronary syndromes treated with percutaneous interventions. J Am Coll Cardiol 2006; 47: 522–8.
52. Kiemeneij F, Laarman GJ, Slagboom T, van der Wieken R. Outpatient coronary stent implantation. J Am Coll Cardiol 1997; 29: 323–7.
53. Mann T, Cubeddu G, Bowen J et al. Stenting in acute coronary syndromes: a comparison of radial versus femoral access sites. J Am Coll Cardiol 1998; 32: 572–6.
54. Saito S, Tanaka S, Hiroe Y et al. Comparative study on transradial approach vs. transfemoral approach in primary stent implantation for patients with acute myocardial infarction: results of the test for myocardial infarction by prospective unicenter randomization for access sites (TEMPURA) trial. Catheter Cardiovasc Interv 2003; 59: 26–33.
55. Philippe F, Larrazet F, Meziane T, Dibie A. Comparison of transradial vs. transfemoral approach in the treatment of acute myocardial infarction with primary angioplasty and abciximab. Catheter Cardiovasc Interv 2004; 61: 67–73.
56. Louvard Y, Ludwig J, Lefevre T et al. Transradial approach for coronary angioplasty in the setting of acute myocardial infarction: a dual-center registry. Catheter Cardiovasc Interv 2002; 55: 206–11.

57. Malenka DJ, Leavitt BJ, Hearne MJ et al. Comparing long-term survival of patients with multivessel coronary disease after CABG or PCI: analysis of BARI-like patients in northern New England. Circulation 2005; 112: I371–6.
58. Mercado N, Wijns W, Serruys PW et al. One-year outcomes of coronary artery bypass graft surgery versus percutaneous coronary intervention with multiple stenting for multisystem disease: a meta-analysis of individual patient data from randomized clinical trials. J Thorac Cardiovasc Surg 2005; 130: 512–19.
59. Mehran R, Dangas GD, Kobayashi Y et al. Short- and long-term results after multivessel stenting in diabetic patients. J Am Coll Cardiol 2004; 43: 1348–54.
60. Klein LW. Are drug-eluting stents the preferred treatment for multivessel coronary artery disease? J Am Coll Cardiol 2006; 47: 22–6.
61. Ijsselmuiden AJ, Ezechiels J, Westendorp IC et al. Complete versus culprit vessel percutaneous coronary intervention in multivessel disease: a randomized comparison. Am Heart J 2004; 148: 467–74.
62. Ambrose JA, D'Agate DJ. Classification of systemic therapies for potential stabilization of the vulnerable plaque to prevent acute myocardial infarction. Am J Cardiol 2005; 95: 379–82.

6

Patients with impaired hemostasis requiring cardiac catheterization and coronary intervention

Nicolai Mejevoi, Jean-Bernard Durand, and Marc Cohen

American College of Cardiology/American Heart Association guidelines for antithrombotic therapy during percutaneous coronary intervention • Rescue percutaneous coronary intervention • Percutaneous coronary intervention in patients on chronic oral anticoagulation • Percutaneous coronary intervention in patients with chronic liver disease or congenital coagulopathy • Percutaneous coronary intervention in patients with renal insufficiency • Percutaneous coronary intervention in patients with thrombocytopenia or disorders of platelet function • Summary

In patients undergoing percutaneous coronary intervention (PCI), adjunctive therapy with anticoagulation and inhibitors of platelet activation and/or aggregation is indispensable in protecting against acute thrombosis of the treated vessel, improving survival, reducing periprocedural myocardial infarction (MI), and the need for urgent target vessel revascularization. At the same time, aggressive anticoagulant and antiplatelet therapy may be associated with increased risk of bleeding, especially in older patients and patients with renal insufficiency. Balancing between the prevention of ischemic events versus minimizing serious bleeding is a key challenge the interventional cardiologist faces on a case-by-case basis. This issue becomes even more challenging in patients referred for PCI who have pre-existent congenital or acquired coagulation and/or platelet abnormalities. This real-life scenario gives an excellent example of such a situation:

> A 46 year old man with a history of hypertension, hyperlipidemia and hemophilia A is admitted to hospital with typical intermittent angina pain of one-day duration, ST segment depression in precordial leads on electrocardiogram (ECG) and mildly elevated troponin I. He also has a history of severe bleeding, last occurring 3 months ago. Coronary arteriography reveals one-vessel disease, with a discrete severe mid-left anterior descending artery stenosis, associated with some haziness. Coronary intervention is indicated.

> What would be the ideal approach to the management of this patient prior to, during, and after the PCI?

The goal of this chapter will be to assess the antiplatelet and anticoagulation options in different patients subsets, all of whom are at increased risk for bleeding: patients requiring rescue PCI post-failed thrombolysis, and planned/emergent

PCI in patients on chronic anticoagulation, or with a history of bleeding diathesis and thrombocytopenia.

AMERICAN COLLEGE OF CARDIOLOGISTS/AMERICAN HEART ASSOCIATION GUIDELINES FOR ANTITHROMBOTIC THERAPY DURING PERCUTANEOUS CORONARY INTERVENTION

Optimal antithrombotic therapy during PCI is continuously evolving. Current guidelines and updates are outlined in Table 6.1.[1-4] The traditional approach to the antiplatelet therapy in PCI includes:

1. aspirin in doses of 300–325 mg given at least 2 h (ideally 24 h) prior to procedure and then daily
2. clopidogrel (as ticlopidine was virtually eliminated) 300 mg bolus at least 6 h prior to procedure (consider 600 mg if less then 6 h, and ideally at a dose of 75 mg daily started at least 10 days before procedure). Ticlopidine can be used if there is an allergy to clopidogrel
3. glycoprotein IIb/IIIa inhibitors (GPI) including abciximab, eptifibatide, and tirofiban, with abciximab and eptifibatide being better studied. Eptifibatide has also been shown to provide additional benefits in 'high-risk acute coronary syndrome (ACS)' patients, when started upstream. Aspirin and clopidogrel are always combined unless contraindicated. All three groups can be used together for improving outcome in 'high-risk' patients, although more aggressive therapy may be associated with increased bleeding.

Anticoagulation usually consists of one of the following: (1) unfractionated heparin (UFH) weight-adjusted bolus followed by a continuous intravenous (IV) infusion, to achieve goal partial thromboplastin time (PTT) and/or activated clotting time (ACT). UFH is dosed to an ACT greater than 300 s without GPI use, or more than 200 s when GPI are used; (2) low-molecular-weight heparin (LMWH), primarily enoxaparin (Lovenox) subcutaneously, 1 mg/kg every 12 h with additional dose given if PCI performed more than 8 h after last dose; (3) direct thrombin inhibitors – hirudin, argatroban and bivalirudin (Angiomax) are also effective anticoagulants administered as an IV bolus followed by maintenance IV infusions; (4) more recently, the selective factor Xa inhibitor – fondaparinux, was studied in OASIS-5 and 6 (Organization to Assess Strategies in Acute Ischemic Syndromes) trials.[5,6] Unfortunately because of an increased incidence of catheter-related thrombus, IV UFH was recommended to be used as an adjunct to the fondaparinux therapy, and the role of fondaparinux in PCI is at best uncertain.

RESCUE PERCUTANEOUS CORONARY INTERVENTION

The most recent studies show a survival benefit of rescue PCI with/without stent placement compared to conservative treatment in patients with failed thrombolysis.[7] The Rescue angioplasty after failed thrombolytic therapy for acute myocardial infarction (REACT) study included 427 patients with failed thrombolysis divided into three groups: rescue PCI, repeated thrombolysis, and conservative treatment. Statistically significant benefits were achieved in combined endpoints of death, recurrent MI, cerebrovascular event, and severe heart failure. Antiplatelet and anticoagulant therapy

Table 6.1   Adjunctive antithrombotic therapy recommended for percutaneous coronary intervention

Medication name	Specific conditions	Class of recommendation	Level of evidence
Aspirin	Used prior to PCI	I	A
Aspirin	Aspirin naive	I	C
Clopidogrel	All PCIs	I	A
Abciximab	UA/NSTEMI no clopidogrel	I	A
	UA/NSTEMI + clopidogrel	IIA	B
	STEMI	IIA	B
	Elective PCI	IIA	B
Eptifibatide	UA/NSTEMI no clopidogrel	I	A
	UA/NSTEMI + clopidogrel	IIA	B
	STEMI	IIB	C
	Elective PCI	IIA	B
Tirofiban	UA/NSTEMI no clopidogrel	I	A
	UA/NSTEMI + Clopidogrel	IIA	B
	STEMI	IIB	C
	Elective PCI	IIA	B
Unfractionated heparin	All PCIs	I	C
Low-molecular-weight heparin	UA/NSTEMI	IIA	B
	STEMI	IIB	B
Bivalirudin	Low-risk PCI	IIA	B
Bivalirudin and argatroban	PCI in patients with HIT	I	B

NSTEMI, non-ST elevation myocardial infarction; PCI, percutaneous coronary intervention; STEMI, ST elevation myocardial infarction; UA, unstable angina.

were used in a standard fashion, and included GPI (abciximab) in 43.4% of PCI patients, UFH was used in the first 24 h of treatment, and could later be changed to LMWH. Although aspects of anticoagulant and antiplatelet therapy were not a goal of this study, analysis of bleeding complications showed no statistically significant difference in major bleeding, with no bleeding-related deaths in the PCI group. The rate of minor sheath-related bleeding was significantly increased in the PCI group as expected; no related life-threatening conditions were reported.[8]

Thus, dual or triple antiplatelet therapy with standard anticoagulation has been used independently of thrombolytic agent administered. Bleeding is more common after thrombolytic use; however, the benefit of aggressive antiplatelet/anticoagulant therapy in this high-risk patients outweighs the risk of bleeding complications.

Most of the bleeding occurred at the arterial puncture site, raising a question of alternative access, such as radial access to decrease the rate and gravity of arterial bleeding.[9] Another way to decrease this type of bleeding might be the use of a micropuncture technique, vascular closure devices,[10] and longer than usual (by 20–30 min) pressure applied after sheath removal. Reports of pulmonary hemorrhage and hemoptysis have been published in patients receiving both GPI and thrombolytic therapy.[11]

PERCUTANEOUS CORONARY INTERVENTION IN PATIENTS ON CHRONIC ORAL ANTICOAGULATION

Much less studied is the approach to patients presenting with a therapeutic international normalized ratio (INR), on chronic anticoagulation due to chronic atrial fibrillation, recurrent deep vein thrombosis, or inherited thrombophilias. If PCI is an elective procedure, in such a patient, a common approach would be to stop oral anti-coagulant 3–4 days prior to procedure, and switch to IV UFH or subcutaneous LMWH. Enoxaparin is widely recommended as an easy-to-use and effective agent, administered subcutaneously with dose adjustments made for reduced creatinine clearance; using 1 mg/kg subcutaneous injections every 12 h, or every 24 h in the case of creatinine clearance less than 30 ml/min. An alternative with enoxaparin in patients with normal renal function is 1.5 mg/kg subcutaneous injection every 24 h. Alternatively UFH continuous IV infusion with PTT and later ACT (intraprocedu-rally) measurements for dose adjustment can be used. Antiplatelet therapy should be used as in any other PCI, with aspirin and clopidogrel. GPIs would be used depend-ing on the clinical and angiographic criteria, such as: presence of intraluminal throm-bus, residual coronary dissection, or suboptimal result. Use of GPIs in elective procedure in patient without ACS would not be routinely recommended.

Oral anticoagulant can be restarted 1–2 days after the procedure, and heparin stopped when therapeutic INR is achieved.

Patients with ACS, who require urgent or emergent procedures, would be man-aged in essentially the same manner with aspirin, clopidogrel, GPIs and intrapro-cedural IV UFH to achieve the desired ACT. Of course, the possibility of bleeding complications may be increased, especially at the arterial puncture site during sheath withdrawal if the INR is elevated. While vitamin K can reverse the INR, this would take a minimum of 6 h or more. Therefore, the safest approach would be to deploy an arterial closure device immediately after the sheath is removed.

If, after the procedure, the INR is less than 1.6, the sheath can be removed when the ACT falls below 150 s. It is important to keep in mind that INR/PT can be signif-icantly changed by the previous use of streptokinase and direct thrombin inhibitors, independently of previous oral anticoagulant use. Fresh-frozen plasma (FFP) can always be given as needed to deal with active bleeding related to the puncture site.

PERCUTANEOUS CORONARY INTERVENTION IN PATIENTS WITH CHRONIC LIVER DISEASE OR CONGENITAL COAGULOPATHY

Patients with chronic liver disease with synthetic insufficiency can present with impaired coagulation. This may also be confounded by thrombocytopenia if there is a concomitant hypersplenism. The prevalence of coronary artery disease (CAD) in this group is no less common than in the general population. These patients may have an increased risk of bleeding. Elevation of PT/INR in these patients is not an equivalent of warfarin-induced coagulopathy, as in most cases it is not as easily cor-rectable by vitamin K administration. Interestingly, in an observational study, cardiac catheterization was not associated with significantly increased risk of bleeding in this group even in the absence of prophylactic FFP or platelets infusion.[12] Data regarding adjunctive therapy for PCI in patients with advanced liver disease are lacking. In patients with impaired hemostasis secondary to liver disease, the approach to antiplatelet therapy is also difficult to optimize. Aspirin should be given very cautiously and may be contraindicated due to gastrointestinal (GI) problems. Clopidogrel can cause hepatotoxicity in rare cases, but is the preferred antiplatelet medication for patients at risk of GI bleeding. GPIs are not well-studied in this group, and should be given in the highest thrombotic risk patients only, with possible preference to eptifibatide – the one that is less affected by liver metabolism, and more quickly cleared and reversible. UFH and LMWH are relatively safely used in this group of patients for associated venous thrombosis, which allows their use for anticoagulation in PCI. Although direct thrombin inhibitors (DTIs) have been promoted as being associated with decreased risk of bleeding, additional data regarding their use are needed, especially since bivalirudin is mainly renally excreted and could pose a liability in patients with renal insufficiency. Argatroban, which is metabolized by the liver, would also be relatively contraindicated in patients with chronic liver disease.

Inherited deficiencies of all identified clotting factors are described with those most prone to bleeding disorders. Most common are sex-linked disorders: hemophilia A – deficiency of factor VIII and seven times less frequent is hemophilia B – deficiency of factor IX. Patients with both types undergoing PCI are described in the literature.

Neither disorder affects platelet function directly, and both cause increased PTT with bleeding tendency. The activity of both factor VIII and IX can be checked and monitored while a patient is undergoing therapy with recombinant factors, cryoprecipitate, or FFP. Most important is to follow and maintain the level of deficient factor at about 80% or normal. The suggested protocol of medication therapy for PCI will include aspirin and clopidogrel in usual doses.[13] GPIs should be reserved for very-high-risk patients only. Anticoagulation can be achieved by UFH, LMWH or bivalirudin. Bivalirudin appears to be an attractive option with shorter length of action, less associated bleeding, and no need for PTT control.[14]

PERCUTANEOUS CORONARY INTERVENTION IN PATIENTS WITH RENAL INSUFFICIENCY

The risks of ischemic and bleeding complications are both increased in patients with renal impairment, providing additional challenges to the antiplatelet treatment and anticoagulation regimens during PCI. Aspirin and clopidogrel should be used in the usual doses. All GPIs are associated with increased bleeding in patients with renal impairment. All three available agents can be used with reasonable safety in this high-risk group although there is no sufficient data for preferential use of one over another in this setting.

In the do Tirofiban and ReoPro Give Similar Efficacy Outcome (TARGET) trial, 4623 patients were randomized to tirofiban or abciximab. In this analysis, patients were grouped in creatinine clearance (CrCl) quartiles (<70, 70–90, 90–114, >114 ml/min), and analyzed for efficacy and bleeding risk. Both ischemic and bleeding complications were highest in the lowest creatinine clearance quartile of patients treated with GPIs. Although tirofiban is renally cleared and abciximab is not, there was no interaction between these GPIs and creatinine clearance regarding ischemic or bleeding events.[15]

Abciximab is not renally excreted, and there are no data for dose adjustment. Both, eptifibatide and tirofiban are given initially in a weight-adjusted bolus, followed by continuous infusion adjusted for calculated CrCl.

In the Enhanced Suppression of the Platelet IIb/IIIa Receptor with Integrilin Therapy (ESPRIT) trial, patients were randomly assigned to placebo or eptifibatide as an adjunct to stent implantation (1755 patients with CrCl ≥60 ml/min and 289 patients with CrCl <60 ml/min). Treatment effect trended towards a greater magnitude in patients with lower CrCl (60 ml/min) compared with those with higher CrCl (90 ml/min). An accompanying increase in bleeding risk also was not apparent with lower CrCl. The treatment effect of eptifibatide is seen regardless of renal function, and tends toward being greater in patients with mild renal impairment.[16] Currently, the official package insert for eptifibatide mandates reducing the infusion by 50% in patients with a CrCl <60 ml/min. There is no sufficient data for dose adjustment and safety of GPIs in patients with end-stage renal disease on hemodialysis, however their use for selected patients is not precluded: abciximab is cleared by the reticuloendothelial system and therefore preferred, Tirofiban is used in 50% dose and can be removed by hemodialysis, eptifibatide is contraindicated.[17]

Anticoagulation can be safely achieved by CrCl dose-adjusted enoxaparin, PTT/ACT-controlled UFH, and by CrCl dose-adjusted bivalirudin. The dose adjustment of the above-mentioned agents for CrCl is well established, and presented in Table 6.2.

PERCUTANEOUS CORONARY INTERVENTION IN PATIENTS WITH THROMBOCYTOPENIA OR DISORDERS OF PLATELET FUNCTION

Optimal antiplatelet and anticoagulation therapy in patients with congenital or acquired platelet disorders needing PCI or thrombolysis is another challenging arena. The best-established management exists for the patients with heparin-induced thrombocytopenia (HIT). All three DTIs: hirudin, argatroban, and bivalirudin can be used during PCI in the setting of HIT.

ATBAT, the Anticoagulant Therapy with Bivalirudin to Assist in the performance of percutaneous coronary intervention in patients with heparin-induced Thrombocytopenia study was an open-labeled prospective study of bivalirudin in 52 consecutive patients requiring PCI with HIT with or without acute thrombosis syndrome. Bivalirudin was administered in two regimens: 'high-dose' standard PCI protocol dose, or 25% decreased bolus with 30% decreased infusion rate. Procedural success rate was 98%. One patient died 46 h after uneventful PCI. In the whole group there was only one case of major bleeding associated with bypass surgery; there were seven cases of minor bleeding. There were no cases of significant thrombocytopenia.[18]

Lewis et al studied argatroban (25 μg/kg/min (350 μg/kg initial bolus), adjusted to achieve an ACT of 300–450 s) in 91 patients undergoing 112 PCIs. Of these, 94.5% had a satisfactory outcome of the procedure, and 97.8% achieved adequate anticoagulation. Death (none), myocardial infarction (four patients), or revascularization (four patients) at 24 h after PCI occurred in seven (7.7%) patients overall. Only one patient (1.1%) experienced periprocedural major bleeding. Overall, argatroban is a good option in this setting, and is Food and Drug Administration (FDA) approved for this indication.[19] The work-up for HIT, looking for platelet factor 4-heparin complex antibodies is time consuming, and not very specific or sensitive, so in severe reaction even without bleeding or evidence of thrombo-occlusive disease heparin should be stopped and potentially substituted by DTI – bivalirudin or argatroban.

Aspirin and clopidogrel are not contraindicated in HIT, and should be used unless the patient has a critically low platelet count. The dose of direct thrombin inhibitors (bivalirudin and argatroban) used for PCI is higher than the one for the treatment of HIT, and so can be decreased 4 h after procedure and continued at the level of HIT treatment if needed.

Table 6.2 Antithrombotic therapy during percutaneous coronary intervention, standard and renal dosing

Medication	Standard dose	Dose adjustment for CrCl
Aspirin	300–325 mg, followed by 162–325 mg daily	Hemodialysis: give dose after dialysis
Clopidogrel	300–600 mg oral bolus, followed by 75 mg daily	No adjustment
Abciximab	Bolus 0.25 mg/kg IV 10–60 min prior to PCI; 0.125 µg/kg/min × 18–24 h; max: 10 µg/min	No adjustment
Eptifibatide	180 µg/kg IV bolus (max: 22.6 mg/bolus) just prior to PCI, then begin 2 µg/kg/min IV × 18–24 h, repeat 180 µg/kg IV bolus 10 min after first load (max bolus 22.6 mg, max infusion 15 mg/h)	CrCl < 50 ml/min: 180 µg/kg × 1, then 1 µg/kg/min, max bolus 22.6 mg, max infusion 7.5 mg/h; no repeated bolus
Tirofiban	Start IV infusion at 0.4 µg/kg/min × 30 min., then continue at 0.1 µg/kg/min × 12–24 h	CrCl <30 ml/min: decrease infusion rate by 50%
Unfractionated heparin	60–70 units/kg IV bolus (maximum 5000 units), then 12–15 units/kg/h IV infusion (maximum 1000 units/h), repeated boluses under PTT/ACT control	No adjustment
Enoxaparin	1 mg/kg subcutaneous twice every 12 h, additional 0.3 mg/kg IV once if last dose > 8 h prior to procedure	CrCl < 30 ml/min: decrease dose to 30 mg SC daily
Bivalirudin	0.75 mg/kg IV bolus, then: 1.75 mg/kg/h IV up to 4 hours, then may continue at: 0.2 mg/kg/h IV up to 20 h; ACT 5 min after bolus and give additional 0.3 mg/kg IV bolus if needed	CrCl < 30 ml/min: usual bolus, then infusion 1 mg/kg/h IV up to 4 h; hemodialysis: usual bolus, then infusion 0.25 mg/kg/h IV up to 4 h; ACT control
Argatroban	350 mcg/kg IV bolus then 25 mcg/kg/min IV; if next ACT < 300 sec give 150 mcg/kg bolus, then 30 mcg/kg/min; if next ACT > 450 sec, decrease to 15 mcg/kg/min	No adjustment

ACT, activated clotting time; CrCl, creatinine clearance; PCI, percutaneous coronary intervention; PTT, partial thromboplastin time; SC, subcutaneous.

Other causes of acquired thrombocytopenia include: idiopathic (immune) thrombocytopenic purpura (ITP), medication-induced thrombocytopenia, thrombotic thrombocytopenic purpura, and hemolytic-uremic syndrome, connective tissue disease, leukemia, cancer, AIDS and other chronic infections.

In patients with known thrombocytopenia undergoing elective PCI, there is time to plan the procedure and, if necessary, correct the disorder. None from the above-mentioned disorders by itself is an absolute contraindication to antiplatelet therapy, so the use of aspirin and clopidogrel is warranted. This is especially important to consider if stent placement is planned with a need for aspirin/clopidogrel therapy for 1–6 months, depending on the type of stent.

Interesting data were obtained by Sarkiss et al (personal communication) in a retrospective study of aspirin therapy in cancer patients with thrombocytopenia and ACS. Seventy patients with cancer who were diagnosed with ACS and referred for cardiology consultation were divided into two groups on the basis of platelet count: ($>100\ \mu\times10^9$/l and $<100\times10^9$/l). Data on the use of aspirin therapy, bleeding complications, and survival rates in each group were collected. Thirty-nine per cent of the patients with ACS had concomitant thrombocytopenia (platelets $<100\times10^9$/l): those who did not receive aspirin had a survival rate of 6% within the first month compared with 90% in those who did receive aspirin ($P<0.0001$). Patients with a platelet count ($>100\times10^9$/l) who received aspirin had a 30-day survival rate of 88% compared with 45% in those who did not receive aspirin ($P=0.0096$). Overall, the rate of bleeding in patients who received aspirin was not significant. There were no incidences of acute GI bleeding, intracranial hemorrhage, or fatal bleed. No cases of fatal bleeding or intracranial hemorrhage were reported. The incidence of minor bleeding was also similar among patients with thrombocytopenia who received or did not receive aspirin therapy. A few high-risk patients with ACS and thrombocytopenia requiring early coronary intervention tolerated aspirin and clopidogrel without bleeding complications.

These data suggest that among patients with cancer and ACS, the presence of thrombocytopenia is associated with a worse outcome. However, aspirin therapy in these patients may greatly influence outcome and is associated with improved survival at 7 and 30 days post-treatment, without significantly increasing the incidence of bleeding complications. Thrombocytopenia is usually associated with decreased ability to form thrombi, which is an underlying cause of ACS. The reason for this paradox of coronary thrombosis in thrombocytopenic patients is unclear. One possibility is the presence of a paraneoplastic syndrome in which platelets may be activated by substances released from tumor cells. These activated platelets, even in the presence of thrombocytopenia, may be hypercoagulable as a compensatory mechanism, and may predispose to thrombotic complications. Despite a low platelet count in these clinical settings, platelets may be highly susceptible to activation and aggregation. Platelet activation in cancer is mediated by a variety of mechanisms, ranging from increased expression of platelet adhesion molecules to direct platelet activation by contact with molecules on the surface of the tumor cell membrane. When compared to healthy controls, patients with cancer have higher levels of fibrinogen, von Willebrand factor and soluble P-selectin (a marker of increased platelet activation).

ITP is not uncommon, and is an autoimmune disorder where platelets are opsonized by antiplatelet auto-antibodies and prematurely destroyed by phagocytic cells; the rescued platelets are hyperfunctioning. There are reported cases of acute MIs in patients with ITP, treated with intravenous immunoglobulin (IVIG) and/or steroids.[20] Hyperactivation of the remaining platelets in settings of PCI increases the risk of thrombotic complications and should be addressed.

A reasonable approach to a stable patient would be a combined pretreatment with steroids for ITP, aspirin, and clopidogrel for antiplatelet effect, and use of bivalirudin during PCI for anticoagulation, as a treatment with the lowest reported risk of bleeding. In case of severe exacerbation of ITP with low platelet count and recent bleeding and/or petechiae co-existing with ACS, lower doses of aspirin (75–100 mg) should be considered, individual risk for bleeding should be assessed, and if 1 month of clopidogrel therapy is not feasible, PCI without stent implantation should be planned. Again bivalirudin appears to be the first choice for anticoagulation. Any surgical/vascular procedure will require a platelet count of >40–50 cells $\times 10^9$/l which warrants platelet transfusion in case of emergency, and IVIG use in ITP, as an agent with the faster action compared to steroids.

Medications are by far the most common cause of thrombocytopenia in hospital settings, ranging from mild to severe. Sometimes it is difficult to identify a single agent causing a problem. Consider the following scenario:

> A patient was admitted with ACS-unstable angina and started on aspirin, clopidogrel, UFH and eptifibatide, as an angiogram with possible PCI is planned, he was also given famotidine for prophylaxis, and is dropping his platelet count from 200 cells/µl to 60 cells $\times 10^9$/l in 6 h. Any of the above-mentioned medications can cause thrombocytopenia.

This patient might have HIT from previous heparin use, or more likely GPI (eptifibatide)-mediated thrombocytopenia. Unless active bleeding is present, aspirin and clopidogrel should be continued, in fact in this acute scenario with aspirin and clopidogrel once-daily administration, there will be time to re-assess the patient clinically and for platelet count. It is important to plan long-term aspirin/clopidogrel use considering stent implantation. Platelet transfusion might be indicated in the case of bleeding or need for emergent PCI with inadequate platelet count.

Rare cases of ACS with PCI are reported in patients with von Willebrand disease.[21] Desmopressin, or replacement therapy with plasma concentrate/recombinant or von Willebrand factor alone, or combined with factor VIII and VII, and FFP are routinely used for treatment or prophylaxis of bleeding in patients with von Willebrand disease, requiring surgery. The same approach is warranted for PCI. Every patient should be assessed separately in relation to the bleeding and treatment history, and a von Willebrand factor activity assay might be needed.[22] Aspirin and clopidogrel do not directly affect platelet adhesion, which is a defect in von Willebrand disease and they can be given. Any of the standard anticoagulation therapies can be used with possible benefits from DTI, associated with less bleeding.

A number of congenital disorders can present with altered platelet function and/or thrombocytopenia. They are uncommon and are extremely rarely associated with coronary disease, requiring intervention.[23] Glanzmann's thrombasthenia is a rare autosomal recessive congenital bleeding disorder caused by deficiency or dysfunction of the platelet surface glycoprotein (GP) IIb/IIIa receptor. It remains the predominant disorder of platelet function and is probably followed in prevalence by Bernard–Soulier Syndrome.[24] Bernard–Soulier syndrome, caused by absent or reduced expression of the platelet GP Ib–IX receptor is a rare autosomal recessive bleeding disorder characterized by platelet dysfunction, the presence of giant platelets, and a prolonged bleeding time. Both disorders are characterized by severely impaired platelet aggregation, which practically precludes the use of antiplatelet therapy in these patients. The suggested approach to anticoagulation for PCI would be the use of DTIs – bivalirudin or argatroban in a short-term infusion. Platelets and FFP should be ready in case of bleeding.

SUMMARY

Patients undergoing PCI require adjunctive antithrombotic therapy to decrease the risk of ischemic complications. The presence of impaired hemostasis increases the risk of bleeding complications. Standard antiplatelet and anticoagulation therapy should be provided unless absolutely contraindicated, demonstrating overall benefit, especially in patients with ACS. The risk of bleeding can be significantly decreased with an individualized approach, considering the level of emergency of the procedure; the mechanism of the pre-existing hemostasis disorder; careful monitoring and correction of the deficient factors; the mechanism of action, half-life, metabolism, excretion route with respective dose-adjustment and specific indications for the antithrombotic medications, avoiding routine use of GPIs. Additional attention must be given to the arterial puncture site, with longer manual pressure applied after sheath removal, appropriate use of an arterial closure device, or planning of alternative vascular (radial) access for PCI.

REFERENCES

1. Smith SC Jr, Feldman TE, Hirshfeld JW Jr et al. ACC/AHA/SCAI 2005 guideline update for percutaneous coronary intervention a report of the American College of Cardiology/American Heart Association Task Force on Practice Guidelines (ACC/AHA/SCAI Writing Committee to Update the 2001 Guidelines for Percutaneous Coronary Intervention). J Am Coll Cardiol 2006; 47: e1–121.
2. Smith SC Jr, Feldman TE, Hirshfeld JW Jr et al. ACC/AHA/SCAI 2005 guideline update for percutaneous coronary intervention: a report of the American College of Cardiology/American Heart Association Task Force on Practice Guidelines (ACC/AHA/SCAI Writing Committee to Update 2001 Guidelines for Percutaneous Coronary Intervention). Circulation 2006; 113: 156–75.
3. Popma JJ, Berger P, Ohman EM et al. Antithrombotic therapy during percutaneous coronary intervention: the Seventh ACCP Conference on Antithrombotic and Thrombolytic Therapy. Chest 2004; 126(3 Suppl): 576S–599S
4. Silber S, Albertsson P, Aviles FF et al. Guidelines for percutaneous coronary interventions. The Task Force for Percutaneous Coronary Interventions of the European Society of Cardiology. Eur Heart J 2005; 26: 804–47.
5. Yusuf S, Mehta SR, Chrolavicius S et al. Comparison of fondaparinux and enoxaparin in acute coronary syndromes. N Engl J Med 2006; 354: 1464–76.
6. Yusuf S, Mehta SR, Chrolavicius S et al. Effects of fondaparinux on mortality and reinfarction in patients with acute ST-segment elevation myocardial infarction: the OASIS-6 randomized trial. JAMA 2006; 295: 1519–30.
7. Shavelle DM, Salami A, Abdelkarim M et al. Rescue percutaneous coronary intervention for failed thrombolysis. Catheter Cardiovasc Interv 2006; 67: 214–20.
8. Gershlick AH, Stephens-Lloyd A, Hughes S et al. Rescue angioplasty after failed thrombolytic therapy for acute myocardial infarction. N Engl J Med 2005; 353: 2758–68.
9. Louvard Y, Benamer H, Garot P et al. Comparison of transradial and transfemoral approaches for coronary angiography and angioplasty in octogenarians (the OCTOPLUS study). Am J Cardiol 2004; 94: 1177–80.
10. MacDonald LA, Beohar N, Wang NC et al. A comparison of arterial closure devices to manual compression in liver transplantation candidates undergoing coronary angiography. J Invasive Cardiol 2003; 15: 68–70.
11. Orford JL, Fasseas P, Holmes DR et al. Alveolar hemorrhage associated with periprocedural eptifibatide administration. J Invasive Cardiol 2004; 16: 341–2.
12. Vaitkus PT, Dickens C, McGrath MK. Low bleeding risk from cardiac catheterization in patients with advanced liver disease. Catheter Cardiovasc Interv 2005; 65: 510–12.

13. Girolami A, Randi ML, Ruzzon E et al. Myocardial infarction, other arterial thrombosis and invasive coronary procedures, in hemaophilia B: a critical evaluation of reported cases. J Thromb Thrombolysis 2005; 20: 43–6.
14. Arora UK, Dhir M, Cintron G et al. Successful multi-vessel percutaneous coronary intervention with bivalirudin in a patient with severe hemophilia A: a case report and review of literature. J Invasive Cardiol 2004; 16: 330–2.
15. Berger PB, Best PJ, Topol EJ et al. The relation of renal function to ischemic and bleeding outcomes with 2 different glycoprotein IIb/IIIa inhibitors: the do Tirofiban and ReoPro Give Similar Efficacy Outcome (TARGET) trial. Am Heart J 2005; 149: 869–75.
16. Reddan DN, O'Shea JC, Sarembock IJ et al. Treatment effects of eptifibatide in planned coronary stent implantation in patients with chronic kidney disease (ESPRIT Trial). Am J Cardiol 2003; 91: 17–21.
17. Jeremias A, Bhatt DL, Chew DP et al. Safety of abciximab during percutaneous coronary intervention in patients with chronic renal insufficiency. Am J Cardiol 2002; 89: 1209–11.
18. Mahaffey KW, Lewis BE, Wildermann NM et al. The anticoagulant therapy with bivalirudin to assist in the performance of percutaneous coronary intervention in patients with heparin-induced thrombocytopenia (ATBAT) study: main results. J Invasive Cardiol 2003; 15: 611–16.
19. Lewis BE, Matthai WH Jr, Cohen M et al. Argatroban anticoagulation during percutaneous coronary intervention in patients with heparin-induced thrombocytopenia. Catheter Cardiovasc Interv 2002; 57: 177–84.
20. Fruchter O, Blich M, Jacob G. Fatal acute myocardial infarction during severe thrombocytopenia in a patient with idiopathic thrombocytopenic purpura. Am J Med Sci 2002; 323: 279–80.
21. James PR, de Belder AJ, Kenny MW. Successful percutaneous transluminal coronary angioplasty for acute myocardial infarction in von Willebrand's disease. Haemophilia 2002; 8: 826–7.
22. Arjomand H, Aquilina P, McCormick D. Acute myocardial infarction in a patient with von Willebrand disease: pathogenetic dilemmas and therapeutic challenges. J Invasive Cardiol 2002; 14: 615–18.
23. Ryckman JG, Hall S, Serra J. Coronary artery bypass grafting in a patient with Glanzmann's thrombasthenia. J Card Surg 2005; 20: 555–6.
24. Nurden AT, Nurden P. Inherited disorders of platelets: an update. Curr Opin Hematol 2006; 13: 157–62.

7

ST elevation acute myocardial infarction admitted in a distant location

Marc C Newell, David M Larson,
and Timothy D Henry

Timely access to primary percutaneous coronary intervention • Transfer of ST elevation myocardial infarction patients • Is transfer for primary percutaneous coronary intervention a feasible strategy? • Real-life models • Key components of an integrated, co-ordinated system of transfer for ST elevation myocardial infarction patients • Future challenges • Conclusion

While primary percutaneous coronary intervention (PCI) is the preferred method of reperfusion for ST elevation myocardial infarction (STEMI), timely access to PCI continues to be a challenge throughout the world. This chapter will address the issue of transfer of STEMI patients from hospitals without cardiac catheterization laboratories for primary PCI. We will discuss the data supporting transfer for primary PCI, the safety and feasibility of transferring STEMI patients, the barriers that must be overcome, and ongoing challenges for management of STEMI patients presenting to rural and community hospitals.

TIMELY ACCESS TO PRIMARY PERCUTANEOUS CORONARY INTERVENTION

It has become increasingly clear that PCI is the preferred reperfusion strategy for STEMI patients if done in a timely manner at high-volume centers.[1-3] However, the vast majority of patients with STEMI present to hospitals without cardiac catheterization laboratories (CCL). Less than 25% of hospitals in the United States (US) have PCI capability,[4] however, the majority of US patients are within 60 min of a PCI center.[5] The majority of data suggest that prolonging the door-to-balloon time decreases the benefits of primary PCI.[6-8] Therefore, both the American College of Cardiology/American Heart Association (ACC/AHA) and European Society of Cardiology (ESC) guidelines set a door-to-balloon time of 90 min as the goal.[1,2] This goal is especially challenging in patients who present to hospitals without PCI capability.

The current ACC/AHA guidelines recommend primary PCI if done in a timely fashion (90 min) by experienced providers (class I-A). For patients in cardiogenic shock or with contraindications to thrombolytics, the guidelines also recommend PCI as the optimal reperfusion strategy (class I-A).[1] The European guidelines recently indicated primary PCI as the recommended treatment for STEMI if performed by an experienced team < 90 min after first medical contact (class I-A).[2]

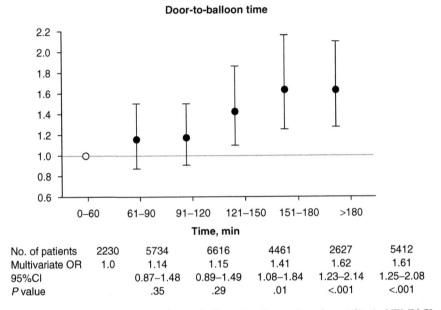

Figure 7.1 Relationships between door-to-balloon time intervals and mortality in NRMI.[6] CI, confidence interval; OR, odd ratio.

These recommendations are based on trials comparing primary PCI to fibrinolysis. In an analysis of 23 randomized trials, Keeley et al demonstrated that primary PCI is the preferred method of reperfusion based on a significant reduction in mortality, reinfarction, and stroke.[3] The combined major adverse cardiac event (MACE) rate occurred in 14% of fibrinolytic-treated patients versus 8% of those receiving PCI ($P < 0.0001$). Support for the 90 min door-to-balloon time in both the ACC/AHA and ESC guidelines comes from the National Registration of Myocardial Infarction (NRMI)-2 database, which demonstrates a direct relationship between mortality and door-to-balloon times (the time from initial hospital presentation to the infarct-related artery patency) (Figure 7.1).[6] Further analysis of the 23 trials used in the Keeley analysis indicates the benefit of primary PCI over thrombolysis may be lost if the PCI-related time delay versus the door-to-drug time (the time from initial presentation to administration of fibrinolytic) exceeds 90 min (Figure 7.2).[7] It is worth noting that only two of the studies had delays greater than 60 min, thus the data beyond 60 min in Figure 7.2 are an extrapolation.[7] Also, one must keep in mind that the 90 min 'cut-off' is the delay beyond the door-to-drug time, which is typically around 30 min. Thus, the theoretical loss of benefit of PCI over thrombolysis suggested in this study probably occurs >120 min from patient presentation.

TRANSFER OF ST ELEVATION MYOCARDIAL INFARCTION PATIENTS

The benefits of primary PCI over fibrinolysis stimulated a number of reports describing transfer of high-risk STEMI patients to PCI centers.[9,10] These initial reports led to a number of randomized clinical trials comparing transfer of STEMI patients for

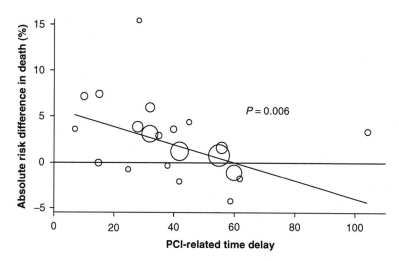

Figure 7.2 Absolute risk reductions in mortality rates with primary PCI as it relates to PCI-related time delay.[7] The circle size reflects the sample size of the individual study.

primary PCI to fibrinolysis.[11-14] The PRimary Angioplasty in patients transferred from General community hospitals to specialized PTCA Units with or without Emergency thrombolysis (PRAGUE) study was a multi-center, randomized, controlled trial designed to determine the best reperfusion strategy in 300 STEMI patients presenting to community hospitals without PCI capability. The results showed a significant reduction in death, myocardial infarction (MI), and stroke at 30 days in patients transferred directly for primary PCI (8% vs. 15% in facilitated PCI group vs. 23% in community hospital streptokinase group; $P < 0.02$).[11] Of note, there were no transfer deaths, and the mean door-to-balloon time was 95 min in the PCI group. The PRAGUE-2 study was a larger nationwide trial in the Czech Republic comparing streptokinase versus transfer for primary PCI in 850 STEMI patients presenting to hospitals without PCI capability. The primary endpoint (30-day mortality) showed a trend favoring transfer for PCI (6.8% in the PCI and 10% in the streptokinase groups, $P = 0.12$). The MACE rate at 30 days was significantly reduced in the PCI group (8.4% vs. 15.2% in the streptokinase group, $P < 0.003$).[12] Of note, two patients died during transfer in this study.

The Danish Multicenter Randomized Study on Fibrinolytic Therapy versus Acute Coronary Angioplasty in Acute Myocardial Infarction (DANAMI-2) was a Danish national, multicenter, randomized controlled trial comparing primary PCI with front-loaded tissue plasminogen activator (tPA) in STEMI patients.[13] Twenty-four referral hospitals without PCI capability, and five PCI centers were involved in the study. Transfer distances ranged from 35 to 95 miles. The results showed an overall statistically significant reduction of the primary endpoint of death, reinfarction, and stroke at 30 days for patients treated with primary PCI (8.0% primary PCI versus 13.7% for tPA, $P < 0.001$). The endpoint was driven by a difference in reinfarction. Of note, the results clearly supported transfer for primary PCI in patients who presented initially to the referral hospitals (8.5% primary endpoint in transfer for PCI patients vs. 14.2% for tPA, $P = 0.002$). There were no deaths during transfer in this study.

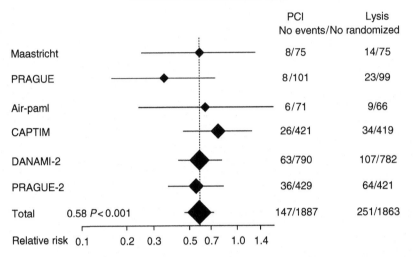

Death/re-infarction/stroke

Figure 7.3   Meta-analysis results of patients transferred for PCI compared with patients treated with fibrinolysis.[15]

The only randomized transfer for PCI in STEMI trial in the US was the Air-PAMI study.[14] This study showed only a trend toward fewer MACE events in the primary PCI group at 30 days compared to fibrinolytic (8.4% vs. 13.6%, $P=0.33$). Unfortunately the trial was underpowered since it stopped early due to poor enrolment. In addition, the average door-to-balloon time was 174 min (±80 min), which is considerably longer than the European trials. This was despite an average transfer distance of 32 ± 36 miles. No patients died during transfer. A recent meta-analysis of six randomized trials (3750 patients) demonstrates transfer for PCI (door-to-balloon was <3 h for all patients) resulted in a 42% reduction in the combined cardiac endpoint of death, reinfarction, or stroke versus patients treated with fibrinolysis and an overall trend toward decreased mortality (Figure 7.3).[15]

The shorter door-to-balloon times in the European trials probably reflect organized transfer systems with short transfer distances. Unfortunately for STEMI patients, these clinical trials may not reflect the real-world situation. The recent data from the NRMI-3/4 database indicate the median door-to-balloon time in STEMI patients transferred for PCI is 180 min in the US, with only 4.2% of patients achieving times less than 90 min, and only 16.2% less than 120 min.[16]

IS TRANSFER FOR PRIMARY PERCUTANEOUS CORONARY INTERVENTION A FEASIBLE STRATEGY?

While the data from randomized trials support the transfer of STEMI patients for primary PCI, there are a number of challenges to implementing this strategy.[17–19]

First, there is the lack of an integrated system of healthcare. For example, the US has a highly fragmented healthcare delivery system, requiring many 'handoffs' in the management of a STEMI patient being transferred for primary PCI. Poor or slow communication between healthcare workers and physicians often leads to inefficiency and delays. Secondly, the lack of standardized STEMI treatment protocols results in variability in time to treatment and the method of reperfusion, as well as beneficial adjunctive therapies such as aspirin, beta-blockers, angiotensin-converting enzyme (ACE) inhibitors, and lipid-lowering agents. While just 20 years ago STEMI treatment options were limited, we now have multiple treatment strategies, which often lead to confusion for primary non-cardiology physicians. In addition, despite a wealth of data on STEMI treatment and extensive guidelines, implementation of these guidelines has been at best disappointing. Despite recommendations that all hospitals have standardized protocols, standing orders and quality assurance programs, this is still not the case.[20] Thirdly, hospital overcrowding is frequently an issue. Many tertiary centers are experiencing critical shortages in staffing and bed capacity. Having to spend time arranging beds, nurses, and a receiving hospital limit efficient patient transfer. Fourthly, the lack of an organized system for interfacility transfer is frequently an issue. The variability in the real-world setting of interhospital transfers is staggering. In the US, certain governmental regulations, such as the Emergency Medical Treatment and Labor Act (EMTALA), also cause unintentional delays. Reimbursement strategies are a fifth major challenge to rapid transfer of STEMI patients. There are many economic barriers to transfer that have not been well studied and vary from country to country. These include implications for the referral hospital in loss of revenue by transferring patients, and transport systems competing for patient transfers, as well as tertiary centers competing for patients. Finally, lifestyle issues and staffing a PCI-capable hospital 24 hours a day, 7 days a week for primary PCI certainly takes a significant commitment on the part of the interventional cardiologists and CCL staff at the PCI hospital.

REAL-LIFE MODELS

A number of institutions around the world have demonstrated that STEMI patients can be transferred from community hospitals to tertiary cardiac centers in a timely and efficient manner. Dudek and colleagues reported successful transfer of STEMI patients from remote locations, first in a cohort of 200 patients, and recently in 669 STEMI patients using facilitated PCI with a door-to-balloon time of 151 minutes.[21,22] The Level 1 Heart Attack program at the Minneapolis Heart Institute in Minnesota, recently reported a median first door-to-balloon time of 97 min in 11 hospitals up to 60 miles from the PCI center, using a standardized protocol and integrated transfer system for primary PCI. The median total door-to-balloon time was 117 min using a facilitated PCI protocol in 17 hospitals up to 60–210 miles from the PCI center.[18,23] The development and success of the Level 1 Heart Attack Program at the Minneapolis Heart Institute is based on an organized system for interhospital transfer, with integration and collaboration of medical personnel, including cardiologists, emergency department (ED) physicians, nurses, emergency medical providers and transporters, as well as other ancillary medical personnel.[24]

KEY COMPONENTS OF AN INTEGRATED, CO-ORDINATED SYSTEM OF TRANSFER FOR ST ELEVATION MYOCARDIAL INFARCTION PATIENTS

Standardized protocol

The most important step in development of a regional transfer program is the use of a standardized STEMI protocol that is agreed upon by the cardiologists, ED, and primary care physicians within the system. Delays occur when the ED physician has to discuss the reperfusion strategy or which adjunctive regimen to use with the on-call cardiologist. Each hospital should have written institution-specific protocols for STEMI that include appropriate lab and diagnostic studies, and adjunctive medications such as antiplatelet and antithrombin regimens, beta-blockers, nitrates, and pain control medications. Key details of the protocol should be available in checklists and standing orders in the ED. Tools such as laminated cards or posters with details of the standardized protocol are helpful.

Empower the emergency department physician

The ACC/AHA and ESC guidelines recommend the ED physician should be responsible for making the initial diagnosis of STEMI and treatment decisions. The ED physician should be able to activate the transfer protocol with a single phone call leading to a page which will mobilize the entire system including the interventional cardiologist and CCL staff to be available within 30 min. Non-diagnostic electrocardiograms (ECGs) or diagnostic dilemmas can be discussed with the cardiologist, but should be the exception rather than the rule.

Individualize transfer agreements

Each community hospital will have unique transfer issues based on distance and availability of air or ground ambulance. Therefore an individualized transfer plan should be developed for each community hospital including pre-arranged transfer agreements with local ambulance or helicopter companies. Helicopter transport services need to be instructed to use a trauma transfer approach which includes 10 min turnaround times and 'hot loads' (keeping the rotors running).

Direct admission to the cardiac catheterization laboratory

Since the initial evaluation has been performed at the community or rural hospital, the patient should be taken directly to the CCL and not re-evaluated in the ED or intensive care unit/coronary care unit (ICU/CCU) at the receiving hospital. Patients can be pre-admitted based on the initial demographic data from the community hospital. Key clinical and laboratory data collected at the community hospital along with the ECG should be faxed directly to the CCL while the patient is being transferred.

Education/training

Education is an essential component to a successful transfer program. This includes education and training of the transport personnel, nursing, and ancillary staff with the community and PCI hospital (ED, CCU and CCL), primary care and ED physicians regarding ECG diagnosis, and details of the standardized protocol in order to facilitate rapid diagnosis and initial stabilization prior to transfer. This training should be facilitated by cardiovascular staff from the PCI hospital. Teamwork at the community and PCI hospitals is essential to achieve the goal of 90 min door-to-balloon times.

Feedback and quality improvement

After a patient is transferred, it is essential that the community or rural hospital physician receive feedback from the PCI hospital. This includes the ED physician, nursing staff, and primary care physicians. Communication fosters a sense of team-work, and the immediate clinical and angiographic correlation will sharpen the diagnostic skills of the ED physician. We have adopted a system where the inter-ventional cardiologist calls the ED physician following the procedure, the attend-ing cardiologist calls the primary care physician, and the Level 1 MI nurse co-ordinator calls the community ED nursing staff. Cumulative data are provided quarterly to each community hospital. A STEMI database is utilized to follow trends in time to treatment, protocol compliance, and clinical outcomes.[18] These data can be used for continuous quality improvement activities, as well as to meet hospital accreditation requirements. When considering the suitability of a rural or community hospital for transfer of STEMI practices for primary PCI, we utilize a 30–30–30 min goal. This includes 30 min in door–out door at the referral hospital, 30 mins interhospital transfer time, and 30 min door-to-balloon time at the PCI center. The primary benefit of a standardized regional transfer system is to improve time to treatment, which will improve outcomes in STEMI patients. The overall improvement in outcomes results not only from improvements in time to treatment but improved adherence to guidelines such as lipid-lowering agents and antiplatelet agents. Other benefits include the opportunity to rapidly implement new research results and guidelines, and to measure outcomes and trends in this high-risk patient population.[25]

While there are clearly challenges to the development of an integrated, co-ordinated transfer system, the benefits justify the time and effort required to improve timely access to primary PCI for all STEMI patients.

FUTURE CHALLENGES

A major unresolved issue is the treatment of STEMI patients transferred from longer distances or with significant transfer delays. While fibrinolytics are a reasonable option in this setting, two other strategies may increase availability for PCI, and deserve consideration. Facilitated PCI (described here as partial- or full-dose fibri-nolytics in conjunction with PCI) has recently been a widely debated topic. In the Assessment of the Safety and Efficacy of a New Treatment Strategy for Acute Myocardial Infarction (ASSENT-4 PCI) trial, 829 STEMI patients receiving full-dose tenecteplase prior to PCI were compared with 838 patients receiving primary PCI alone. The primary endpoint of congestive heart failure, death, and shock at 90 days occurred in 19% of facilitated PCI patients compared to 13% of primary PCI patients $(P=0.0045)$.[26] ASSENT-4 did not test the hypothesis regarding transfer delays, as 45% of patients were enrolled in PCI centers and randomization to balloon was only 115 min. In addition, there were a number of trial design issues including inadequate antiplatelet and antithrombin regimens due to the concern for bleeding with full-dose fibrinolytic.

Unfortunately, there are almost no data regarding the use of facilitated PCI in patients with long delays or transfer distances. Data from single-center studies suggest the facilitated approach may offset the time delays.[21-23] In 200 patients, Dudek et al found 86% of patients had Thrombolysis In Myocardial Infarction (TIMI) grade 2 or 3 flow using a facilitated PCI approach with abciximab and reduced-dose alteplase from remote locations.[21] Mortality was 3.5% at 30 days, despite 21% of patients requiring treatment for arrhythmia or hypotension during transfer. The same group recently reported their results in 669 STEMI patients using facilitated PCI with door-to-balloon times of 151 min. These patients had no significant difference in PCI success, mortality, reinfarction, or revascularization at 12 months compared with patients presenting to the tertiary center.[22] In the Minneapolis Heart Institute Level 1 Heart Attack Program, patients transferred from distances of 60–210 miles receive half-dose tenecteplase in addition to aspirin, clopidogrel, and heparin.[18] We recently reported 72% pre-PCI TIMI 2 or 3 flow with a 3.8% 30-day mortality in 176 consecutive facilitated PCI patients compared to pre-PCI TIMI 2 or 3 flow rate of 31% and 6.3% 30-day mortality ($P <0.0001$ and not significant, respectively) at the PCI center.[27]

The other option for increasing availability of PCI in STEMI patients with long delays or transfer distances is the liberal use of rescue PCI. In the French multicenter Comparison of Angioplasty and Prehospital Thrombolysis in Acute Myocardial Infarction (CAPTIM) trial, 840 STEMI patients were randomized to prehospital fibrinolysis with alteplase versus primary PCI.[28] The primary endpoint (death, non-fatal reinfarction, or stroke) was reached in 6.2% of PCI patients versus 8.2% of the prehospital fibrinolysis group ($P=0.29$). Rescue PCI was utilized in 26% of fibrinolytic-treated patients. There was no significant difference in 12-month MACE rates (16.4% fibrinolysis vs. 14% PCI). Recently, the Rescue Angioplasty versus Conservative Treatment or Repeat Thrombolysis (REACT) trial, a multicentered trial in the UK, randomized 427 STEMI patients with failed reperfusion to repeat fibrinolysis, conservative treatment, or rescue PCI. The trial results support the strategy of aggressive rescue PCI, as the composite endpoint of death, reinfarction, stroke, or severe heart failure within 6 months favored rescue PCI (rescue PCI 15.3%, conservative 29.8%, repeat fibrinolysis 31%, $P <0.01$).[29]

CONCLUSION

Primary PCI is the preferred reperfusion strategy in STEMI patients if performed in a timely manner at high-volume centers. Availability is the major limitation to this strategy, and can be addressed using an efficient co-ordinated system of transfer for primary PCI. Facilitated PCI and liberal use of rescue PCI in patients presenting to non-PCI centers are alternative approaches to increase the number of patients benefiting from PCI in STEMI.

REFERENCES

1. Antman EM, Anbe DT, Armstrong PW et al. ACC/AHA guidelines for the management of patients with ST-elevation myocardial infarction – executive summary: a report of the American College of Cardiology/American Heart Association Task Force on Practice Guidelines (Writing Committee to Revise the 1999 Guidelines for the Management of Patients With Acute Myocardial Infarction). Circulation 2004; 110: 588–636.

2. Van de Werf F, Ardissino D, Betriu A et al. Management of acute myocardial infarction in patients presenting with ST-segment elevation. The Task Force on the Management of Acute Myocardial Infarction of the European Society of Cardiology. Eur Heart J 2003; 4: 28–66.
3. Keeley E, Boura J, Grines CL. Primary angioplasty versus intravenous thrombolytic therapy for acute myocardial infarction: a quantitative review of 23 randomized trials. Lancet 2003; 361: 13–20.
4. Wennberg DE, Lucas FL, Siewers AE et al. Outcomes of percutaneous coronary interventions performed at centers without and with onsite coronary artery bypass graft surgery. JAMA 2004; 292: 1961–8.
5. Nallamothu BK, Bates ER, Wang Y et al. Driving times and distances to hospitals with percutaneous coronary intervention in the United States. Circulation 2006; 113: 1189–95.
6. Cannon CP, Gibson CM, Lambrew CT et al. Relationship of symptom-onset-to-balloon time and door-to-balloon time with mortality in patients undergoing angioplasty for acute myocardial infarction. JAMA 2000; 283: 2941–7.
7. Nallamothu BK, Bates ER. Percutaneous coronary intervention versus fibrinolytic therapy in acute myocardial infarction: is timing (almost) everything? Am J Cardiol 2003; 92: 824–6.
8. Zijlstra F. Angioplasty vs thrombolysis for acute myocardial infarction: a quantitative overview of the effects of interhospital transportation. Eur Heart J 2003; 24: 21–3.
9. Zijlstra F, van't Hof AW, Liem AL et al. Transferring patients for primary angioplasty: a retrospective analysis of 104 selected high risk patients with acute myocardial infarction. Heart 1997; 78: 333–6.
10. Straumann E, Yoon S, Naegeli B et al. Hospital transfer for primary coronary angioplasty in high risk patients with acute myocardial infarction. Heart 1999; 82: 415–19.
11. Widimsky P, Groch L, Zelizko M et al. Multicentre randomized trial comparing transport to primary angioplasty vs immediate thrombolysis vs combined strategy for patients with acute myocardial infarction presenting to a community hospital without a catheterization laboratory. The PRAGUE study. Eur Heart J 2000; 21: 823–31.
12. Widimsky P, Budesinsky T, Vorac D et al. Long distance transport for primary angioplasty vs immediate thrombolysis in acute myocardial infarction. Final results of the randomized national multicentre trial – PRAGUE-2. Eur Heart J 2003; 24: 94–104.
13. Andersen HR, Nielsen TT, Rasmussen K et al. A comparison of coronary angioplasty with fibrinolytic therapy in acute myocardial infarction. N Engl J Med 2003; 349: 733–42.
14. Grines CL, Westerhausen D, Weaver WD et al. A randomized trial of transfer for primary angioplasty versus on-site thrombolysis in patients with high-risk myocardial infarction: the Air Primary Angioplasty in Myocardial Infarction study. J Am Coll Cardiol 2002; 39: 1713–19.
15. Dalby M, Bouzamondo A, Lechat P et al. Transfer for primary angioplasty versus immediate thrombolysis in acute myocardial infarction: a meta-analysis. Circulation 2003; 108: 1809–14.
16. Nallamothu BK, Bates ER, Herrin J et al. Times to treatment in transfer patients undergoing primary percutaneous coronary intervention in the United States: National Registry of Myocardial Infarction (NRMI)-3/4 analysis. Circulation 2005; 111: 761–7.
17. Henry TD, Atkins JM, Cunningham MS et al. ST elevation myocardial infarction: recommendations on triage of patients to cardiovascular centers of excellence. J Am Coll Cardiol 2006; 47: 1339–45.
18. Henry TD, Unger BT, Sharkey SW et al. Design of a standardized system for transfer of patients with ST-elevation myocardial infarction for percutaneous coronary intervention. Am Heart J 2005; 150: 373–84.
19. Rathore SS, Epstein AJ, Nallamothu BK et al. Regionalization of ST-segment elevation acute coronary syndrome care. J Am Coll Cardiol 2006; 47: 1346–9.
20. Larson DM, Sharkey SW, Unger BT, Henry TD. Implementation of acute myocardial infarction guidelines in community hospitals. Acad Emerg Med 2005; 12: 522–7.

21. Dudek D, Zmudka K, Kaluza G et al. Facilitated percutaneous coronary intervention in patients with acute myocardial infarction transferred from remote hospitals. Am J Cardiol 2003; 91: 227–9.
22. Dudek D, Dziewierz A, Siudak Z et al. Percutaneous coronary interventions after 150 minutes transfer delay in patients with ST-elevation acute myocardial infarction. Circulation 2005; 112: II–621.
23. Henry TD, Sharkey SW, Graham KJ et al. Transfer for direct percutaneous coronary intervention for ST-elevation myocardial infarction: the Minneapolis Heart Institute Level 1 Myocardial Infarction Program. Circulation 2005; 112: II–620.
24. Larson DM, Henry TD. Regional transfer programs for primary percutaneous coronary intervention. In: Cannon CP, O'Gara PT (eds) Critical Pathways in Cardiovascular Medicine. Philadelphia, PA: Lippincott Williams & Wilkins, 2006 (in press).
25. Newell MC, Henry CR, Sigakis CJG et al. Comparison of safety and efficacy of sirolimus-eluting stents versus bare metal stents in patients with ST-segment elevation myocardial infarction. Am J Cardiol 2006; 97: 1299–302.
26. Assessment of the Safety and Efficacy of a New Treatment Strategy with Percutaneous Coronary Intervention (ASSENT-4 PCI) investigators. Primary versus tenecteplase-facilitated percutaneous coronary intervention in patients with ST-segment elevation acute myocardial infarction (ASSENT-4 PCI): randomised trial. Lancet 2006; 367: 569–78.
27. Larson DM, Menssen KM, Newell MC et al. Long distance transfer for direct percutaneous coronary intervention: a facilitated approach. J Am Coll Cardiol 2006; 47: 174A.
28. Bonnefoy E, Lapostolle F, Leizorovicz A et al. Primary angioplasty versus prehospital fibrinolysis in acute myocardial infarction: a randomised study. Lancet 2002; 360: 825–9.
29. Gershlick AH, Stephens-Lloyd A, Hughes S et al. Rescue angioplasty after failed thrombolytic therapy for acute myocardial infarction. N Engl J Med 2005; 353: 2758–68.

8

Stable obstructive coronary disease and very low left ventricular function

Pedro de Araújo Gonçalves,
and Ricardo Seabra-Gomes

Patients with depressed left ventricular function as a high-risk group for revascularization procedures • Accurate selection of patients for revascularization • Use of devices to protect against distal embolization • Use of assist devices for supported angioplasty

Primum non nocere. (Hippocrates)

The last 20 years have seen dramatic advances in the field of percutaneous coronary interventions (PCI). Not only has the progressive development of new devices made the procedures more effective and safe, but it has also allowed operators to treat a wider range of patients and more complex lesions. High-risk populations now represent a substantial number of patients treated in everyday practice, and one such example are those with a very depressed left ventricular (LV) function.

PATIENTS WITH DEPRESSED LEFT VENTRICULAR FUNCTION AS A HIGH-RISK GROUP FOR REVASCULARIZATION PROCEDURES

The severity of LV dysfunction and heart failure symptoms is closely related to the rate of major adverse cardiac events (MACE) after revascularization procedures in patients with coronary artery disease (CAD).

In the field of surgical revascularization, a depressed LV function is an independent risk factor across different score systems.[1] In the widely used European System for Cardiac Operative Risk Evaluation (EUROSCORE), 'LV ejection fraction (EF) <30%' is one of the most important risk factors for operative mortality. In this score, the relative weight attributed to low EF was the same as for 'critical preoperative state' and 'active endocarditis' at the time of surgery.[2]

The comparison between coronary artery bypass surgery (CABG) and medical treatment for patients with chronic stable angina from randomized controlled trials (RCTs) conducted many years ago showed an absolute benefit of surgery among patients with an abnormal ejection fraction (EF).[3] The 5-year mortality was 13.3% for normal and 25.2% for abnormal LV function, with significantly better results under surgical treatment ($P=0.02$) for those with abnormal function.[3] Since then, surgery was considered preferable if there was depressed LV function and those patients were excluded from trials.

The 'first-generation' RCT of CABG versus PCI included mainly low-risk patients and only a very small proportion (~20%) with low EF. No RCT was large enough and had sufficient power to detect benefits, with either treatment, in patients with depressed LV function. CABG has remained preferable for high-risk patients such as those with severe LV dysfunction.

Stenting PCI has shown to be superior to balloon PCI in patients with ischemic LV dysfunction. In a long-term follow-up study, patients with EF ≤40% had better survival at 5 years if they received a stent compared with balloon alone (76% vs. 53%, P <0.05), suggesting that the more durable revascularization provided by stenting could improve survival.[4]

Using the Mayo Clinic risk score, symptomatic heart failure with New York Heart Association (NYHA) class ≥III was one of the eight independent predictors of complications after PCI defined as either death, Q-wave myocardial infarction, emergent or urgent coronary artery bypass graft surgery, or cerebrovascular accident.[5]

Patients with severely depressed LV function have also been excluded from the major drug-eluting stents (DES) trials. Nevertheless, DES are commonly used off-label in these patients, and in a recent study, a low EF was pointed out as one independent predictor of DES thrombosis in a large cohort of 'real-world' practice patients.[6]

ACCURATE SELECTION OF PATIENTS FOR REVASCULARIZATION

Patients with LV dysfunction have a large area of myocardium that fails to contract. Fortunately, for many of these patients, a substantial amount of this myocardium is not a true scar but rather part of the process of hibernation or stunning. As these two types of processes represent viable myocardium, revascularization can improve the contractile function by recruiting blood to these regions.[7]

The accurate selection of patients likely to benefit from the revascularization procedure is based on the identification of a suitable pathological substrate where viable myocardium represents a significant proportion of the total non-contracting myocardium. This can be achieved by stress echocardiography, nuclear myocardial perfusion imaging, and cardiac magnetic resonance imaging.

In a meta-analysis of nine studies using an empirical Bayes random effects model, it was determined that there was a statistically significant interaction of viability and treatment (by CABG or PCI) allocation (odds ratio (OR) of 2.76) with regard to long-term mortality. However, due to several limitations and biases of this type of analysis, RCT should be undertaken.[8]

Two ongoing trials are addressing the role of revascularization in patients with depressed LV function. The Heart Failure Revascularization Trial (HEART) trial was designed to determine whether coronary revascularization improves the survival of patients with heart failure who have evidence of dysfunctional but viable myocardium on stress-induced ischemia, and who are already receiving optimal medical treatment.[9] The Surgical Treatment for Ischemic Heart Failure (STICH) trial is enrolling patients with ischemic cardiomyopathy, and is evaluating the benefit of coronary revascularization over optimal medical therapy and whether this benefit can be enhanced by ventricular restoration surgery.[10]

Another important issue in the selection of patients for a revascularization procedure is the assessment of the level of risk, aiming for a favorable risk–benefit ratio. Besides using the aforementioned risk scores, there are some angiographic characteristics that help in the prediction of the procedural risk.

If the target vessel for the procedure is responsible for a significant amount of the remaining viable myocardium, there will be a considerable risk of hemodynamic collapse during balloon inflation, in a case of acute vessel closure or occurrence of 'no reflow' phenomenon. Although usually associated with the thromboembolic nature of acute coronary syndromes, the 'no reflow' is also associated with elective procedures, due to microembolization of atherosclerotic debris, especially in degenerated venous graft interventions and with the use of rotational atherectomy.[11] The knowledge of the expected level of complications is crucial to the selection of the proper combination of experienced operators, adjunctive pharmacologies, distal protection, and LV assist devices.[12]

USE OF DEVICES TO PROTECT AGAINST DISTAL EMBOLIZATION

One of the most popular controversies in the field of interventional cardiology has been the issue of cardiac enzyme elevation after successful angioplasty as an independent predictor of adverse outcomes. Patients with significantly depressed baseline LV systolic function represent a subgroup where this does not seem to constitute a controversy, because of a lower tolerance to an additional loss of viable myocytes.[13] As compared to patients with normal LV function, it is reasonable to consider that the relative contribution of the same absolute amount of myocardial damage translated by the creatine kinase (CK)-MB (muscle and brain subunits) rise, is higher for patients with very low LV function.

Many pharmacological interventions have proved to be of value in reducing the myocardial injury associated with PCI. Distal protection devices are now well established as adjuncts to PCI in vein grafts or thrombus-containing lesions, preventing microembolization.[14]

Although the use of these devices can increase the complexity of the procedure, as in other fields of medicine, *proactive is better than reactive.*

USE OF ASSIST DEVICES FOR SUPPORTED ANGIOPLASTY

The intra-aortic balloon pump (IABP) is the most widely used hemodynamic support device. It works through counterpulsation, augmenting the diastolic pressure and consequently the coronary perfusion pressure and reducing the afterload, leading to an increase in the cardiac output. In the Benchmark registry, the most frequent indication for use of IABP was to provide hemodynamic support during or after cardiac catheterization, and in many of these patients the use was prophylactic in the context of high-risk PCI.[15]

The most important limitations of IABP are the inability to provide adequate support in patients with severely compromised LV function, as well as in patients with very rapid and irregular heart rates. In the face of these limitations, new intravascular devices have been developed, extending the concept of LV assistance from the surgical arena to the catheterization laboratory, and thus allowing the expansion of mechanical circulatory support indications. These devices have been evaluated in patients with hemodynamic collapse due to cardiogenic shock, acute myocarditis, transplant rejection, or postcardiotomy.[16]

Recently, with the advent of less invasive assist devices, they are now being used also for short-term support during high-risk elective procedures.[17–19]

The IMPELLA Recover LP 2.5 is the smallest assist device being used in this context. It has an easy percutaneous insertion through a 12F sheath and is positioned

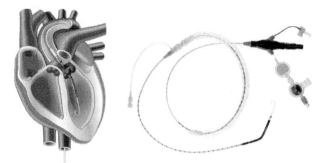

Figure 8.1   IMPELLA Recover LP 2.5.

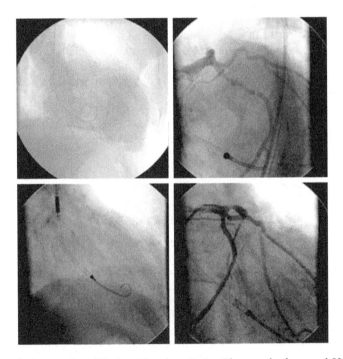

Figure 8.2   Case example: a 77-year-old male patient with severely depressed LV function, occluded left anterior descending coronary artery and significant lesions in the remaining left circumflex artery (LCx) and intermediate branch. Treated with two DES, during IMPELLA Recover LP 2.5 support.

in the LV where it pumps blood to the aorta, just above the aortic valve (Figure 8.1). It can be used for up to 5 days, and has a maximal output of 2.5 l/min. It has a pressure sensor that guides the correct position of the device.

   In Figures 8.2 and 8.3, two case examples of Impella-supported high-risk PCI in patients with severely depressed LV function are shown.

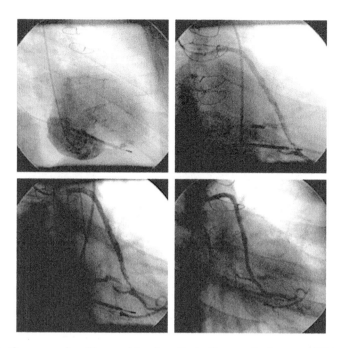

Figure 8.3 Case example: a 74-year-old male patient with severely depressed LV function and an implantable cardioverter defibrillator (ICD) with significant lesions in the proximal and distal segments of a vein graft to an obtuse marginal branch. Treated with three DES, during IMPELLA Recover LP 2.5 support.

Another percutaneous ventricular assist device is the TANDEMHEART pVAD, that delivers a left atrial-to-femoral artery bypass assistance.

This device assists the LV by removing oxygenated blood from the left atrium and delivering it to the femoral artery. A trans-septal puncture is needed to advance the inflow 21F canula into the left atrium, and the outflow canula in the femoral artery is between 9 and 14F (Figure 8.4). It can be used up to 18 days and has a maximal output of 4.0 l/min.

A comparison of the main characteristics of these two percutaneous LV assist devices is shown in Table 8.1.

Assist devices, although adding complexity, represent a favourable trade-off in face of the added efficacy and safety of the procedure. Once again, *proactive is better than reactive.*

PCI in the setting of chronic stable angina pectoris is usually an elective procedure often performed immediately after diagnostic coronary angiography. The presence of a depressed LV function may not support this decision, particularly if there is multivessel coronary disease and involvement of the left anterior descending coronary artery or the left main. Surgery could then be considered the best alternative with established benefits according to the guidelines.[20]

However, each patient should be considered individually. Patient preferences, comorbidities, tolerance to double antiplatelet regimens, and guarantee of adherence, as well as training and competence of operators, existence of IABP or the new assist devices, surgical backup, etc, may turn the decision to the less invasive PCI procedure.

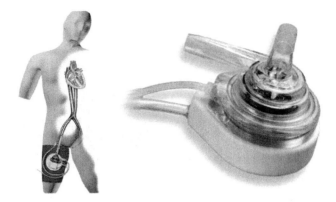

Figure 8.4   TANDEMHEART pVAD™.

Table 8.1   Comparison of the main characteristics of two percutaneous LV assist devices

	Vascular access	Inflow/ outflow	Trans-septal puncture	Output Up to 2.5	Duration of support
IMPELLA Recover LP 2.5	Femoral artery 12F	LV/aorta	No	Up to 2.5 l/min	Up to 5 days
TANDEMHEART pVAD	Femoral vein 21F; femoral artery 9–14F	Left atrium/ femoral artery	Yes	Up to 4.0 l/min	Up to 18 days

This practice may never be sufficiently large to allow RCT between PCI and CABG. In this context, stenting is better than balloon PCI, and DES are the preferable stents to use. Prophylactic percutaneous assist devices should be used if hemodynamic collapse could be expected. They can increase safety for patients and a more relaxed performance for the operators. The aim should be to make the procedure quick and safe.

In a professionally responsible way, each interventional cardiologist should weigh the risk and benefit of PCI in the context of severely depressed LV function, and always ask himself if it should be done, even if he knows that it can be done.

REFERENCES

1. Geissler HJ, Hölzl P, Marohl S et al. Risk stratification in heart surgery: comparison of six score systems. Eur J Cardiothorac Surg 2000; 17: 400–6.
2. Nashef SAM, Roques F, Michel P et al, for the EuroSCORE study group. European system for cardiac operative risk evaluation (EuroSCORE). Eur J Cardiothorac Surg 1999; 16: 9–13.

3. Rihal CS, Raco DL, Gersh BJ et al. Implications for coronary artery bypass surgery and percutaneous coronary intervention in chronic stable angina. Review of the evidence and methodological considerations. Circulation 2003; 108: 2439–45.
4. Lipinski MJ, Martin RE, Cowley MJ et al. Improved survival for stenting vs. balloon angioplasty for the treatment of coronary artery disease in patients with ischemic left ventricular dysfunction. Catheter Cardiovasc Interv 2005; 66: 547–53.
5. Singh M, Rihal CS, Selzer F et al. Validation of Mayo Clinic risk adjustment model for in-hospital complications after percutaneous coronary interventions, using the National Heart, Lung, and Blood Institute Dynamic Registry. J Am Coll Cardiol 2003; 42: 1722–8.
6. Iakovou I, Schmidt T, Bonizzoni E et al. Incidence, predictors, and outcome of thrombosis after successful implantation of drug-eluting stents. JAMA 2005; 293: 2126–30.
7. Wijns W, Vatner SF, Camici PG. Hibernating myocardium. N Engl J Med 1998; 339: 173–81.
8. Bourque JM, Hasselblad V, Velazquez EJ et al. Revascularization in patients with coronary artery disease, left ventricular dysfunction, and viability: a meta-analysis. Am Heart J 2003; 146: 621–7.
9. Cleland JGF, Freemantle N, Ball SG et al. The heart failure revascularisation trial (HEART): rationale, design and methodology. Eur J Heart Failure 2003; 5: 295–303.
10. Joyce D, Loebe M, Noon GP et al. Revascularization and ventricular restoration in patients with ischemic heart failure: the STICH trial. Curr Opin Cardiol 2003; 6: 454–7.
11. Klein LW, Kern MJ, Berger P et al, on behalf of the Interventional Cardiology Committee of the Society of Cardiac Angiography and Interventions. Suggested management of the no-reflow phenomenon in the cardiac catheterization laboratory. Cathet Cardiovasc Intervent 2003; 60: 194–201.
12. De Feyter PJ, McFadden E. Risk score for percutaneous coronary intervention: forewarned is forearmed. J Am Coll Cardiol 2003; 42: 1729–30.
13. Cutlip DE, Kuntz RE. Cardiac enzyme elevation after successful percutaneous coronary intervention is not an independent predictor of adverse outcomes. Circulation 2005; 112: 916–21.
14. Baim DS, Wahr D, George B et al. Randomized trial of a distal embolic protection device during percutaneous intervention of saphenous vein aorto-coronary bypass grafts. Circulation 2002; 105: 1285–90.
15. Ferguson JJ, Cohen M, Freedman RJ et al. The current practice of intra-aortic balloon counterpulsation: results from the Benchmark Registry. J Am Coll Cardiol 2001; 38: 1456–62.
16. Siegenthaler MP, Brehm K, Strecker T et al. The Impella Recover microaxial left ventricular assist device reduces mortality for postcardiotomy failure: a three-center experience. J Thorac Cardiovasc Surg 2004; 127: 812–22.
17. Vranckx P, Foley DP, de Feyter PJ et al. Clinical introduction of the Tandemheart, a percutaneous left ventricular assist device, for circulatory support during high-risk percutaneous coronary intervention. Int J Cardiovasc Intervent 2003; 5: 35–9.
18. Bonvini RF, Hendiri T, Camenzind E et al. High-risk left main coronary stenting supported by percutaneous left ventricular assist device. Catheter Cardiovasc Interv 2005; 66: 209–12.
19. Valgimigli M, Steendijk P, Sianos G et al. Left ventricular unloading and concomitant total cardiac output increase by the use of percutaneous Impella Recover LP 2.5 assist device during high-risk percutaneous intervention. Catheter Cardiovasc Interv 2005; 65: 263–7.
20. Gibbons RJ, Abrams J, Chatterjee K, et al. ACC/AHA 2002 guideline update for the management of patients with chronic stable angina: a report of the American College of Cardiology/American Heart Association Task Force on Practice Guidelines (Committee to Update the 1999 Guidelines for the Management of Patients with Chronic Stable Angina). 2002. Available at www.acc.org/clinical/guidelines/stable/stable.pdf.

9

Multivessel disease in patients with acute myocardial infarction and high-risk unstable angina: culprit versus non-culprit intervention

Francesco Saia and David Antoniucci

Multivessel disease in patients with acute coronary syndromes • The 'vulnerable' patient • Multivessel percutaneous coronary intervention in patients with ST elevation myocardial infarction • Multivessel percutaneous coronary intervention in patients with left ventricular dysfunction or cardiogenic shock • Multivessel percutaneous coronary intervention in patients with unstable angina non-ST elevation myocardial infarction • Conclusions

The definition 'acute coronary syndromes' (ACS) includes three different clinical entities, i.e. ST elevation acute myocardial infarction (STEMI), unstable angina (UA), and non-ST elevation myocardial infarction (NSTEMI), which share a common underlying pathophysiological mechanism, i.e. atherosclerotic plaque rupture or erosion, with differing degrees of superimposed thrombosis and distal embolization, and enhanced vasoreactivity. Hence, ACS are most of the time triggered by a single 'culprit' lesion, although sometimes there are multiple lesions which could be equally responsible for the clinical event.

Coronary angiography is now generally recommended in the early phase of STEMI and high-risk ACS, and percutaneous coronary intervention (PCI) has gained a pivotal role for the subsequent treatment.[1-4] Despite the fact that usually there is just one culprit lesion, a considerable proportion of patients presenting with ACS exhibit a severe disease of more than one major epicardial vessel at coronary angiography, namely multivessel disease (MVD) (Figure 9.1). When PCI is performed, a common clinical dilemma for the interventional cardiologist is whether it is wiser to treat the culprit lesion and postpone the treatment of other lesions/vessels to a second elective procedure, or to pursue complete coronary revascularization in a single stage. However, especially in the past, PCI in the acute phase of ACS was associated with an increased risk of periprocedural complications and adverse cardiovascular events. As a direct consequence, a strategy of immediate angioplasty of the culprit lesion and deferred treatment of other non-culprit lesions was proposed by many as a possible way to reduce untoward events.[5,6] In recent years, technological advances coupled with high acute success rates and lower complication rates have increased the use of PCI in patients with ACS. Stenting and the use of adjunctive platelet glycoprotein IIb/IIIa inhibitors have further broadened the use of PCI by improving both the safety and the efficacy of these procedures. Complete revascularization of both culprit and

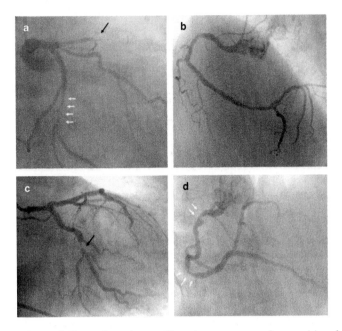

Figure 9.1 Multivessel disease in patients with acute coronary syndromes. (a) and (b) Patient with STEMI. (a) Caudal right anterior oblique view showing the culprit lesion on the left anterior descending coronary artery (black arrow), which is totally occluded, and another tight lesion in the circumflex coronary artery (white arrows); (b) right coronary artery of the same patient, showing mild parietal atheromasia. (c) and (d) Patient with non-Q-wave myocardial infarction. (c) Caudal right anterior oblique view showing the culprit lesion on the left circumflex artery (black arrow); (d) right coronary artery of the same patient, showing two non-culprit severe lesions (white arrows).

non-culprit lesions and vessels in a single procedure has progressively become more appealing than it was previously, but much controversy still remains. In addition, some important differences do exist between STEMI and non-ST elevation ACS patients, which may justify a different therapeutic approach.

The purpose of this chapter is to review the available evidence on multivessel PCI in patients presenting with ACS, and to describe the factors that may help the choice of culprit versus non-culprit vessel intervention.

MULTIVESSEL DISEASE IN PATIENTS WITH ACUTE CORONARY SYNDROMES

In recent clinical trials on patients admitted with a diagnosis of STEMI, the incidence of multivessel disease was around 50%, and this figure is consistent with the findings of real-world registries.[7–10]

Multivessel disease predicts an increased risk of reduced global left ventricular function and both in-hospital and long-term mortality after AMI.[11–13] Similarly, the absence of significant disease in the non-infarct territory was a significant predictor of improved survival.[14] In a report from the Thrombolysis and Angioplasty in Myocardial Infarction (TAMI) study group, the angiographic findings of 855 patients consecutively enrolled in five phases of the TAMI study were correlated with their in-hospital outcome.[12] All patients received intravenous thrombolytic therapy and underwent cardiac catheterization within 90 min of the initiation of therapy. When compared with the group of patients with single-vessel disease, patients with MVD had a lower global left ventricular ejection fraction, albeit the severity of the infarct zone dysfunction was similar in the two groups. This difference was driven by a significant difference in the function of the non-infarct zone, which was hyperkinetic in the group with minimal or single-vessel disease, and hypocontractile or dyskinetic in those with MVD.[12] In an analysis of 1009 consecutive patients with ST elevation AMI treated by primary PCI in Florence,[10] patients with MVD had higher rates of 5-year all cause mortality (28% vs. 12%; $P=0.0001$) (Figure 9.2), cardiac death (23% vs. 8%; $P=0.0001$), revascularization procedure (26% vs. 15%; $P=0.0001$), and hospitalization for heart failure (6% vs. 3%; $P=0.048$) than did patients with single vessel disease. Non-fatal reinfarction rates were similar (6% vs. 5%, $P=0.700$) between the two groups. At multivariate analysis, the presence of MVD was independently associated with a twofold increase of cardiac mortality (hazard ratio [HR] 2.059, 95% confidence interval (CI) 1.404–3.019; $P=0.0002$). Other variables significantly related to mortality were age, cardiogenic shock, and previous myocardial infarction (MI).

Data from the Thrombolysis In Myocardial Infarction (TIMI) IIIB and Fragmin and fast Revascularization during InStability in Coronary artery disease (FRISC II) show that 44–59% of patients with UA/NSTEMI have MVD.[15,16] In this setting, patients with MVD as well as those with left main stenosis are at higher risk of serious cardiac events.[1,2] In patients undergoing only culprit lesion angioplasty for UA,[17] MVD was a predictor of late ischemic events both in the pre-stent era, and in the stent era.[18] Remarkably, the extent and severity of coronary artery disease is closely correlated with the TIMI risk score, which predicts adverse clinical outcomes in patients with non-ST elevation ACS.[19]

MVD as a marker of severe and diffuse atherosclerotic coronary artery disease, accounts for the poorer clinical outcome. Clearly, a more aggressive therapeutic strategy might be helpful to reduce the increased risk associated with this condition. Immediate treatment of severe lesions in non-culprit vessels holds a number of potential benefits. Treatment of non-culprit lesions with specific characteristics of vulnerability (e.g. complicated and rupture-prone plaques) might help to prevent recurrent cardiac events. However, as previously mentioned, the issue of appropriateness and timing of non-culprit simultaneous revascularization of severe lesions in non-culprit vessels is debated.[10,20,21]

THE 'VULNERABLE' PATIENT

According to current pathophysiological concepts, ACS are triggered by acute atherosclerotic plaque complication. Plaque rupture is the most common type of plaque complication and accounts for approximately 70% of fatal acute MIs and/or sudden coronary deaths.[22] The rupture of the fibrous cap leads to the exposure of the thrombogenic material of the atherosclerotic plaque, with subsequent activation of the clotting cascade and platelet adhesion, activation, and aggregation. This leads to thrombosis with an abrupt luminal compromise, which is responsible for sudden cardiac events.[23,24] The conversion of a stable, asymptomatic lesion to an unstable, ruptured plaque involves many processes, the most studied of which

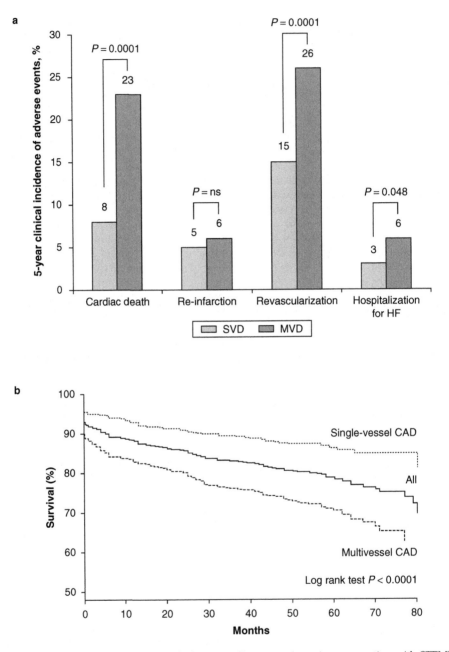

Figure 9.2   Long-term incidence of adverse cardiac events in patients presenting with STEMI treated with primary angioplasty according to the angiographic patterns of single-vessel disease (SVD) and multivessel disease (MVD). (a) Five-year incidence of single adverse events (HF = heart failure; ns = not significant); (b) cumulative long-term survival. From Parodi G, Memisha G, Valenti R et al. Five year outcome after primary coronary intervention for acute ST elevation myocardial infarction: results from a single centre experience. Heart 2005; 91: 1541–4 with permission.[10]

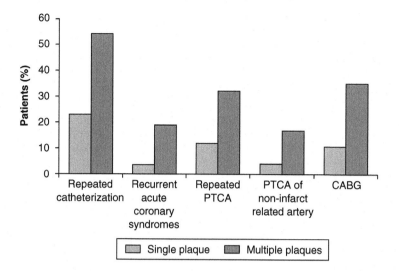

Figure 9.3 Outcome within one year after myocardial infarction in patients with multiple complex plaques or single complex plaques. PTCA, percutaneous transluminal coronary angioplasty; and CABG coronary-artery bypass grafting. $P < 0.001$ for all comparison between groups. From Goldstein JA, Demetriou D, Grines CL et al. Multiple complex coronary plaques in patients with acute myocardial infarction. N Engl J Med 2000; 343: 915–22, with permission.[35]

are inflammation, cellular breakdown, and expansion of the acellular, lipid-rich, necrotic core. Excessive mechanical stress in combination with local inflammation and excessive extracellular matrix degradation due to macrophage proteasis secretion and activation is considered the most important mechanism of plaque rupture.[25–28] The terms 'high-risk', 'vulnerable' or 'thrombosis-prone' plaque can be used as synonyms to describe a plaque that is at increased risk of thrombosis and rapid stenosis progression which often leads to symptomatic disease.[29] Angiographically, ischemia-related arteries in unstable angina and Q-wave acute MI are characterized by eccentric stenosis with overhanging edges or irregular borders.[30] These lesions probably represent either disrupted atherosclerotic plaques or partially occlusive or lysed thrombi, or both. Recent studies have shown widespread coronary inflammation in ACS patients, challenging the hypothesis of a single vulnerable plaque in this condition.[31,32] Patients with acute MI have evidence of systemic inflammation as reflected by activated circulating neutrophils, lymphocytes and monocytes, increased concentration of pro-inflammatory cytokines (IL-1, IL-6),[33] and elevated levels of C-reactive and amyloid proteins.[34] Inflammation could affect endothelial function, and activate the metalloproteases and collagenases responsible for endothelial-cell detachment and lysis of the plaque capsule at the sites where it is weakest, generating a multifocal process.[31] Thus, the concept of pan-coronary vulnerability in ACS has been developed, shifting attention from the single plaque to the 'vulnerable patient'.[22] Indeed, multiple angiographically complex plaques have been demonstrated in around 40% of patients with acute MI, and the presence of multiple complex plaques was associated with an increased incidence of recurrent acute coronary syndromes, repeated angioplasty, particularly of non-infarct-related lesions, and coronary-artery bypass graft surgery (Figure 9.3).[35]

In patients with acute myocardial infarction, multiple plaque rupture has been associated with systemic inflammation and poor prognosis.[36] The presence of more than one vulnerable plaque in ACS patients has been observed also at necropsy examination,[37] with intravascular ultrasound (IVUS),[38] IVUS-palpography,[39] and coronary angioscopy.[40]

Thus, patients with ACS may harbour multiple vulnerable plaques that are associated with adverse clinical outcomes, and this may have implications for management. Treatment of these plaques, even when they are not recognized as the culprit ones, might carry acute and long-term benefits that outweigh the risks of periprocedural events and restenosis. To further tangle the controversy, it should be noted that the lesions underlying an ACS may be either stenotic or non-stenotic. However, non-stenotic lesions are far more frequent than stenotic plaques, and account for the majority of culprit ruptured plaques.[41] Thus, treatment of non-culprit non-stenotic lesions with peculiar characteristics of high risk for complication and consequent triggering of a new ACS has also been evoked as a possible future scenario to reduce the late risk of events,[42] especially since the risk of restenosis has been dramatically reduced by the introduction in clinical practice of drug-eluting stents (Figure 9.4).[43–47] However, research in this field is in a very early phase, and at present such an approach cannot be considered in clinical practice.

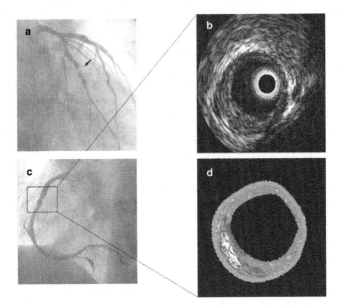

Figure 9.4   Clinical examples of possible vulnerable plaques in non-culprit vessels in patients with acute coronary syndromes. (a) Right anterior oblique view showing the culprit lesion on the left circumflex artery (black arrow); (b) right coronary artery of the same patient, showing a moderate proximal stenosis (box); (c) cross-sectional IVUS examination of the lesion highlighted in (b), showing an eccentric plaque; (d) virtual histology of the plaque in (c) showing the colour-coded plaque composition (calcium = white; fibrous tissue = green; fibrolipid = greenish-yellow; lipid core = red). The presence of a calcific-necrotic core within the plaque (white and red), and of a lipid core in close contact with the lumen are suggestive of plaque vulnerability.

MULTIVESSEL PERCUTANEOUS CORONARY INTERVENTION IN PATIENTS WITH ST ELEVATION MYOCARDIAL INFARCTION

Rationale

Primary PCI for STEMI is effective in securing and maintaining the patency of the infarct-related artery (IRA), and reported rates of achieving TIMI 3 flow range from 70% to 90% of cases. In randomized trials, primary PCI has been demonstrated to be more effective than thrombolytic therapy for the treatment of STEMI, by reducing overall short- and long-term incidence of death, non-fatal re-infarction, and stroke.[48] Accordingly, this strategy is now recommended as a class I treatment by both the European Society of Cardiology's and the American Heart Association (AHA)/ American College of Cardiology (ACC) guidelines for the management of patients with ST elevation AMI.[3,4] Thus, a growing number of patients are acutely referred to the catheterization laboratory for coronary angiography and, when indicated, for primary PCI.

As previously mentioned, about half of the patients admitted with acute MI have MVD at presentation,[20] and MVD in this setting confers an increased risk of morbidity and mortality after reperfusion therapy.[49] Nevertheless, treatment of non-culprit lesions at the time of primary PCI in patients with MVD is generally not indicated in the absence of hemodynamic compromise.[4]

The hypothetical benefits of multivessel PCI in the setting of ACS comprise:

- acute improvement of left ventricular mechanical function
- reduction of early ischemic events
- reduction of arterial access site complications
- cost saving by reducing the need for staged revascularization procedures.

These benefits of multivessel PCI may be mitigated, however, by an increased risk of periprocedural problems such as:

- technical complications and reperfusion events
- adverse reactions to contrast medium and volume loading
- In addition, multiple stenting increases the risk of mid-term restenosis, and subacute stent thrombosis, which are well-recognized drawbacks when considering the treatment of lesions not causing ischemia and/or symptoms.[50,51]

Clinical experiences

To date, multivessel PCI in the setting of AMI has been addressed only by a few observational and retrospective studies. Early reports suggested that a strategy of primary PCI directed at the IRA with staged intervention of the non-IRA is associated with good procedural success and favorable long-term outcome.[21] However, contrasting data are available regarding safety, efficacy, and costs of complete versus only IRA revascularization.

In a retrospective study, 506 patients with STEMI and MVD were subdivided into three groups on the basis of the revascularization strategy: (1) patients undergoing PCI of the IRA only (*n*=354); (2) patients undergoing PCI of both the IRA and non-IRA(s) during the initial procedure (*n*=26); and (3) patients undergoing PCI of the IRA followed by staged, in-hospital PCI of the non-IRA(s) (*n*=126).[20] In patients with MVD, compared with PCI restricted to the IRA only, multivessel PCI (groups 2 and 3) was associated with higher rates of re-infarction (13.0% vs. 2.8%, $P < 0.001$), revascularization (25% vs. 15%, $P = 0.007$), and major adverse cardiac events (MACE) (40% vs. 28%, $P = 0.006$). Multivessel PCI was an independent predictor of MACE at 1 year (odds ratio (OR) = 1.67, $P = 0.01$). Patients undergoing multivessel PCI during the initial procedure had a higher in-hospital mortality rate (19% vs. 2.4% staged MV PCI vs. 5.6% IRA-only PCI; $P = 0.003$), and a trend toward higher 30-day mortality. However, this difference was not statistically significant at 1-year follow-up and, importantly, no additional deaths were observed in this group after hospital discharge. Thirty days and 1 year after primary PCI, patients undergoing staged, in-hospital PCI had higher re-infarction rates compared to the other groups ($P < 0.001$).[20] The authors conclude that PCI should be directed at the IRA only, with decisions about PCI of non-culprit lesions guided by objective evidence of residual ischemia at late follow-up.

In another small study, compared with patients undergoing culprit artery PCI, patients undergoing simultaneous multivessel PCI had a higher risk of death (25% vs. 16.4%; $P = $ not significant (NS)), re-infarction (8.8% vs. 1.6%; $P = 0.07$), coronary artery bypass graft (CABG) (4.4% vs. 0%; $P = 0.10$), and stroke (10.3% vs. 0%; $P = 0.01$).[52] However, this study had several limitations and a clear selection bias for high-risk characteristics may have influenced the outcomes of the multivessel PCI group, and may not have been accounted for.[52]

Recently, however, another retrospective study showed similar procedural success and did not show an excess risk of death or of combined death, MI, CABG or target vessel revascularization up to 3 years, comparing multivessel PCI ($n = 239$ patients, PCI within 7 days after acute MI) and PCI of IRA only ($n = 1145$ patients), in patients with MVD.[53] Conversely, there was a trend toward better outcomes after multivessel PCI, although the difference was not statistically significant. In this study, both patients with ST elevation and non-ST elevation were included.[53]

In a small prospective randomized multicentre study, 69 MVD patients with STEMI < 12 h after symptom onset undergoing primary angioplasty, were randomized between culprit lesion treatment only ($n = 17$) and complete multivessel treatment ($n = 52$).[54] A similar low incidence of in-hospital major adverse cardiac events was observed. In the culprit treatment group there was an increase in the incidence of new revascularization at 12-month follow-up (35 vs. 17%, $P = 0.247$), that was not statistically significant but was sufficient to compensate the initial higher in-hospital costs of multivessel PCI, with a similar 12-month hospital cost in the two groups. The conclusion of this study was that a more aggressive approach in multivessel patients is not associated with any clinical or economic advantage, and that when only the culprit lesion was initially treated, the need for subsequent clinically driven revascularization remained low.[54]

In the 2000–2001 New York State Angioplasty Registry database, the in-hospital clinical outcome of patients with MVD who underwent either multivessel PCI ($n = 632$) or IRA-PCI ($n = 1350$) within 24 h of acute MI was assessed. In-hospital mortality was three-fold lower (0.8 vs. 2.3%, $P = 0.018$) in the multivessel PCI group. No differences were observed in other ischemic complications, renal failure, or length of stay. After multivariate analysis, multivessel PCI remained a significant predictor of lower in-hospital death (OR = 0.27, 95% CI = 0.08–0.90, $P = 0.03$). Importantly, patients with previous MI, angioplasty, bypass surgery, or cardiogenic shock were excluded. Therefore, this study suggests that a strategy of multivessel angioplasty during acute MI may be safe and effective in selected patients.[55]

MULTIVESSEL PERCUTANEOUS CORONARY INTERVENTION IN PATIENTS WITH LEFT VENTRICULAR DYSFUNCTION OR CARDIOGENIC SHOCK

Patients with MVD and hemodynamic compromise represent a group who might particularly benefit from complete revascularization. In fact, the acute mechanical dysfunction of the infarct area is normally compensated by hypercontractility of the non-infarct segments, provided they are not ischemic *per se*.[12] This compensatory mechanism can be crucial in critically ill patients. In addition, it has been shown that during acute MI, coronary flow slows globally, both in culprit and in non-culprit arteries, and this is correlated with hemodynamic changes, wall motion abnormality, and clinical outcome, including mortality.[56] In the setting of significant non-culprit coronary artery stenosis, such hemodynamic perturbations could lead to areas of jeopardized myocardium remote from the infarct zone. The delayed non-culprit artery flow may also be the result of more extensive necrosis in shared microvasculature, or shared territories of injury, and increased circulating catecholamine levels. Among the multiple variables associated with slower non-culprit artery flow, there is a larger territory infarcted and, of course, the presence of tighter stenoses within these arteries.[56] Hence, relief of tight stenoses in non-culprit arteries might improve the clinical outcome, especially in larger MIs.

In a preliminary analysis, patients with AMI complicated by cardiogenic shock or congestive heart failure exhibit improved 6-month mortality rate when complete revascularization was performed compared with incomplete revascularization (Telanya JM, personal communication, Transcatheter Cardiovascular Therapeutics (TCT) 2002). Indeed, a secondary analysis of the SHould we emergently revascularize Occluded Coronaries for cardiogenic shocK (SHOCK) trial suggested that surgery should be considered in shock patients with multivessel disease not amenable to relatively complete percutaneous revascularization.[57] However, it should be remembered that excessive contrast volume loading may be harmful in patients with a fragile hemodynamic state.

The risk of contrast-induced nephropathy

Contrast-induced acute renal failure (ARF) after PCI is associated with significant in-hospital and long-term morbidity and mortality.[58,59] Independent predictors of ARF following PCI have been reported. Besides baseline creatinine clearance and diabetes, a strong correlation has been found between this untoward event and acute MI,[59] shock,[59,60] and contrast dose.[58–60] Patients undergoing primary PCI may be at higher risk of ARF because of hemodynamic instability and unfeasibility of adequate prophylaxis.[61] In this setting, a single-center experience found age >75 years (OR = 5.28), anterior infarction (OR = 2.17), time-to-reperfusion >6 h (OR = 2.51), contrast agent volume >300 ml (OR = 2.80), and use of intraaortic balloon (OR = 15.51) to be independent correlates of ARF.[61] Patients developing ARF had longer hospital stay, more complicated clinical course, and significantly higher mortality rate (31% vs. 0.6%; $P < 0.001$).[61]

The obvious conclusion of these observation is that preventive strategies are needed. Multivessel PCI in the setting of STEMI may expose these patients to high volumes of contrast, and therefore further increase their risk of developing ARF. Therefore, decisions to perform multivessel PCI should take into account the patients' baseline characteristics and the expected contrast dose to complete the procedure.

The 'unfriendly' milieu

Notably, it has been suggested that significant exaggeration of non-culprit lesion stenosis severity may occur at infarct angiography,[62] and this may affect revascularization decision making in an appreciable number of MVD patients. Potential causes for the dynamic component of non-culprit stenosis include vasoconstriction, thrombus, plaque regression at follow-up, or changes in reference segment vessel tone. In light of these findings, immediate PCI of non-culprit lesions may expose the patient to unnecessary risks of both acute complications and restenosis.[62]

Bioactivity of several important coronary vasoconstricors, including serotonin, endothelin, angiotensin, and thromboxane, is increased during MI,[63,64] whereas oxidant stress reduces the vasodilatory effects of nitric oxide, adenosine, and prostacyclin.[65] These data suggest that revascularization of a non-culprit vessel should be avoided in such an unfriendly milieu, because it may increase the risk–benefit ratio after PCI.

Drug-eluting stents

One of the drawbacks of multivessel PCI is the late occurrence of restenosis and the need for repeat interventions. This has been advocated as a major reason to avoid percutaneous treatment of lesions which have not been demonstrated to cause ischemia and/or symptoms (i.e. the oculo-stenotic reflex), especially in patients presenting with ACS.

Recently, drug-eluting stents have been introduced in clinical practice, and they have been associated with a dramatic reduction in restenosis and need for further revascularizations compared to bare-metal stents in a number of randomized trials.[43–47] In a large single-centre registry, the use of drug-eluting stents in the setting of ACS was shown to be safe at 30 days.[66] At long-term follow-up of patients with STEMI, MVD did not emerge as an independent predictor of adverse events at multivariate analysis,[9] supporting the hypothesis that drug-eluting stent utilization might effectively open up new horizons in the treatment of MVD in patients with ACS. However, this hypothesis should be tested in dedicated clinical trials.

MULTIVESSEL PERCUTANEOUS CORONARY INTERVENTION IN PATIENTS WITH UNSTABLE ANGINA/NON-ST ELEVATION MYOCARDIAL INFARCTION

In patients with UA/NSTEMI, risk stratification is critically important because it determines the choice of treatment strategy and provides specific prognostic information. Guidelines for risk-stratification were published by the ACC and AHA,[1] and by the European Society of Cardiology (ESC).[2] Risk stratification should take into account clinical factors, electrocardiogram (ECG) and serum markers, evidence of spontaneous or inducible ischemia, measures of left ventricular function, and coronary anatomy. The risk for subsequent events should be assessed early, at the time of admission to the hospital, and it should later be modified in the light of additional information collected.[2] Patients at low risk can be discharged early. Patients at intermediate risk may either receive initial medical therapy and be closely monitored for high-risk features, or undergo early angiography with a view to revascularization. Patients at high risk should undergo early angiography and revascularization if their anatomy is suitable. Similarly to STEMI patients, around 50%

of the UA/NSTEMI patients show MVD and/or left main stenosis.[1,2] Coronary revascularization (PCI or CABG) in these patients is carried out to improve prognosis, relieve symptoms, prevent ischemic complications, and improve functional capacity. Motivation for an early revascularization strategy may depend on the perceived risk of progression to MI or death, and there is some evidence showing that patients can be discharged earlier and that readmissions are reduced.

In general, recommendations for the choice of a revascularization procedure in unstable angina are similar to those for elective revascularization procedures.[1,2] Complete revascularization should be pursued because it is associated with reduced need for future CABG, a trend toward better survival, and no difference in repeat PCI.[67,68] In some patients, a staged procedure may be considered, with immediate balloon angioplasty and stenting of the culprit lesion, and subsequent reassessment of the need for treatment of other lesions.

The rationale and the risks for immediate complete revascularization versus culprit lesion treatment only are the same as for STEMI patients. However, there are a number of remarkable differences. In general, patients with UA/NSTEMI did not have a direct link between PCI delay and myocardial damage as for STEMI patients. Therefore, in most cases there is enough time to evaluate the clinical condition of the patient and to administer a full medical treatment. Pretreatment with thienopyridines and glycoprotein IIb/IIIa inhibitors reduces the early hazard associated with PCI in a high-risk setting. Careful clinical evaluation allows prediction of the risk of developing contrast-induced acute renal failure and adoption of preventive measures. Similarly, the risks of volume loading may be weighed in the light of patient hemodynamic parameters. The likelihood of reperfusion events and major arrhythmias is to some extent lower than in STEMI patients, and short periods of procedure-related MI may be better tolerated.

On the other hand, there is no clear evidence that a strategy of immediate complete revascularization offers a clinical advantage over culprit-lesion revascularization only, in unselected patients with UA.[5,69] In addition, PCI may be associated with periprocedural MI due to obstruction of branch vessels or distal embolization of plaque material and microvascular injury, or both. These phenomena are more common in patients with non-ST elevation acute coronary syndromes than in those who are undergoing elective interventions,[17] therefore treatment of a coronary stenosis should be always motivated by a documentation or a very high likelihood of related myocardial ischemia. This offers a good rationale for early culprit lesion/artery intervention and subsequent ischemia re-evaluation. However, with modern techniques, an invasive physiological evaluation may help appropriate decision making based on the functional significance of the coronary stenosis detected at the angiogram.[70]

Once again, however, it should be noted that PCI may not treat the unstable plaques that cause the clinical syndrome, which may be non-flow limiting and multiple.[35,71] This aspect is now attracting much attention in the search for reliable diagnostic methods to identify and treat vulnerable plaques in the catheterization laboratory.[22]

In conclusion, since the definition UA/NSTEMI encompasses a heterogeneous spectrum of patients with different prognoses, it would be appropriate to stratify and to treat patients according to their different risk. Revascularization is not recommended unless the benefits are likely to outweigh the risks, and a decision about the revascularization strategy must be made on a case-by-case basis. Complete revascularization should probably be pursued immediately in UA/NSTEMI patients when they do not present very complex lesions that may expose them to excessive procedural times, X-ray and contrast volume exposition. From a clinical point of view, patients with diabetes mellitus or poor left ventricular function, patients with cardiogenic shock, patients with a large quantity of viable myocardium at risk, and patients in whom a clear identification of the culprit lesion is not possible from the coronary angiography, are most likely to benefit from such an approach.

CONCLUSIONS

Multivessel coronary disease is a common finding in patients with acute coronary syndromes, and it is independently associated with a worse clinical outcome. However, treatment and timing of non-culprit lesion percutaneous coronary intervention is a matter of controversy because there is a lack of conclusive clinical data about the safety and effectiveness of this procedure.

In STEMI patients, according to current guidelines, primary or rescue PCI should be limited to the culprit artery, unless the patient presents severe hemodynamic instability.[4] The introduction in clinical practice of stents first and drug-eluting stents afterwards, glycoprotein IIb/IIIa inhibitors, intra-aortic balloon pump, non-ionic contrast agents, and a general improvement of technologies and periprocedural medications may encourage an immediate complete revascularization strategy in more patients, although the safety and efficacy of this approach should be evaluated in dedicated trials.

In UA/NSTEMI patients, the decision about culprit versus non-culprit vessel intervention may be more liberal, and follows the general rules that apply for elective patients. A decision should be made on a patient-by-patient basis, taking into account risks and benefits of the revascularization procedure, albeit a complete revascularization may be cost-effective in most patients. In some patients, a staged procedure may be considered, with immediate balloon angioplasty and stenting of the culprit lesion, and subsequent reassessment of the need for treatment of other lesions. Patients without a clearly identifiable culprit lesion, and patients at higher risk of adverse events such as those with diabetes mellitus, poor left ventricular function, and a large amount of viable myocardium at risk should probably be treated more aggressively in the first instance, unless contraindications are identified (e.g. anticipated high volume of contrast medium in patients with significant chronic renal insufficiency).

REFERENCES

1. Braunwald E, Antman EM, Beasley JW et al. ACC/AHA 2002 guideline update for the management of patients with unstable angina and non-ST segment elevation myocardial infarction – summary article: a report of the American College of Cardiology/American Heart Association task force on practice guidelines (Committee on the Management of Patients With Unstable Angina). J Am Coll Cardiol 2002; 40: 1366–74.
2. Bertrand ME, Simoons ML, Fox KA et al. Management of acute coronary syndromes in patients presenting without persistent ST segment elevation. Eur Heart J 2002; 23: 1809–40.
3. Van de Werf F, Ardissino D, Betriu A et al. Management of acute myocardial infarction in patients presenting with ST segment elevation. The Task Force on the Management of Acute Myocardial Infarction of the European Society of Cardiology. Eur Heart J 2003; 24: 28–66.
4. Antman EM, Anbe DT, Armstrong PW et al. ACC/AHA guidelines for the management of patients with ST elevation myocardial infarction; a report of the American College of Cardiology/American Heart Association Task Force on Practice Guidelines (Committee to Revise the 1999 Guidelines for the Management of patients with acute myocardial infarction). J Am Coll Cardiol 2004; 44: E1–E211.

5. de Feyter PJ, Serruys PW, Arnold A et al. Coronary angioplasty of the unstable angina related vessel in patients with multivessel disease. Eur Heart J 1986; 7: 460–7.
6. Wohlgelernter D, Cleman M, Highman HA et al. Percutaneous transluminal coronary angioplasty of the 'culprit lesion' for management of unstable angina pectoris in patients with multivessel coronary artery disease. Am J Cardiol 1986; 58: 460–4.
7. Stone GW, Grines CL, Cox DA et al. Comparison of angioplasty with stenting, with or without abciximab, in acute myocardial infarction. N Engl J Med 2002; 346: 957–66.
8. Andersen HR, Nielsen TT, Rasmussen K et al. A comparison of coronary angioplasty with fibrinolytic therapy in acute myocardial infarction. N Engl J Med 2003; 349: 733–42.
9. Lemos PA, Saia F, Hofma SH et al. Short- and long-term clinical benefit of sirolimus-eluting stents compared to conventional bare stents for patients with acute myocardial infarction. J Am Coll Cardiol 2004; 43: 704–8.
10. Parodi G, Memisha G, Valenti R et al. Five year outcome after primary coronary intervention for acute ST elevation myocardial infarction: results from a single centre experience. Heart 2005; 91: 1541–4.
11. Kahn JK, O'Keefe HJ, Jr., Rutherford BD et al. Timing and mechanism of in-hospital and late death after primary coronary angioplasty during acute myocardial infarction. Am J Cardiol 1990; 66: 1045–8.
12. Muller DW, Topol EJ, Ellis SG et al. Multivessel coronary artery disease: a key predictor of short-term prognosis after reperfusion therapy for acute myocardial infarction. Thrombolysis and Angioplasty in Myocardial Infarction (TAMI) Study Group. Am Heart J 1991; 121: 1042–9.
13. Ottervanger JP, Van't Hof AW, Reiffers S et al. Long-term recovery of left ventricular function after primary angioplasty for acute myocardial infarction. Eur Heart J 2001; 22: 785–90.
14. Grines CL, Topol EJ, Califf RM et al. Prognostic implications and predictors of enhanced regional wall motion of the noninfarct zone after thrombolysis and angioplasty therapy of acute myocardial infarction. The TAMI Study Groups. Circulation 1989; 80: 245–53.
15. Effects of tissue plasminogen activator and a comparison of early invasive and conservative strategies in unstable angina and non-Q-wave myocardial infarction. Results of the TIMI IIIB Trial. Thrombolysis in Myocardial Ischemia. Circulation 1994; 89: 1545–56.
16. Invasive compared with non-invasive treatment in unstable coronary-artery disease: FRISC II prospective randomised multicentre study. FRagmin and Fast Revascularisation during InStability in Coronary artery disease Investigators. Lancet 1999; 354: 708–15.
17. de Feyter PJ, Suryapranata H, Serruys PW et al. Coronary angioplasty for unstable angina: immediate and late results in 200 consecutive patients with identification of risk factors for unfavorable early and late outcome. J Am Coll Cardiol 1988; 12: 324–33.
18. Marzocchi A, Ortolani P, Piovaccari G et al. Coronary stenting for unstable angina: predictors of 30-day and long-term clinical outcome. Coron Artery Dis 1999; 10: 81–8.
19. Garcia S, Canoniero M, Peter A et al. Correlation of TIMI risk score with angiographic severity and extent of coronary artery disease in patients with non-ST-elevation acute coronary syndromes. Am J Cardiol 2004; 93: 813–16.
20. Corpus RA, House JA, Marso SP et al. Multivessel percutaneous coronary intervention in patients with multivessel disease and acute myocardial infarction. Am Heart J 2004; 148: 493–500.
21. Kahn JK, Rutherford BD, McConahay DR et al. Results of primary angioplasty for acute myocardial infarction in patients with multivessel coronary artery disease. J Am Coll Cardiol 1990; 16: 1089–96.
22. Naghavi M, Libby P, Falk E et al. From vulnerable plaque to vulnerable patient: a call for new definitions and risk assessment strategies: Part I. Circulation 2003; 108: 1664–72.
23. Falk E. Plaque rupture with severe pre-existing stenosis precipitating coronary thrombosis. Characteristics of coronary atherosclerotic plaques underlying fatal occlusive thrombi. Br Heart J 1983; 50: 127–34.
24. Davies MJ, Thomas AC. Plaque fissuring—the cause of acute myocardial infarction, sudden ischaemic death, and crescendo angina. Br Heart J 1985; 53: 363–73.
25. Libby P. Molecular bases of the acute coronary syndromes. Circulation 1995; 91: 2844–50.

26. Lee RT, Schoen FJ, Loree HM et al. Circumferential stress and matrix metalloproteinase 1 in human coronary atherosclerosis. Implications for plaque rupture. Arterioscler Thromb Vasc Biol 1996; 16: 1070–3.
27. Dollery CM, McEwan JR, Henney AM. Matrix metalloproteinases and cardiovascular disease. Circ Res 1995; 77: 863–8.
28. Galis ZS, Sukhova GK, Lark MW et al. Increased expression of matrix metalloproteinases and matrix degrading activity in vulnerable regions of human atherosclerotic plaques. J Clin Invest 1994; 94: 2493–503.
29. Muller JE, Abela GS, Nesto RW et al. Triggers, acute risk factors and vulnerable plaques: the lexicon of a new frontier. J Am Coll Cardiol 1994; 23: 809–13.
30. Ambrose JA, Winters SL, Stern A et al. Angiographic morphology and the pathogenesis of unstable angina pectoris. J Am Coll Cardiol 1985; 5: 609–16.
31. Buffon A, Biasucci LM, Liuzzo G et al. Widespread coronary inflammation in unstable angina. N Engl J Med 2002; 347: 5–12.
32. Spagnoli LG, Bonanno E, Mauriello A et al. Multicentric inflammation in epicardial coronary arteries of patients dying of acute myocardial infarction. J Am Coll Cardiol 2002; 40: 1579–88.
33. Biasucci LM, Liuzzo G, Angiolillo DJ et al. Inflammation and acute coronary syndromes. Herz 2000; 25: 108–12.
34. Liuzzo G, Biasucci LM, Gallimore JR et al. The prognostic value of C-reactive protein and serum amyloid a protein in severe unstable angina. N Engl J Med 1994; 331: 417–24.
35. Goldstein JA, Demetriou D, Grines CL et al. Multiple complex coronary plaques in patients with acute myocardial infarction. N Engl J Med 2000; 343: 915–22.
36. Tanaka A, Shimada K, Sano T et al. Multiple plaque rupture and C-reactive protein in acute myocardial infarction. J Am Coll Cardiol 2005; 45: 1594–9.
37. Burke AP, Farb A, Malcom GT et al. Coronary risk factors and plaque morphology in men with coronary disease who died suddenly. N Engl J Med 1997; 336: 1276–82.
38. Rioufol G, Finet G, Ginon I et al. Multiple atherosclerotic plaque rupture in acute coronary syndrome: a three-vessel intravascular ultrasound study. Circulation 2002; 106: 804–8.
39. Schaar JA, Regar E, Mastik F et al. Incidence of high-strain patterns in human coronary arteries: assessment with three-dimensional intravascular palpography and correlation with clinical presentation. Circulation 2004; 109: 2716–19.
40. Asakura M, Ueda Y, Yamaguchi O et al. Extensive development of vulnerable plaques as a pan-coronary process in patients with myocardial infarction: an angioscopic study. J Am Coll Cardiol 2001; 37: 1284–8.
41. Ambrose JA, Tannenbaum MA, Alexopoulos D et al. Angiographic progression of coronary artery disease and the development of myocardial infarction. J Am Coll Cardiol 1988; 12: 56–62.
42. Hoye A, Lemos PA, Arampatzis CA et al. effectiveness of sirolimus-Eluting stent implantation for coronary narrowings < 50% in diameter. Am J Cardiol 2004; 94: 112–14.
43. Morice MC, Serruys PW, Sousa JE et al. A randomized comparison of a sirolimus-eluting stent with a standard stent for coronary revascularization. N Engl J Med 2002; 346: 1773–80.
44. Moses JW, Leon MB, Popma JJ et al. Sirolimus-eluting stents versus standard stents in patients with stenosis in a native coronary artery. N Engl J Med 2003; 349: 1315–23.
45. Schofer J, Schluter M, Gershlick AH et al. Sirolimus-eluting stents for treatment of patients with long atherosclerotic lesions in small coronary arteries: double-blind, randomised controlled trial (E-SIRIUS). Lancet 2003; 362: 1093–9.
46. Colombo A, Drzewiecki J, Banning A et al. Randomized study to assess the effectiveness of slow- and moderate-release polymer-based paclitaxel-eluting stents for coronary artery lesions. Circulation 2003; 108: 788–94.
47. Stone GW, Ellis SG, Cox DA et al. A polymer-based, paclitaxel-eluting stent in patients with coronary artery disease. N Engl J Med 2004; 350: 221–31.
48. Keeley EC, Boura JA, Grines CL. Primary angioplasty versus intravenous thrombolytic therapy for acute myocardial infarction: a quantitative review of 23 randomised trials. Lancet 2003; 361: 13–20.

49. Shihara M, Tsutsui H, Tsuchihashi M et al. In-hospital and one-year outcomes for patients undergoing percutaneous coronary intervention for acute myocardial infarction. Am J Cardiol 2002; 90: 932–6.
50. Kastrati A, Schomig A, Elezi S et al. Predictive factors of restenosis after coronary stent placement. J Am Coll Cardiol 1997; 30: 1428–36.
51. Orford JL, Lennon R, Melby S et al. Frequency and correlates of coronary stent thrombosis in the modern era: analysis of a single center registry. J Am Coll Cardiol 2002; 40: 1567–72.
52. Roe MT, Cura FA, Joski PS et al. Initial experience with multivessel percutaneous coronary intervention during mechanical reperfusion for acute myocardial infarction. Am J Cardiol 2001; 88: 170–3, A6.
53. Chen LY, Lennon RJ, Grantham JA et al. In-hospital and long-term outcomes of multivessel percutaneous coronary revascularization after acute myocardial infarction. Am J Cardiol 2005; 95: 349–54.
54. Di Mario C, Mara S, Flavio A et al. Single vs multivessel treatment during primary angioplasty: results of the multicentre randomised HEpacoat for cuLPrit or multivessel stenting for Acute Myocardial Infarction (HELP AMI) Study. Int J Cardiovasc Intervent 2004; 6: 128–33.
55. Kong JA, Chou ET, Minutello RM et al. Safety of single versus multi-vessel angioplasty for patients with acute myocardial infarction and multi-vessel coronary artery disease: report from the New York State Angioplasty Registry. Coron Artery Dis 2006; 17: 71–5.
56. Gibson CM, Ryan KA, Murphy SA et al. Impaired coronary blood flow in nonculprit arteries in the setting of acute myocardial infarction. The TIMI Study Group. Thrombolysis in myocardial infarction. J Am Coll Cardiol 1999; 34: 974–82.
57. Webb JG, Lowe AM, Sanborn TA et al. Percutaneous coronary intervention for cardiogenic shock in the SHOCK trial. J Am Coll Cardiol 2003; 42: 1380–6.
58. McCullough PA, Wolyn R, Rocher LL et al. Acute renal failure after coronary intervention: incidence, risk factors, and relationship to mortality. Am J Med 1997; 103: 368–75.
59. Rihal CS, Textor SC, Grill DE et al. Incidence and prognostic importance of acute renal failure after percutaneous coronary intervention. Circulation 2002; 105: 2259–64.
60. Mehran R, Aymong ED, Nikolsky E et al. A simple risk score for prediction of contrast-induced nephropathy after percutaneous coronary intervention: development and initial validation. J Am Coll Cardiol 2004; 44: 1393–9.
61. Marenzi G, Lauri G, Assanelli E et al. Contrast-induced nephropathy in patients undergoing primary angioplasty for acute myocardial infarction. J Am Coll Cardiol 2004; 44: 1780–5.
62. Hanratty CG, Koyama Y, Rasmussen HH et al. Exaggeration of nonculprit stenosis severity during acute myocardial infarction: implications for immediate multivessel revascularization. J Am Coll Cardiol 2002; 40: 911–16.
63. Fuster V, Stein B, Ambrose JA et al. Atherosclerotic plaque rupture and thrombosis. Evolving concepts. Circulation 1990; 82: II47–59.
64. Stewart DJ, Kubac G, Costello KB et al. Increased plasma endothelin-1 in the early hours of acute myocardial infarction. J Am Coll Cardiol 1991; 18: 38–43.
65. Reilly MP, Delanty N, Roy L et al. Increased formation of the isoprostanes IPF2alpha-I and 8-epi-prostaglandin F2alpha in acute coronary angioplasty: evidence for oxidant stress during coronary reperfusion in humans. Circulation 1997; 96: 3314–20.
66. Lemos PA, Lee C, Degertekin M et al. Early outcome after sirolimus-eluting stent implantation in patients with acute coronary syndromes. Insights from the Rapamycin-Eluting Stent Evaluated At Rotterdam Cardiology Hospital (RESEARCH) registry. J Am Coll Cardiol 2003; 41: 2093–9.
67. McLellan CS, Ghali WA, Labinaz M et al. Association between completeness of percutaneous coronary revascularization and postprocedure outcomes. Am Heart J 2005; 150: 800–6.
68. van den Brand MJ, Rensing BJ, Morel MA et al. The effect of completeness of revascularization on event-free survival at one year in the ARTS trial. J Am Coll Cardiol 2002; 39: 559–64.
69. Mariani G, De Servi S, Dellavalle A et al. Complete or incomplete percutaneous coronary revascularization in patients with unstable angina in stent era: are early and one-year results different? Catheter Cardiovasc Interv 2001; 54: 448–53.

70. Barbato E, De Bruyne B, MacCarthy P et al. Functional assessment of coronary atherosclerosis in the catheterization laboratory: the key role of fractional flow reserve. Ital Heart J 2005; 6: 549–56.
71. Little WC, Constantinescu M, Applegate RJ et al. Can coronary angiography predict the site of a subsequent myocardial infarction in patients with mild-to-moderate coronary artery disease? Circulation 1988; 78: 1157–66.

10

Patients requiring cardiac and non-cardiac surgical procedures following percutaneous coronary interventions

Gary E Lane and David R Holmes Jr

Non-cardiac surgery following percutaneous coronary intervention • Cardiac surgery following percutaneous coronary intervention • Future progress

Advances in percutaneous coronary intervention (PCI) technique and practice have enhanced procedural safety and patient outcomes. Much of this progress can be attributed to stent-based PCI techniques and pharmacological adjuncts. Yet, these important advances influence the dynamic of patient care beyond the revascularization benefits. In particular, mandatory combination antiplatelet therapy complicates the diagnostic or therapeutic management of comorbid conditions and, in an urgent setting, cardiac surgical procedures to correct complications of the PCI procedure.

NON-CARDIAC SURGERY FOLLOWING PERCUTANEOUS CORONARY INTERVENTION

Percutaneous coronary intervention and peri-operative cardiovascular morbidity

Patients with coronary artery disease are at risk for peri-operative myocardial infarction (MI) and death while undergoing non-cardiac surgical procedures. Ischemic complications also adversely affect long-term prognosis. Considerable effort is extended to identify patients in jeopardy by recognizing clinical risk factors (angina, diabetes, prior infarction, heart failure, renal insufficiency, advanced age), evaluating functional capacity, and determining surgical procedure risk.[1] This often results in non-invasive stress testing, with abnormal results leading to coronary angiography and potential revascularization.

The myriad of factors to consider and the paucity of clear decision-facilitating data available is illustrated by the diverse opinions rendered regarding the necessity of revascularization.[2] The ACC/AHA (American College of Cardiology/American Heart Association) guidelines state that it is 'almost never appropriate' to utilize revascularization procedures to reduce the risk of non-cardiac surgery unless otherwise indicated.[1] Clearly patients with extensive (multivessel/left main+/− left ventricular dysfunction) disease should undergo revascularization, not only to reduce their risk of non-cardiac surgery, but also to improve their long-term prognosis.

Guideline-driven risk assessment frequently documents coronary artery disease in the surgical population. However, contemporary information may constrain the use of revascularization to reduce operative risk. Beta-blocker therapy with bisprolol has been shown to considerably decrease the risk of cardiac death (3.4% vs. 17%, $P=0.02$) and non-fatal infarction (0% vs. 17%, $P<0.001$) in 173 patients undergoing vascular surgery with abnormal dobutamine stress echocardiography.[3] A recent trial randomized 510 stable patients with angiographically significant coronary disease to undergo revascularization (PCI=59%, coronary artery bypass graft (CABG)=41%) or medical therapy before major vascular surgery. Patients with significant left main disease or an ejection fraction <0.20 were excluded. Beta-blockers were used in 84% and 86% of both groups. There was no significant difference in the incidence of MI, hospital mortality, or survival over 2.7 years.[4]

Peri-operative medical management emphasizing beta-blockade may effectively mitigate risk for most patients with coronary disease. Nevertheless, there remains a group of patients with multiple clinical risk factors and extensive ischemia who are at high risk for peri-operative events despite beta-blockade, and who should be considered for revascularization.[5]

Percutaneous coronary angioplasty prior to non-cardiac surgery

Retrospective examination has indicated that patients who undergo successful bypass surgery have a reduced risk of peri-operative death and MI with subsequent non-cardiac surgical procedures. In particular, patients in the Coronary Artery Surgery Study (CASS) database with severe angina and multivessel disease requiring high-risk procedures derived a significant advantage with previous surgical revascularization.[1] Nevertheless, the cumulative risk of bypass surgery and an ensuing high-risk non-cardiac surgery must be considered.

Table 10.1 Coronary balloon angioplasty prior to non-cardiac surgery

Author	n	%VS	PTCA → NCS (days)	Peri-operative mortality (%)	Peri-operative MI (%)	Publication Year
Allen et al[6]	148	43	338 (4–1867)	2.7	0.7	1991
Huber et al[7]	50	52	9 (1–115)	1.9	5.6	1992
Elmore et al[8]	14	100	10	0	0	1993
Jones et al[9]	108	91	14.5 (0–41)	0.9	3.8	1993
Gottlieb et al[10]	194	100	11 (3–546)	0.5	0.5	1998
Posner et al[11]	686	0	365 (2–2402)	2.2	2.6	1999
Hassan et al[12]	251	11	750 (365–1380)	0.8	0.8	2001

MI, myocardial infarction; NCS, non-cardiac surgery; PTCA, percutaneous transluminal coronary angioplasty; VS vascular surgery.

Table 10.2   Coronary stenting (BMS) prior to non-cardiac surgery

Author	*n*	PCI → NCS (days)	Perioperative mortality (%)	Perioperative MI (%)	Major bleeding (%)	Publication year
Kaluza et al[13]	40	13 (1–39)	20	17.5	27.5	2000
Sharma et al[14]	47	(0–90)	17	13	17	2004
Wilson et al[15]	207	(1–60)	3	1	1	2003
Reddy et al[16]	16	(0–42)	25	37.5	19	2005

BMS, bare-metal stent; MI, myocardial infarction; NCS, non-cardiac surgery; PCI, percutaneous coronary intervention (stenting).

Several retrospective reports described the use of preoperative balloon angioplasty to attenuate the risk of non-cardiac surgery. Seven small studies (Table 10.1) reported low rates of peri-operative infarction and mortality at least comparable to the benefits seen in patients who had undergone prior bypass surgery.[6-12] Yet the lack of controls and diverse factors related to type of surgical procedures, timing of angioplasty and risk variability limit confidence regarding the benefit of pre-operative angioplasty. In the Bypass Angioplasty Revascularization Investigation (BARI) trial of patients with multivessel disease, a consistently low risk of peri-operative cardiac events was noted for both patients who underwent preoperative angioplasty or bypass surgery.[12] A retrospective cohort study by Posner et al did not demonstrate a reduction in the risk of peri-operative mortality or infarction although angina and congestive heart failure (CHF) were reduced in patients undergoing angioplasty.[11] No benefit was seen for patients undergoing angioplasty <90 days before non-cardiac surgery. The heterogeneity of these investigations contributes to the uncertainty regarding the timing of angioplasty. Non-cardiac surgery conducted within days or weeks of balloon angioplasty could expose the patient to an increased risk of an ischemic event due to a surgery-induced prothrombotic effects upon an acutely injured vessel. Likewise delay can negate gain if restenosis occurs before surgery.

Coronary stenting prior to non-cardiac surgery

The safety and durability of PCI procedures has been significantly enhanced by the widespread adoption of stents. High-pressure deployment and antiplatelet therapy including uniform thienopyridine therapy has minimized the risk of stent thrombosis. Adherence to these requirements is mandatory to avoid stent thrombosis with an associated mortality as high as 40–50%. However, the advance of stent-based PCI complicates and may increase the hazards of revascularization prior to non-cardiac surgery. This peril has been detailed in published series of non-cardiac surgery after PCI with bare-metal stents (BMS) (Table 10.2).

Kaluza et al reported a striking risk of catastrophic outcomes in 40 patients undergoing non-cardiac surgery <6 weeks after stent implantation.[13] All deaths (8/25, 32%) and infarctions (7/25, 28%) occurred in 25 patients operated on within a 2-week period after the stent procedure. Five patients underwent surgery the next day and four died. All of these complications were presumed to be due to stent thrombosis (angiographic documentation or infarction in the region supplied by stented artery). One or both antiplatelet drugs were 'typically' interrupted 1 or 2 days before surgery. Bleeding complications were also significant and highlighted by the deaths of three out of five patients who did not discontinue ticlopidine prior to surgery.

This sentinel report was followed by three other series. Sharma et al identified 47 patients operated on within 90 days of stent placement.[14] Thienopyridines were discontinued >4 pre-operative days in 7/27 patients operated within 3 weeks. Six of the seven patients died after surgery. In contrast, 1/20 patients continued on a thienopyridine through surgery died suddenly. In the group ($n=20$) operated on >3 weeks after PCI, there was one death and two infarctions. Peri-operative bleeding risk did not appear to be related to thienopyridine treatment. Wilson et al documented a lower incidence of major adverse events, but the period of risk appeared to persist for 6 weeks.[15] No events occurred in patients operated >6 weeks after stent placement. The report of Reddy et al also documented a risk extending to 6 weeks in 16 patients, with 38% sustaining infarction and a 25% mortality.[16] Of the patients with these events, 60% were receiving clopidogrel during surgery. All patients who developed major bleeding ($n=3$) were receiving clopidogrel. No patient ($n=40$) operated on >6 weeks after PCI experienced a major adverse event or bleeding.

Although these retrospective reports of heterogeneous groups and circumstances may limit conclusions, clearly there is a distinct early hazard to proceeding with non-cardiac surgery up to 6 weeks after BMS placement. This interval coincides with the risk period for stent thrombosis expected after BMS placement due to need for re-endothelialization and healing of the vascular surface. The surgical procedure promotes thrombosis by systemic effects including sympathetic activation, release of neuroendocrine hormones, inhibition of fibrinolysis, increase of plasma procoagulant factors, and induction of a hypercoagulable state.[15] This risk may be partially mitigated by continuation of antiplatelet therapy (including thienopyridines) in the peri-operative period. Nevertheless, a hazard remains even on antiplatelet therapy, and these drugs also increase the likelihood of hemorrhage.

The progress of drug-eluting stents

Drug-eluting stent (DES) technology has dramatically reduced restenosis and target vessel revascularization. In the US, >80% of stented patients receive a DES.[17] The effect of antiproliferative drugs delays re-endothelialization and prolongs the risk for stent thrombosis. The Food and Drug Administration (FDA)-approved recommendation for dual antiplatelet therapy is 3 months for the sirolimus-eluting stent, and 6 months for the paclitaxel-eluting stent.[18]

Currently there is controversy regarding the late safety profile of DES. Meta-analysis of randomized trials and registries that led to approval of these devices indicate that DES do not increase the risk of stent thrombosis (up 1 year) compared to BMS.[19,20] However a study of 2229 consecutive 'real-world' patients identified a significantly higher risk (1.3%) at 9 months.[21] Notably, thrombosis occurred in 29% of patients with premature discontinuation of dual antiplatelet therapy. Late (>30 days) DES stent thrombosis has recently been reported in case studies and small series. Late stent thrombosis occurred commonly in conjunction with non-cardiac surgery in (3/4), (3/4), (2/8) and (2/2) patients in four small series.[17,22-24] These events happened after discontinuing antiplatelet therapy (including aspirin) in the surgical patients, although events occurred an average of 382 (49–927) days after stent placement. Only one event (49 days) occurred within the recommended dual antiplatelet therapy interval. These reports challenge the current recommended treatment duration for antiplatelet therapy after DES, and further complicate the conduct of even temporally remote surgery for these patients.

Late stent thrombosis is a known significant complication of coronary brachytherapy. It has also been reported 33–270 days after BMS deployment.[25] These events after BMS placement may partially explain the benefit of prolonged dual antiplatelet therapy after PCI reported the PCI-CURE (Clopidogrel in Unstable Angina to prevent Recurrent Events) and CREDO (Clopidogrel for Reduction of Events During Observation) trials.[26,27]

Hemorrhagic risk of antiplatelet therapy

Withdrawal of antiplatelet therapy contributes to the peri-operative thrombotic events that can occur in stented patients undergoing non-cardiac surgery. These agents are discontinued due to concern regarding potential bleeding complications. Increased blood loss has been reported with pre-operative aspirin in general surgical, urological and gynecological procedures, However, in a series of patients undergoing emergency abdominal surgery there was no increased bleeding risk.[28] More extensive data are available for patients undergoing cardiac surgery, and pre-operative aspirin is associated with increased blood loss and need for early re-operation but without a deleterious effect on operative mortality.[28,29]

There is little information available regarding the utilization of thienopyridines and non-cardiac surgery. The series from Kaluza and colleagues identified five patients who continued ticlopidine and three out of five suffered bleeding complications and death after surgery which occurred within 3 days of stenting.[13] Among 18 patients on clopidogrel before surgery in the report of Reddy et al, three patients developed major bleeding.[16] In contrast, the two series reported by Wilson et al, and Sharma et al did not find any relationship between continuation of antiplatelet therapy and perioperative hemorrhage.[14,15] Nevertheless there are an increasing number of reports documenting increased blood loss and need for re-operation when clopidogrel is received within 5 days of coronary bypass surgery.[28,30]

Non-cardiac surgery following percutaneous coronary intervention: strategic approach

A plethora of issues must be considered when a patient with coronary artery disease requires non-cardiac surgery. Consultative assessment and selective non-invasive testing can exclude most patients from revascularization consideration. The effectiveness of medical management with beta-blockade must be considered as an effective deterrent for ischemic events in the relatively short peri-operative interval. Yet, patients with recent unstable symptoms, multiple clinical risk factors in combination with large areas of ischemia, or survival-limiting anatomy remain revascularization candidates.

With the requirements of contemporary PCI procedures, the interventionalist's task becomes even more complex. A comprehensive assessment of the patient's

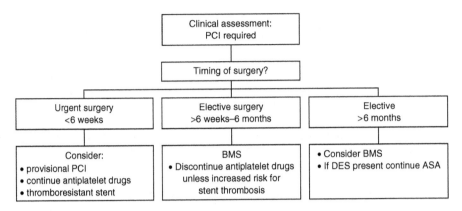

Figure 10.1　Strategy for management of patients requiring non-cardiac surgery following PCI. ASA, aspirin; BMS, bare-metal stent; DES, drug-eluting stent.

status must be incorporated into procedural planning. In presurgical patients, integrative management with an emphasis on the temporal aspects demands skilful communication before and during the intervention. Recommendations regarding the most appropriate approach are limited by the paucity and retrospective nature of the data available (Figure 10.1).

Clearly non-cardiac surgical procedures should be avoided if at all possible for at least 6 weeks after PCI. Patients who must undergo urgent surgery (< 4–6 weeks) may be considered for a provisional stenting approach to PCI, although this is probably feasible in only a minority of patients. Depending upon the surgical procedure it may be possible to continue dual antiplatelet therapy in the peri-operative period, accepting some increased risk of bleeding. However the systemic insult from the surgical procedure may still increase the risk for an ischemic event. A stent incorporating a thromboresistant surface (heparin-coated or phosphorylcholine) may be utilized in this situation to mitigate the risk of stent thrombosis. A large registry has demonstrated a reduction in stent thrombosis with the heparin-coated stent.[31] Furthermore in the HOPE (HEPACOTE and Antithrombotic Regimen of Asprin Alone) study, a low thrombosis rate was found with only aspirin after heparin-coated stent placement.[32]

If a patient requires surgery in the near-term (1–6 months) and can be delayed >6 weeks, then a BMS can be implanted and surgery can proceed with discontinuation of antiplatelet therapy. However, caution may be necessary for patients with conditions (longer stents, bifurcations, diabetes, renal failure) that increase the risk of stent thrombosis.

Utilization of a DES prior to non-cardiac surgery significantly complicates management. Certainly, DES placement should be strictly avoided if surgery is planned within 3–6 months. If a patient requires non-cardiac surgery before the end of the obligatory dual antiplatelet therapy period, if at all possible this therapy should continue in the peri-operative interval. If major hemorrhage occurs, platelet transfusion may be necessary. There is still uncertainty regarding patients with DES who undergo surgery after the period of essential antiplatelet therapy. Caution is advised in view of the reports of late stent thrombosis in conjunction with non-cardiac surgery. More investigation is needed to determine the risk of these events.

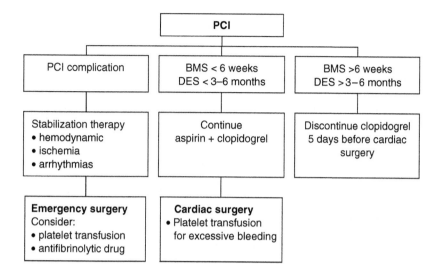

Figure 10.2   Strategy for management of patients requiring cardiac surgery following PCI. BMS, bare-mental stent; DES, drug-eluting stent.

Consideration should be given to continuing at least aspirin therapy in this setting, particularly with increased risk factors for stent thrombosis or the consequences of this event, such as diabetes, renal failure, bifurcations, lengthy stented segments, left main, or other critical anatomical locations.[21]

CARDIAC SURGERY FOLLOWING PERCUTANEOUS CORONARY INTERVENTION

Cardiac surgery may closely follow PCI procedures for acute failure or complications of PCI, recurrent restenosis after PCI, as definitive therapy for severe multivessel disease following 'culprit' PCI, and as part of a hybrid cardiac procedure. The subsequent cardiac surgical procedure is complicated by the PCI-mandated adjunctive antiplatelet therapy and, in an emergent situation, acute ischemia, and possible hemodynamic instability (Figure 10.2).

Emergency coronary bypass surgery after percutaneous coronary intervention

The incidence of emergency bypass surgery for failed PCI has markedly declined. This is exemplified in a report from the Mayo Clinic demonstrating a significant decrease from 2.9% in the 'pre-stent' era (1979–1994), to 0.3% in the 'current stent' era (2000–2003) ($P < 0.001$).[33] Nevertheless the mortality rate for emergency bypass surgery has remained similar (12% and 10%).

The interventional team must provide prompt multifaceted and comprehensive management for these patients. Early communication with the surgical team regarding an evolving complication is vital. Treatment of ischemia (medical and/or balloon counterpulsation) and the manifestations (pain, arrhythmias, and hemo-dynamic compromise) are paramount. Perforation therapy may require mani-pulation within the vessel (balloon inflation, covered stent), and pericardiocentesis. The interventional operator must assist in transport logistics and management of antithrombotic therapy. Platelet function is impaired from coronary bypass sur-gery due to the effects of the extracorporeal circuit, hypothermia, and mechanical filtering. The common utilization of antiplatelet therapy for PCI augments the platelet defect of bypass surgery increasing the risk of severe bleeding, the con-sequences of transfusion, and re-operation which is associated with an increased hospital mortality.[29]

Glycoprotein IIb/IIIa inhibitors significantly reduce MI, urgent revascularization, and death after PCI. Concern remains regarding the potential for increased peri-operative hemorrhage from these drugs. Although major trials testing abciximab for PCI did not indicate an increased risk for major hemorrhage, single-center series have shown a modest increase in hemorrhage when bypass surgery occurs within 12 h of administration.[28] The bleeding risk of abciximab can be mollified by platelet transfusion. The drug has a short plasma half-life and a high receptor affinity allow-ing transfused platelets to be effective. Platelet transfusion can be given after discon-tinuation of extracorporeal circulation and heparin neutralization for excessive bleeding. The small-molecule competitive IIb/IIIa inhibitors (eptifibatide, tirofiban) have low receptor affinity and the amount of unbound drug makes platelet transfu-sion ineffective. However the effects of these drugs subside within 4–6 h, and bleed-ing risk is not increased with emergency bypass surgery.[34]

Aspirin is an essential therapy for patients with acute ischemic syndromes and PCI. Early studies reported increased blood loss and re-operation when aspirin was continued within a few days of bypass surgery. More contemporary observations indicate there is no increase in hemorrhage, and pre-operative aspirin appears to decrease peri-operative infarction and mortality.[30]

Although at many institutions clopidogrel is withheld prior to angiography in patients with acute ischemic syndromes, ACC/AHA guidelines recommend that a loading dose of clopidogrel be given to patients prior to PCI.[18] Early observa-tional studies identified increased bleeding and a resultant 5–10× higher risk for re-operation when clopidogrel is administered within 5–7 days of bypass surgery. Recent reports are more mixed regarding the bleeding risk. Overall, in the CURE trial predominantly moderate rather than major or life-threatening bleeding was seen in patients who received dual antiplatelet therapy ≤5 days prior to bypass surgery.[30]

Platelet transfusion can be utilized in patients exhibiting hemorrhage after heparin neutralization. Antifibrinolytic therapy with the serine proteinase inhibitor, aprotonin has been shown to decrease postoperative bleeding and transfusion requirements in patients receiving aspirin and clopidogrel.[35] Although meta-analysis of randomized trials of aprotonin and bypass surgery reported no prothrombotic hazard,[36] a recently published observational study ($n=4374$) documented a 200% increased risk of renal failure, 55% increased risk of MI and a 181% increased risk of stroke or encephalopathy.[37] In the same analysis, the antifibrinolytic agents aminocaproic acid and transexamic acid were not associated with increased adverse events compared with no agent. Data are not available regarding the use of these agents after recent stent placement.

Non-urgent or elective coronary bypass surgery

Current ACC/AHA guidelines recommend withholding clopidogrel for 5 days prior to bypass surgery if 'clinical circumstances permit'.[29] Certainly antiplatelet therapy should not be prematurely discontinued before the recommended treatment interval after stent placement. After this interval it is reasonable to discontinue clopidogrel in stable patients, although it seems prudent to continue aspirin in patients at higher risk for stent thrombosis or with a DES.

Surgical bypass (minimally invasive) usually precedes PCI in hybrid coronary revascularization However, initial PCI or same-day procedures have been conducted, and PCI followed by valve surgery has been reported. Antiplatelet therapy should be continued after an initial PCI procedure despite the bleeding risk.

FUTURE PROGRESS

The dynamic interaction of surgery and PCI will continue to evolve. Investigation should address the management (platelet transfusions and antifibrinolytic agents) of potential hemorrhage in non-cardiac surgery. More information is especially needed regarding the risk of DES stent thrombosis and surgery. Stents combining both antiproliferative and thromboresistant drug coatings will have the potential to minimize the risk of subsequent surgical procedures.

REFERENCES

1. Eagle KA, Berger PB, Calkins H et al. ACC/AHA guideline update for perioperative cardiovascular evaluation for noncardiac surgery – executive summary a report of the American College of Cardiology/American Heart Association Task Force on Practice Guidelines (Committee to Update the 1996 Guidelines on Perioperative Cardiovascular Evaluation for Noncardiac Surgery). Circulation 2002; 105: 1257–67.
2. Pierpont GL, Moritz TE, Goldman S et al. Disparate opinions regarding indications for coronary artery revascularization before elective vascular surgery. Am J Cardiol 2004; 94: 1124–8.
3. Poldermans D, Boersma E, Bax JJ et al. The effect of bisoprolol on perioperative mortality and myocardial infarction in high-risk patients undergoing vascular surgery. Dutch Echocardiographic Cardiac Risk Evaluation Applying Stress Echocardiography Study Group. N Engl J Med 1999; 341: 1789–94.
4. McFalls EO, Ward HB, Moritz TE et al. Coronary-artery revascularization before elective major vascular surgery. N Engl J Med 2004; 351: 2795–804.
5. Boersma E, Poldermans D, Bax JJ et al. Predictors of cardiac events after major vascular surgery: Role of clinical characteristics, dobutamine echocardiography, and beta-blocker therapy. JAMA 2001; 285: 1865–73.
6. Allen JR, Helling TS, Hartzler GO. Operative procedures not involving the heart after percutaneous transluminal coronary angioplasty. Surg Gynecol Obstet 1991; 173: 285–8.
7. Huber KC, Evans MA, Bresnahan JF et al. Outcome of noncardiac operations in patients with severe coronary artery disease successfully treated preoperatively with coronary angioplasty. Mayo Clin Proc 1992; 67: 15–21.
8. Elmore JR, Hallett JW, Jr., Gibbons RJ et al. Myocardial revascularization before abdominal aortic aneurysmorrhaphy: effect of coronary angioplasty. Mayo Clin Proc 1993; 68: 637–41.
9. Jones SE, Raymond RE, Simpfendorfer CC et al. Cardiac outcome of major noncardiac surgery in patients undergoing preoperative coronary angioplasty. J Invasive Cardiol 1993; 5: 212–18.

10. Gottlieb A, Banoub M, Sprung J et al. Perioperative cardiovascular morbidity in patients with coronary artery disease undergoing vascular surgery after percutaneous transluminal coronary angioplasty. J Cardiothorac Vasc Anesth 1998; 12: 501–6.
11. Posner KL, Van Norman GA, Chan V. Adverse cardiac outcomes after noncardiac surgery in patients with prior percutaneous transluminal coronary angioplasty. Anesth Analg 1999; 89: 553–60.
12. Hassan SA, Hlatky MA, Boothroyd DB et al. Outcomes of noncardiac surgery after coronary bypass surgery or coronary angioplasty in the Bypass Angioplasty Revascularization Investigation (BARI). Am J Med 2001; 110: 260–6.
13. Kaluza GL, Joseph J, Lee JR et al. Catastrophic outcomes of noncardiac surgery soon after coronary stenting. J Am Coll Cardiol 2000; 35: 1288–94.
14. Sharma AK, Ajani AE, Hamwi SM et al. Major noncardiac surgery following coronary stenting: when is it safe to operate? Catheter Cardiovasc Interv 2004; 63: 141–5.
15. Wilson SH, Fasseas P, Orford JL et al. Clinical outcome of patients undergoing non-cardiac surgery in the two months following coronary stenting. J Am Coll Cardiol 2003; 42: 234–40.
16. Reddy PR, Vaitkus PT. Risks of noncardiac surgery after coronary stenting. Am J Cardiol 2005; 95: 755–7.
17. Ong AT, McFadden EP, Regar E et al. Late angiographic stent thrombosis (LAST) events with drug-eluting stents. J Am Coll Cardiol 2005; 45: 2088–92.
18. Smith SC Jr, Feldman TE, Hirshfeld JW Jr et al. ACC/AHA/SCAI 2005 Guideline Update for Percutaneous Coronary Intervention – summary article: a report of the American College of Cardiology/American Heart Association Task Force on Practice Guidelines (ACC/AHA/SCAI Writing Committee to Update the 2001 Guidelines for Percutaneous Coronary Intervention). Circulation 2006; 113: 156–75.
19. Bavry AA, Kumbhani DJ, Helton TJ et al. What is the risk of stent thrombosis associated with the use of paclitaxel-eluting stents for percutaneous coronary intervention?: a meta-analysis. J Am Coll Cardiol 2005; 45: 941–6.
20. Bavry AA, Kumbhani DJ, Helton TJ et al. Risk of thrombosis with the use of sirolimus-eluting stents for percutaneous coronary intervention (from registry and clinical trial data). Am J Cardiol 2005; 95: 1469–72.
21. Iakovou I, Schmidt T, Bonizzoni E et al. Incidence, predictors, and outcome of thrombosis after successful implantation of drug-eluting stents. JAMA 2005; 293: 2126–30.
22. Nasser M, Kapeliovich M, Markiewicz W. Late thrombosis of sirolimus-eluting stents following noncardiac surgery. Catheter Cardiovasc Interv 2005; 65: 516–19.
23. McFadden EP, Stabile E, Regar E et al. Late thrombosis in drug-eluting coronary stents after discontinuation of antiplatelet therapy. Lancet 2004; 364: 1519–21.
24. Rodriguez AE, Mieres J, Fernandez-Pereira C et al. Coronary stent thrombosis in the current drug-eluting stent era: insights from the ERACI III trial. J Am Coll Cardiol 2006; 47: 205–7.
25. Casserly IP, Goldstein JA, Lasala JM. Late stent thrombosis in the nonbrachytherapy population: a real phenomenon? Catheter Cardiovasc Interv 2003; 59: 504–8.
26. Mehta SR, Yusuf S, Peters RJ et al. Effects of pretreatment with clopidogrel and aspirin followed by long-term therapy in patients undergoing percutaneous coronary intervention: the PCI-CURE study. Lancet 2001; 358: 527–33.
27. Steinhubl SR, Berger PB, Mann JT, 3rd et al. Early and sustained dual oral antiplatelet therapy following percutaneous coronary intervention: a randomized controlled trial. JAMA 2002; 288: 2411–20.
28. Merritt JC, Bhatt DL. The efficacy and safety of perioperative antiplatelet therapy. J Thromb Thrombolysis 2004; 17: 21–7.
29. Eagle KA, Guyton RA, Davidoff R et al. ACC/AHA 2004 guideline update for coronary artery bypass graft surgery: summary article: a report of the American College of Cardiology/American Heart Association Task Force on Practice Guidelines (Committee to Update the 1999 Guidelines for Coronary Artery Bypass Graft Surgery). Circulation 2004; 110: 1168–76.
30. Cannon CP, Mehta SR, Aranki SF. Balancing the benefit and risk of oral antiplatelet agents in coronary artery bypass surgery. Ann Thorac Surg 2005; 80: 768–79.

31. Gupta V, Aravamuthan BR, Baskerville S et al. Reduction of subacute stent thrombosis (SAT) using heparin-coated stents in a large-scale, real world registry. J Invasive Cardiol 2004; 16: 304–10.
32. Mehran R, Aymong ED, Ashby DT et al. Safety of an aspirin-alone regimen after intracoronary stenting with a heparin-coated stent: final results of the HOPE (HEPACOAT and an Antithrombotic Regimen of Aspirin Alone) study. Circulation 2003; 108: 1078–83.
33. Yang EH, Gumina RJ, Lennon RJ et al. Emergency coronary artery bypass surgery for percutaneous coronary interventions: changes in the incidence, clinical characteristics, and indications from 1979 to 2003. J Am Coll Cardiol 2005; 46: 2004–9.
34. Cheng DK, Jackevicius CA, Seidelin P et al. Safety of glycoprotein IIb/IIIa inhibitors in urgent or emergency coronary artery bypass graft surgery. Can J Cardiol 2004; 20: 223–8.
35. van der Linden J, Lindvall G, Sartipy U. Aprotinin decreases postoperative bleeding and number of transfusions in patients on clopidogrel undergoing coronary artery bypass graft surgery: a double-blind, placebo-controlled, randomized clinical trial. Circulation 2005; 112: 1276–80.
36. Sedrakyan A, Treasure T, Elefteriades JA. Effect of aprotinin on clinical outcomes in coronary artery bypass graft surgery: a systematic review and meta-analysis of randomized clinical trials. J Thorac Cardiovasc Surg 2004; 128: 442–8.
37. Mangano DT, Tudor IC, Dietzel C. The risk associated with aprotinin in cardiac surgery. N Engl J Med 2006; 354: 353–65.

11

Invasive treatment (percutaneous coronary intervention) of patients at high surgical risk

Douglass A Morrison

Key issues • Which patients are most likely to benefit from coronary artery bypass grafts? • Which patients are most likely to die or suffer major morbidity from coronary artery bypass graft? • Specific subsets that could perhaps be excluded from the traditional anatomical approach: acute myocardial infarction and post-coronary artery bypass graft • Which patients are most likely to benefit from percutaneous coronary intervention? • Coronary anatomical features • The revascularization paradox: from anatomical to clinical components of risk • Patients likely to benefit from revascularization (medically refractory myocardial ischemia) are increasingly 'high risk' • Summary

KEY ISSUES

- Traditionally, the choice between coronary artery bypass graft (CABG) surgery and medical therapy has been made largely based upon coronary artery anatomy. Based upon < 5000 randomly allocated patients from three trials of stable angina and two trials of unstable patients, patients with left main disease and three-vessel disease (especially with mild/moderate left ventricular systolic dysfunction) have been largely directed to CABG.
- Because of compelling registry data regarding operative mortality, patients with acute myocardial infarction (MI) were directed to a period of medical stabilization (7–30 days) prior to CABG.
- Similarly, because of high-risk of operative mortality, the anatomical dictates for CABG have been relaxed for patients with one or more prior CABG, especially if they had one or more patent grafts from their first operation.
- Because patients with left main or three-vessel disease also have higher short-term procedural mortality (as well as greater long-term gain), they are specific examples of *the revascularization paradox: patients at highest risk of adverse outcome, often have the most to gain from revascularization.*
- Over the past two decades, the best randomized trial data supporting the application of percutaneous coronary intervention (PCI) rather than medical therapy has come from trials of patients with ST-elevation MI (STEMI) and unstable angina/non-STEMI. These trials support the use of PCI emergently or urgently to patients who are *high risk based upon clinical instability, rather than based upon coronary anatomy.*
- Bare metal stents (BMS) and adjunctive drugs, such as glycoprotein IIb/IIIa inhibitors and thienopyridines, have been associated with greatly reduced rates of acute complication with PCI, and with reduced emergency CABG and need for surgical standby.

- Both BMS and drug-eluting stents (DES) have also allowed for application of PCI to far broader anatomical and clinical spectra, while also being associated with improved long-term outcomes.
- As medical therapy has also improved, and the randomized trial data supporting the application of medical therapy to stable patients have accumulated, *'medically refractory ischemia'* has become an even more important criteria for considering CABG or PCI.
- The synthesis of these lines of reasoning requires a more thorough individual risk versus benefit assessment than the traditional, 'left main and three-vessel disease patients go to CABG; one- or two-vessel disease patients go to PCI'.
- Medically refractory ischemia remains the best reason to consider revascularization.
- Acute myocardial infarction, hemodynamic instability, and certain comorbidities (such as pulmonary, cerebrovascular, and hepatic) argue for palliative PCI, whenever technically feasible.

WHICH PATIENTS ARE MOST LIKELY TO DERIVE BENEFIT FROM CORONARY ARTERY BYPASS GRAFT?

Patients with triple vessel disease and left main disease, as well as patients with with ischemic left ventricular (LV) dysfunction were found to benefit from the surgical revascularization relative to medical therapy. Coronary bypass surgery improves long-term survival in a broad spectrum of patients at moderate to high risk with medical therapy, and such benefit appears to be greatest among those at highest risk with medical therapy. Clinical and angiographic markers of risk, including severity of coronary artery disease, LV dysfunction, and myocardial ischemia, can identify patients in various risk strata.

The 2004 ACC/AHA Guideline Update for CABG lists three major trials (Veterans Affairs Cooperative, European Cooperative, and Coronary Artery Surgery Study; all from the 1960–1970s period), and four additional small trials in its summary of randomized trial evidence for CABG versus medical therapy.[1] Table 8 in that document summarizes 1324 patients allocated to CABG, and 1325 allocated to medical therapy. Despite an extensive list of limitations (Table 7 in the guideline update[1] and Table 11.1 of this chapter) which include patient selection, surgical limitations, and limitations of medical therapy relative to current standards, these are the evidence upon which primary anatomical recommendations are derived. The updated guideline gives a Class I recommendation (should; is recommended; is indicated; is beneficial) based upon Class A (data derived from multiple randomized trials and/or meta-analyses) for patients with:

- significant left main coronary artery stenosis
- left main equivalent stenosis (>70% left anterior descending [LAD] and circumflex), three-vessel disease,

with any of the following clinical features:

- asymptomatic or mild angina
- stable angina
- unstable angina/non-ST segment elevation MI (NSTEMI)
- life-threatening ventricular arrhythmias
- poor LV function.

Table 11.1   Limitations of the medical therapy versus CABG 'evidence base'

Patient selection

All of the following groups were *excluded*:
- age >65 years
- women (except for Coronary Artery Surgery Study [CASS])
- LVEF <0.40
- myocardial infarction <30 days
- hemodynamically unstable
- medically refractory ischemia
- unstable ischemia (exceptions are VA Cooperative unstable angina, and National Institute of Health (NIH) unstable angina trials)
- prior CABG or valve.

Medical therapy limitations compared with current medical therapy
- Aspirin not given routinely or early pre-operatively
- Statins not available
- Beta-blockers not routine
- Angiotensin-converting enzyme inhibition and/or angiotensin receptor blockers not available

Surgical therapy limitations compared with current surgical therapy
- Arterial conduits rarely used (CASS 14%)
- Cardioprotection has evolved, but remains heterogeneous
- Less-invasive options not employed

Derived from the ACC/AHA CABG Guideline Update Table 7,[1] and the original trials from which that table was derived.

Several additional points of recommendation from the updated guideline deserve emphasis:

- In all of the above recommendations, there are no caveats regarding symptoms, ischemia, or adequacy of medical therapy. It is simply assumed, based upon the evidence base described (limitations notwithstanding) that in these anatomical subsets (left main, left main equivalent, and three-vessel disease), CABG prolongs life regardless of symptoms, ischemia and adequacy of medical therapy.
- Symptoms, ischemia and adequacy of medical therapy are mentioned regarding CABG for patients with one- or two-vessel disease, who have stable or unstable angina.

WHICH PATIENTS ARE MOST LIKELY TO DIE OR SUFFER MAJOR MORBIDITY FROM CORONARY ARTERY BYPASS GRAFT?

In summary, early mortality after CABG is associated particularly with *advanced age, poor LV function, and the urgency of operation.*

ACC/AHA 2004 Guideline Update for
Coronary Artery Bypass Graft Surgery[1]

Based upon a review of seven series of CABG, which included over 172 000 patients, who were operated on between 1986 and 1994, seven core variables which predicted surgical 30-day mortality were summarized in the updated guideline.[1] The variables were:

- urgency of operation
- age
- prior heart surgery
- gender
- left ventricular ejection fraction (LVEF)
- per cent stenosis of left main coronary
- number of major coronary arteries with >70% stenosis.

Although not as strongly predictive, 13 additional variables added to the strength of the predictive model. Included among these 13 were a number of measures of comorbidity, including diabetes, renal disease, peripheral vascular disease, and cerebrovascular disease. Although most of the core variables apply to the 'revascularization paradox', whereby they are associated with both increased likelihood of benefit and increased likelihood of risk, comorbidities are primarily associated with increased risk.

The CABG guideline emphasizes three specific morbidities associated with CABG: cerebral adverse outcomes, mediastinitis, and renal failure. There are two adverse cerebral outcomes, stroke and diffuse encephalopathy, which are both seen in upwards of 3% of CABG cases. Stroke or diffuse encephalopathy is unusual after PCI. Older age and hypertension are risk factors for higher incidence of either stroke or encephalopathy. Additional risk factors for stroke after CABG include:

- proximal aortic atherosclerosis
- prior neurological disease
- use of intra-aortic balloon pump (IABP)
- diabetes
- unstable angina.

Additional risk factors for CABG-associated encephalopathy include:

- alcohol consumption
- atrial fibrillation
- hypertension
- prior CABG
- peripheral vascular disease
- congestive heart failure (CHF).

Deep sternal wound infection, and/or mediastinitis is said to occur in 1–4% of cases and be associated with as high as 25% mortality. Risk factors for mediastinitis include:

- obesity
- diabetes
- use of bilateral internal mammary arteries (IMA).

The surgical guideline reports that postoperative renal failure occurs in ~7.7% of first-time CABG cases. Among CABG patients without renal failure, 30-day mortality was 0.9%, as opposed to 19% with renal insufficiency who did not require hemodialysis, and 63% among CABG patients who required postoperative dialysis. Risk factors for CABG-associated renal failure included:

- advanced age
- moderate to severe CHF
- prior CABG
- diabetes
- pre-existing renal disease.

For the most part, these risk factors for adverse outcome were also among the exclusions from the medical therapy versus CABG trials, which have been used to suggest survival benefit, among various CAD anatomical subsets. Accordingly, these clinical characteristics can be used to identify subsets that are at higher risk with CABG, *and may have less to gain from CABG. Medically refractory myocardial ischemia in patients with one or more of these characteristics may be reasons to thoroughly consider the risk versus benefits of PCI.*

SPECIFIC SUBSETS WHICH PERHAPS SHOULD BE EXCLUDED FROM THE TRADITIONAL ANATOMICAL APPROACH: ACUTE MYOCARDIAL INFARCTION AND POST-CORONARY ARTERY BYPASS GRAFT (TABLE 11.3)

Within the updated CABG guidelines, there is a major section of caveats regarding surgical approach for patients with ST-elevation MI;[1] this section emphasizes features such as failed angioplasty; or recurrent ischemia; or mechanical defects, such as ventricular septal rupture; or cardiogenic shock. There is additional reference in this section regarding the best timing for surgery after MI, and Table 19 from the updated guideline, based upon a retrospective review of 2296 patients suggests higher operative mortality, stroke rates, peri-procedural MI rates, and atrial fibrillation rates among patients who underwent CABG early after an MI. This section acknowledges that the widespread use of fibrinolytic therapy and more frequent primary PCI have both largely superseded early application of bypass surgery.[1] In point of fact, although none of the >23 trials comparing PCI versus contemporary medical therapy for STEMI specifically excluded the possibility of CABG in selected patients, neither did any randomly allocate any subset between CABG and PCI.

Given the unequivocal demonstration that primary angioplasty is clinically superior to best medical therapy for acute STEMI, and that time to reperfusion is a critical component of outcome, door-to-balloon times have been measured as quality indicators for the care of patients with STEMI. Time to reperfusion is an additional factor (besides the high risk associated with general anesthesia and heart–lung bypass during acute MI) which has been used to explain why in most centers >90% of STEMI revascularization is conducted by PCI. *The majority of patients in all contemporary STEMI PCI versus medicine trials were also revascularized by PCI.*

Bonchek et al, in the most recent American College of Cardiology Self Assessment Program (ACCSAP 6) summarize this issue as follows:

The role of surgery in AMI (acute myocardial infarction) without mechanical complications has been diminished by the increasing success of PCI . . .

Every effort should be made to stabilize the patients with an IABP and pharmaco-logical measures for a minimum of 48 hours before proceeding with CABG. [Ideally we prefer to wait one week after a complicated MI if ischemia can be relieved].

The specific subset with prior CABG is dealt with differently. First, 'disabling angina despite non-surgical therapy' is considered class I. The same anatomical categories (left main, left main equivalent, and three-vessel disease) are again invoked in patients whose grafts have all occluded. Since the Veterans Affairs Cooperative Study #385, the Angina With Extremely Serious Operative Mortality Evaluation (AWESOME) is the only CABG trial to have included patients with prior CABG (with or without patent grafts), and it demonstrated comparable survival and angina relief with PCI, PCI is a proven less-invasive and less-morbid alternative for post-CABG patients.[2-4]

WHICH PATIENTS ARE THE MOST LIKELY TO BENEFIT FROM PCI?

In reviewing the 2005 ACC/AHA/SCA&I PCI Guideline update,[5] it is clear that the evidence base comparing medical therapy with PCI, *among stable patients,* is even more limited than the previously cited medical therapy versus CABG data. Table 12 from that guideline (Table 11.2 in this chapter) summarizes the data that are available.

Table 11.2 Limitations of the medical therapy versus PCI among stable patients' 'evidence base'

Patient selection

All of the following groups were *excluded*:
- acute coronary syndromes
- three-vessel disease
- low LVEF
- prior CABG.

Limitations of medical therapy compared with contemporary therapy

- Statins routine
- Beta-blockers not routine
- Angiotensin-converting enzyme inhibitors or angiotensin receptor blockade not routine
- Dual antiplatelet therapy

Limitations of PCI compared to contemporary therapy

- No stents
- No drug-eluting stents
- No glycoprotein IIb/IIIa inhibitors

Derived from the ACC/AHA CABG Guideline Update Table 12,[1] and the original trials from which that table was derived.

The very best evidence for the benefit of PCI over medical therapy, on clinical outcomes is seen in the STEMI and NSTEMI literatures (Table 19 and Figure 5 in the 2005 PCI Guideline Update[5]). These patients are at higher risk of death or MI with PCI than are stable patients, but *MI is definitely reduced and survival enhanced with PCI rather than medical therapy, among post-MI patients.* There is no evidence that PCI is associated with improved survival compared to medical therapy for stable angina patients.

CORONARY ANATOMICAL FEATURES

Early reports demonstrated that balloon angioplasty could reduce the severity of coronary stenosis and diminish or eliminate objective and subjective manifestations of ischemia. Although angioplasty was clearly feasible and effective, the scope of coronary disease to be treated was quite narrow ... With experience and time, however the cognitive and technical aspects as much as the equipment used to perform angioplasty became more refined ... Observational reports of large numbers of patients confirmed that angioplasty could be applied to broad groups of coronary patients with higher rates of success and lower rates of complications than seen in earlier experiences ... More than 1 000 000 PCI procedures are performed yearly in the United States and it has been estimated that nearly 2 000 000 procedures are performed annually worldwide.

ACC/AHA/SCA&I 2005 Guideline Update for
Percutaneous Coronary Intervention[5]

As documented in other chapters in this text, advances in stent and pharmacological technology have virtually obviated the need for surgical backup for PCI. The application of BMS and, more recently, DES have led to improved short-term and long-term clinical outcomes of many patients with one or more of the following anatomical features, which significantly reduced the application of balloon angioplasty:

- diffuse disease/long lesions (>20 mm)
- small caliber (<2.5 mm)
- ostial lesions
- bifurcation lesions
- chronic total occlusions
- saphenous vein graft lesions.

Additionally, glycoprotein IIb/IIIa inhibitors, thienopyridines, and direct thrombin inhibitors have improved the clinical outcomes of the patients with high thrombus burdens, such as:

- STEMI
- NSTEMI
- Saphenous vein graft lesion.

THE REVASCULARIZATION PARADOX: FROM ANATOMICAL TO CLINICAL COMPONENTS OF RISK

Conceptually, the notion that patients with a higher short-term risk may have a better long-term outcome with revascularization, may appear similar, when one considers the 1970s CABG literature and the 1990s to 2000s PCI literature. However, there is an important distinction. In the 1960s and 1970s, risk to the patient with CAD was thought of primarily in terms of *fixed coronary anatomic narrowings*. In the 1990s and 2000s CAD risk is seen far more as a function of acute plaque rupture and/or erosion with either *hemodynamic, and/or ischemic, and/or arrhythmic instability*.

Table 11.3 Evidence base comparing medical therapy versus PCI among patient with unstable angina/NSTEMI (5 trials with 8880 randomly allocated patients) or STEMI (23 trials with 7739 randomly allocated patients).

Patient selection

All of the following groups were *included*:
- any age
- women
- within hours of acute MI
- STEMI, non-STEMI
- low LVEF
- prior CABG
- Left main vessel
- three-vessel
- two-vessel
- one-vessel.

Medical therapy

Any or all were *included*:
- aspirin
- statins
- beta-blockers
- dual antiplatelet therapy with stents.

PCI therapy

Any or all were *included*:
- bare-metal stents
- dual antiplatelet therapy
- glycoprotein IIb/IIIa inhibitors.

Based upon Table 19 and Figure 5 in the 2005 ACC/AHA CABG Guideline Update,[1] and the trials from which they were derived.

This conceptual shift from anatomy to pathophysiology leads to several changes in approach:

- optimal medical therapy, to reduce myocardial oxygen demand and stabilize plaque, begun immediately, for all CAD patients
- emergency revascularization, primarily by PCI/stenting of STEMI and NSTEMI patients with ongoing ischemia and hemodynamic and/or rhythm compromise
- the decision to proceed to diagnostic angiography in stable patients being more appropriately influenced by patient symptoms, ischemia, and medical refractoriness
- the choice between CABG and PCI for stable patients being made on an individual basis, using a 'team approach'
- including in the individual decision-making process appropriate concern for major comorbidity.

PATIENTS LIKELY TO BENEFIT FROM REVASCULARIZATION (MEDICALLY REFRACTORY MYOCARDIAL ISCHEMIA) ARE INCREASINGLY 'HIGH RISK'

A number of studies have documented that high-risk features are often used to avoid catheterization and revascularization. Given the following factors, it is a certainty that the general level of risk adverse outcomes among patients with clinical indication for revascularization by either CABG or PCI will increase over the next decade:

- aging of the 'baby boom' population
- obesity epidemic
- diabetes epidemic
- general reduction in adult activity levels
- smoking prevalence
- prevalence of hypertension
- prevalence of hyperlipidemia
- survival of acute MI coupled with no decline in MI incidence
- survival of congestive heart failure coupled with increased incidence of CHF
- prevalence of chronic obstructive pulmonary disease (COPD)
- prevalence of peripheral vascular disease
- prevalence of renal failure.

SUMMARY

Most of the randomized trial data supporting the application of CABG over medical therapy demonstrated clinical benefit among 'high-risk' subsets, defined in terms of static coronary anatomy (three-vessel, and left main fixed coronary artery narrowings), and moderate left ventricular systolic dysfunction (left ventricular ejection fractions >0.35 but <0.55). Initially, PCI was applied to patients with rather simple anatomy and stable low-risk features; the randomized trial data supporting this application over medical therapy were even more limited than the trials supporting CABG. Medical therapy has advanced and concordant results from large trials support the increasing application of at least five separate drug categories to coronary artery disease patients for hard clinical outcomes.

The demonstration that most acute coronary syndromes result from dynamic vascular biology, such as plaque rupture and/or erosion has provided theoretical support for major changes in the clinical care of patients with STEMI and NSTEMI. Additionally, the randomized trial data comparing PCI with contemporary medical therapy in these two patient subsets demonstrates hard clinical advantage for PCI. Time to reperfusion, current trial results, and previous registry studies of CABG mortality and morbidity all support the use of PCI rather than CABG for most acute coronary syndrome emergencies.

Comorbidity, particularly cerebrovascular, pulmonary, hepatic, and renal, are all reasons to consider the substantially lower morbidity of PCI relative to CABG. Patients with advanced comorbidity, like patients with hemodynamic and ischemic instability, often shift the risk/benefit comparison of CABG with PCI, toward PCI.

Stable patients with multiple high-grade narrowing, in multiple vessels, or in anatomical configurations which are particularly hard to effectively treat with PCI, continue to benefit from CABG. Acute coronary syndromes, hemodynamic instability, and major comorbidity all constitute high-risk clinical characteristics which foster the consideration of PCI as the revascularization method of first choice.

In summary, an appropriate approach for the decision-making of high-risk patients should follow a careful evaluation of clinical and anatomical characteristics, on a case-by-case basis. An algorithm for revascularization of coming high-risk population is proposed in Table 11.4.

Table 11.4   Proposed revascularization algorithm for the coming high-risk population

Question 1: is this patient likely to benefit from myocardial revascularization?

- Symptoms which probably relate to myocardial ischemia?
- Objective evidence of myocardial ischemia?
- Myocardial ischemia in multiple anatomical distributions?

Question 2: does this patient have an acute coronary syndrome (ACS)?

- STEMI constitutes a yes answer to all the above and exits to cardiac catheterization laboratory in <90 minutes.
- NSTEMI constitutes a yes answer to first two parts of question 1, and to question 2. It identifies patients who probably have plaque rupture or erosion and local coronary prothrombotic state, if not actual thrombus and/or distal embolization. Trials have demonstrated objective clinical benefit from both antiplatelet and antithrombin anticoagulation in these subsets. Widespread ischemia, the presence of arrhythmia, and/or the presence of hemodynamic compromise all constitute reasons to consider urgent coronary angiography for the NSTEMI patient.

Question 3: is there any subset of patient with coronary artery disease which has not been shown to benefit from smoking cessation, lipid lowering with statins, blood pressure control, aspirin, diabetes control, and regular physical activity?

- All CAD patients should receive these treatments, whether they will undergo coronary angiography, PCI, CABG, transplant, implantable cardioverter-defibrillator (ICD), or medical therapy.

Question 4: does this patient have medically refractory myocardial ischemia?

- Medically refractory (including rapid risk factor modification efforts) ischemia is a strong reason to consider coronary angiography for patients with unstable angina, stable angina or atypical symptoms or silent ischemia
- Enough beta-blocker to have resting bradycardia; relatively contraindicated by severity of LV dysfunction or COPD or atrioventricular block
- Blood pressure to 'goal': enough beta-blocker, nitrate, calcium blocker to have resting blood pressure <120 mmHg systolic; relatively contraindicated
- Optimal low-density lipoprotein
- Optimal hemoglobin A_{1c}
- Smoking cessation effort
- Adequate investigation and treatment of 'secondary causes' (anemia, thyrotoxicosis, fever, etc)

Question 5: having established a potential clinical benefit for revascularization before sending the patient for coronary angiography, now consider the coronary anatomy

- Left main stenosis; diffuse, osteal or distal; calcified; severe; bifurcation or trifurcation
- Three-vessel versus two-vessel or one-vessel; severe; proximal; branch only
- Large enough caliber vessels to 'comfortably' attempt bypass
- Total occlusion that probably cannot be crossed with wire/balloon/stent
- So heavily calcified, likely to need rotablator; unapproachable
- Extreme tortuosity; unapproachable
- Prior CABG; patent grafts; patent left internal mammary artery (LIMA); no grafts

Question 6: what is the patient's current level of left ventricular systolic and diastolic function?

- In the past, authorities and guidelines have argued that mild/moderate left ventricular (LV) systolic dysfunction was an additional reason to do coronary angiography and

Table 11.4 Continued

consider revascularization. For the most part, patients with severe LV dysfunction were considered exceptions, unless they had clear symptoms and/or reversible ischemia.

- As above, medically refractory ischemia and symptoms make benefit more likely but acute or long-term complications carry higher risk of death among patients with more severe LV dysfunction. Accordingly the answer to this question can influence strategies, for example whether to employ intra-aortic balloon counterpulsation or left ventricular assist device (LVAD) or even cardiopulmonary support.
- The level of diastolic dysfunction can influence dye dose, use of supportive hemodynamic monitoring, and choice between CABG and PCI.

Question 7: does this patient have significant comorbidities which influence the relative choice between CABG and PCI as a means of either acute or long-term revascularization?

All of the following prompt consideration of palliative PCI for even patients with complex coronary anatomic configurations:

- dementia
- cerebrovascular accident
- cerebrovascular disease
- COPD necessitating continuous oxygen or chronic steroid administration
- severe skeletal deformity
- significant neuromuscular impairment
- renal failure requiring dialysis
- severe liver failure
- severe coagulopathy
- cancer, with limited life span.

REFERENCES

1. Eagle KA, Guyton RA, Davidoff R et al. ACC/AHA 2004 Guideline update for coronary artery bypass graft surgery: a report of the American College of Cardiology/American Heart association Task force on Practice Guidelines (Committee to update the 1999 Guidelines for Coronary Bypass Graft Surgery). Circulation 2004; 110: e340–437.
2. Morrison DA, Sethi G, Sacks J, et al. Percutaneous coronary intervention versus coronary artery bypass graft surgery for patients with medically refractory myocardial ischemia and risk factors for adverse outcomes with bypass: a multicenter, randomized trial. Investigators of the Department of Veterans Affairs Cooperative Study #385, the Angina With Extremely Serious Operative Mortality Evaluation (AWESOME). J Am Coll Cardiol 2001; 38: 143–9.
3. Morrison DA, Sethi G, Sacks J, et al. Percutaneous coronary intervention versus coronary bypass graft surgery for patients with medically refractory myocardial ischemia and risk factors for adverse outcomes with bypass: The VA AWESOME multicenter registry: comparison with the randomized clinical trial. J Am Coll Cardiol 2002; 39: 266–73.
4. Morrison DA, Sethi G, Sacks J, et al. Percutaneous coronary intervention versus repeat bypass surgery for patients with medically refractory myocardial ischemia: AWESOME randomized trial and registry experience with post-CABG patients. J Am Coll Cardiol 2002; 40: 1951–4.
5. Smith SC, Feldman TE, Hirshfeld JW Jr et al. ACC/AHA/SCA&I 2005 Guideline Update for Percutaneous Coronary Intervention: a report of the American College of Cardiology/American Heart Association Task Force on Practice Guidelines (ACC/AHA/SCA&I Writing Committee to Update the 2001 Guidelines for Percutaneous Coronary Intervention). Circulation 2006; 113: e166–286.

12

Percutaneous coronary intervention for patients with multivessel disease

Andrew TL Ong and Patrick W Serruys

Revascularization for coronary artery disease • Practical considerations in the treatment of multivessel disease • Cost-effectiveness and quality of life • The future • Limitations • Conclusion

The management of coronary artery disease has rapidly evolved over the last 30 years. As a result of multiple large, rigorous, scientific trials, percutaneous coronary intervention (PCI) using stents has been shown to afford a similar mortality outcome as coronary artery bypass surgery in multivessel disease, and in selected cases has replaced surgery as the preferred revascularization strategy. Drug-eluting stents have revolutionized PCI, and new devices to treat chronic total occlusions (CTOs) have been developed, resulting in improved recanalization rates, and reduced restenosis rates. This chapter will summarize the extensive literature available on multivessel stenting and provide an evidence-based guide on this commonly encountered, and difficult clinical dilemma. Finally, the future direction of multivessel stenting will be discussed.

REVASCULARIZATION FOR CORONARY ARTERY DISEASE

Coronary artery bypass surgery was introduced in 1968 and rapidly established itself as the gold standard for treatment.[1] Two important early randomized studies demonstrated the survival benefit with revascularization (coronary artery bypass grafting (CABG)) over medical therapy for the treatment of significant left main stem disease,[2] for three-vessel disease and for two- or three-vessel disease involving the proximal left anterior descending artery.[3] Percutaneous coronary intervention (PCI) began in 1977 with the first percutaneous transluminal coronary angioplasty (PTCA) performed by Andreas Gruentzig as a non-surgical alternative.[4] The development of coronary stents, initially as an emergent device to control acute vessel closure following balloon angioplasty was a huge advancement for PCI. Two landmark studies, the Belgium Netherlands Stent (BENESTENT) Study, and the Stent Restenosis Study (STRESS) subsequently demonstrated that, in single lesion disease, elective stent placement resulted in better clinical and angiographic outcomes than standard coronary angioplasty.[5,6]

These two trials, together with improvements in antiplatelet therapy, led to the era of stenting, as the preferred method of PCI.

Stenting versus coronary artery bypass surgery

The four largest and most contemporary, multicenter, randomized studies comparing PCI to surgery involve coronary stents and were conducted in the mid to late 1990s (Table 12.1). They were the Arterial Revascularization Therapy Study (ARTS),[7] the Surgery or Stent (SoS) Trial,[8] Argentinean Randomized Study: Coronary Angioplasty With Stenting Versus Coronary Bypass Surgery in Patients With Multiple-Vessel Disease (ERACI-2),[9] and Angina With Extremely Serious Operative Mortality Evaluation (AWESOME) trial.[10] The ARTS trial was the largest trial with 1205 patients from 69 centers, and clearly established that in patients with multivessel disease, mortality at 1 year was similar irrespective of whether the patient underwent stent implantation or surgery.[7] This similar mortality rate at 1-year was reinforced in a 3051 patient meta-analysis of ARTS, SoS, ERACI-2 and MASS-2.[11] More recently, the longterm (5-year) results from the ARTS trial continued to demonstrate that mortality was similar for both stenting or CABG.[12] These new findings were a marked improvement over previous reports where surgery was associated with an improved survival rate over balloon angioplasty at 5 years.[13]

In the ARTS trial, the primary endpoint of a composite of freedom from death, myocardial infarction (MI), cerebrovascular accident (CVA) or repeat revascularization at 1 year was lower in the stent group (73.8% vs. 87.8%, $P < 0.001$), due to the increased need for repeat revascularization (21.0% versus 3.8%, $P < 0.001$, Table 12.2). These findings were reproduced in the other trials, and although seminal, are now historical in terms of applicability in contemporary practice due to improvements in both stenting and CABG treatment. Therefore, given the similar survival between stenting and CABG, the major remaining limitation to multivessel stenting is the excess need for repeat intervention, predominantly due to restenosis, in the stent group.

Drug-eluting stents

The management of coronary artery disease has changed following the introduction of drug-eluting stents (DES) in 2002.[14,15] Multiple randomized trials have consistently demonstrated that DES reduce restenosis compared to bare-metal stents in single lesions, with no excess mortality or MI.[16] The efficacy of DES for multivessel disease have been reported in various single center registries.[17,18] The Rapamycin-Eluting Stent Evaluated At Rotterdam Cardiology Hospital (RESEARCH) and Taxus-Stent Evaluated At Rotterdam Cardiology Hospital (T-SEARCH) Registries have shown in an 'all comers' population low re-intervention rates in an unrestricted setting.[19,20]

The first major trial in the era of DES for the treatment of multivessel disease was the Arterial Revascularization Therapies Study Part II trial (ARTS II).[12,21] This 607-patient, 87-center, stratified, non-randomized, open-labeled, single arm PCI study using sirolimus-eluting stents (SES) was seen as an intermediate phase preceding a full-fledged randomized study comparing surgery to DES. In this population, 54% had three-vessel disease, the remainder, two-vessel disease. A mean total length of 73 mm of SES was implanted. At 30 days, there were no deaths, 0.2% suffered a stroke and MI occurred in 0.8% of the cohort. The one-year results demonstrated favorable outcomes in the contemporary DES group with low re-intervention rates: only 6.4% of the population required repeat PCI and 2.1% underwent CABG. These results were the first to demonstrate that multivessel drug-eluting stenting was safe, feasible and associated with low re-intervention rates.

Table 12.1 Summary of the four major contemporary randomized trials comparing stenting to coronary artery bypass surgery for multivessel disease

	ARTS[7]	SoS[8]	ERACI-2[9]	AWESOME[10]
Principal investigator	Patrick W Serruys and Felix Unger	Urlich Sigwart and Rodney H Stables	Alfredo Rodriguez	Douglas Morrison and Stewart Scott
Inclusion criteria	Stable, unstable angina, or silent ischemia	Stable, or unstable angina	Stable, unstable angina, or asymptomatic patients with myocardium at risk (>2 areas with perfusion defects)	Medically refractory myocardial ischemia plus the presence of at least one high-risk factor[a]
	Equivalent revascularization mandatory	Equivalent revascularization not mandatory	Complete functional revascularization	Equivalent revascularization mandatory
Enrolment period	1997–1998	1996–1999	1996–1998	1995–2000
Number of patients	1205	988	450	454
Number of centers	67	53	7	16
Geographical location	Europe, South America, Canada, Australia and New Zealand	Europe and Canada	Argentina	USA
Primary endpoint	MACCE-free survival at 1 year	Rate of repeat revascularization	MACCE at 30 days	Mortality
Baseline characteristics (PCI, CABG)				
age (years)	61, 61	61, 62	62, 61	67, 67
male (%)	77, 76	80, 78	77, 81	100, 100
diabetes (%)	19, 16	14, 15	17, 17	29, 34
three-vessel disease (%)	30, 33	38, 47	55, 58	40, 50
ejection fraction (%)	61, 60	57, 57	Not stated	47, 44
PCI procedural characteristics				
stent use (%)	89 (of lesions)	78 (of lesions)	Not stated	54
glycoprotein IIb/IIIa use (%)	Not stated	8	28	11
Outcomes				
major adverse cardiac and cerebral events at 1 year, PCI vs. CABG (%)	26.2 vs. 12.2	22.5 vs. 12.4	Not reported	Not reported

[a]High-risk factor: prior open heart surgery, age >70 years, left ventricular function <35%, MI in the past week, or use of balloon pump.

Table 12.2 Ranked major adverse cardiac and cerebral events at 1-year, in worst order in the ARTS trial stratified according to extent of revascularization and treatment strategy[44]

Event	Coronary artery bypass grafting (CABG)			Percutaneous coronary intervention (PCI)		
	Complete ($n = 477$)	Incomplete ($n = 90$)	P value within CABG	Complete ($n = 406$)	Incomplete ($n = 170$)	P value within PCI
Death (%)	2.5	4.4	ns	1.7	3.5	ns
Cerebrovascular accident (%)	1.9	0	ns	1.7	1.2	ns
Myocardial infarction (%)	3.4	4.4	ns	4.9	5.9	ns
(Repeat) coronary artery bypass grafting (%)	0.2	1.1	ns	2.0	10.0	<0.05
(Repeat) percutaneous coronary intervention (%)	2.1	2.2	ns	13.1	10.0	ns
Any major adverse cerebral and cardiac event (%)	11.1	12.8	ns	23.4	30.6	<0.05

ns, not significant.

PRACTICAL CONSIDERATIONS IN THE TREATMENT OF MULTIVESSEL DISEASE

As reported in the ARTS II trial, multivessel stenting, in particular with drug-eluting stents is a safe, feasible, and readily accomplished alternative to coronary artery bypass surgery. In considering whether a patient is suitable for multivessel stenting, the following subgroups require further discussion.

Left main stem disease

Surgery has been the gold standard for the treatment of left main stem disease since the publication of the Veteran's Affairs study. Percutaneous treatment of the left main stem with bare stents has been limited by restenosis, occurring in 22% of patients.[22] Consequently, percutaneous treatment has remained confined predominantly to emergency cases as a salvage procedure and for high-surgical risk patients. In the 3 years since the commercialization of DES, with reductions in restenosis rates of up to 80% in clinical trials, there has been renewed interest regarding percutaneous treatment of left main stem disease. The first publication on this topic was promising, and reported a restenosis rate of 8% in a small population of 16 patients.[23] More recently, larger studies have confirmed the beneficial effects of DES in this population.[24-26] Two randomized trials comparing DES implantation to CABG are under way (SYNergy between percutaneous coronary intervention with TAXus and cardiac surgery [SYNTAX] and COMparison of Bypass surgery and AngioplasTy using sirolimus electing stent in patients with left main coronary disease [COMBAT], discussed further on).[27] Pending the release of their results, stenting of the left main should remain an elective procedure, with the available options fully discussed with the patient prior to a decision being made. It should not be performed on an *ad hoc* basis, unless as an emergency, life-saving procedure when CABG is not immediately available.

Patients with diabetes

Diabetic patients undergoing treatment for multivessel disease usually have diffuse disease, and three-vessel disease. With bare-metal stents, the optimal revascularization strategy of diabetic patients with multivessel disease remains coronary artery bypass surgery, due to the markedly increased need for repeat revascularization with bare-metal stenting, based on the long-term outcome from the ARTS randomized trial. In the randomized clinical trials, the relative reduction in restenosis rates with DES is similar in diabetic patients to that in non-diabetic patients, although the absolute incidence of target vessel revascularization (TVR) remains higher in diabetic patients.[28] A real-world study of 293 all-comers diabetic patients of whom 66% had multivessel disease, reported a TVR rate of 10.3% with SES, and 5.9% with paclitaxel-eluting stents (PES), $P=0.2$).[29] Currently in progress is the large Future Revascularization Evaluation in patients with Diabetes Mellitus: Optimal Management of Multivessel Disease (FREEDOM) multicenter study, randomizing diabetic patients with multivessel disease to either DES implantation or CABG.

Chronic total occlusions

With the percutaneous approach, the presence of chronic total occlusions remains the biggest and most important obstacle and technical challenge to achieving total revascularization. CTOs occur relatively frequently, are seen in up to 20% of patients undergoing diagnostic coronary angiography, and comprise 10% of PCIs in the contemporary practice of a tertiary referral catheterization laboratory.[30] Historically, the success rate of crossing CTOs percutaneously approximates 60% using conventional techniques. This success rate is dependent on operator experience, the number of attempts performed, anatomical considerations, and the choice of devices available. In order to overcome this major limitation, new devices and adjunctive methods have been developed to improve the success rate. Multislice computed tomography coronary angiography provides additional information such as occlusion length and severity of calcification, features that predict procedural success are and often underestimated by conventional coronary angiography.[31] The Total Occlusion Trial with Angioplasty by using Laser guidewire (TOTAL) randomized trial did not not show a benefit with laser-tipped guidewires over conventional wires.[32] Local delivery of thrombolytic therapy to the site of occlusion via a specialized catheter to facilitate wire crossing was recently reported with promising results.[33] Japanese device makers have led the development of specialized guidewires allowing a stepwise systematic approach. New devices in development include a blunt dissection catheter,[34] a helical screw-like tipped micro-catheter,[35] and a stand-alone system using optical coherence reflectometry (OCR) together with radiofrequency ablation. OCR is used to direct the tip of a guidewire in a co-axial plane within the lumen, and radiofrequency ablation delivered at the tip is used to enhance forward wire passage; recanalization rates of 51.7% and 54.3% have been reported in patients who had previously failed conventional wire techniques.[36,37] Finally, a technique utilized in peripheral angioplasty has been newly introduced in which a subintimal dissection plane or false lumen is deliberately created parallel to the true lumen containing the CTO.[38] Under the direct vision of an intravascular ultrasound (IVUS) catheter placed in the false lumen, a guidewire is advanced from the false lumen into the true lumen distal to the occlusion site, bypassing the occlusion, and the newly created track is then stented with DES. Following successful recanalization, the placement of DES has been shown to improve the mid-term outcomes of patients with CTOs, by reducing restenosis compared to bare-metal stenting. While no randomized study on CTOs in DES have been published to date, three registries, all with angiographic follow-up, convincingly demonstrate a sustained reduction in restenosis rates, need for reintervention, and occurrence of major adverse cardiac events with drug-eluting compared to bare-metal stents (Table 12.3).[30,39–41]

The goal of multivessel stenting should always be total revascularization, as the overall trend supports it. From a practical treatment point of view, if a patient undergoing PCI for multivessel disease has a CTO, it would be reasonable to first attempt to cross the occlusion, before attempting any other lesion. In that way, if the lesion is unable to be crossed, the patient would then automatically become a surgical candidate, so as to offer him/her optimal revascularization.

Complete revascularization

The concept of completeness of revascularization is made difficult due to a lack of a universal definition. Comparisons between studies must be interpreted with caution as different studies employ different definitions. Two commonly used definitions depend on 'anatomical' or 'functional' considerations. For example, revascularization may be declared complete if all stenotic vessels are revascularized, irrespective

Table 12.3   Summary of studies comparing DES to BMS for the treatment of CTOs

Composition of groups	Hoye et al[30] Consecutive cohort	Hoye et al[30] Historical control	Werner et al[39] Consecutive cohort	Werner et al[39] Matched control	Ge et al[40] Consecutive cohort	Ge et al[40] Historical control
Stent type	SES	BMS	PES	BMS	SES	BMS
Patients (n)	56	28	48	48	122	259
Diabetes (%)	14	7	33	29	28	19
Prior MI	55	46	42	47	55	63
Minimum duration of CTO	1 month	1 month	2 weeks	2 weeks	3 months	3 months
Occlusion >3 months (%)	n/a	n/a	73	65	100	100
CTO length (mm)	11.3	12.7	18±13	16±12	10.4±10.2	9.6±6.9
Reference diameter (mm)	2.35±0.46	2.37±0.50	2.65±0.65	2.57±0.47	3.05±0.44	3.05±0.55
MLD post-procedure (mm)	2.06±0.48	2.18±0.49	2.26±0.36	2.16±0.60	2.67±0.49	2.69±0.53
Late loss (mm)	0.13±0.46	–	0.19±0.62	1.21±0.70	0.28±0.56	1.04±0.87
Binary restenosis rate (%)	9.1	–	8.3	51.1	9.2	33.3
Re-occlusion (%)	1.8	–	2.1	23.4	2.5	6.6
Stent thrombosis within 1 month (%)	1.8	0	0	0	0	0
TLR (%)	n/a	n/a	n/a	n/a	7.4	26.3
MACE (%)	3.6*	17.9[a]	12.4[a]	47.9[a]	16.4[b]	35.1[b]

Columns in bold denote the DES groups.
DES, drug-eluting stents; MLD, minimal luminal diameter; n/a, not available; PES, paclitaxel-eluting stents; SES, sirolimus-eluting stents; TLR, target lesion revascularization.
[a]Clinical follow-up at 12 months; [b]clinical follow-up at 6 months.

of size (anatomical revascularization) and territory supplied, others impose minimum diameter criteria, yet others differentiate between main vessels and branch vessels. Secondly, a functional classification may be used, whereby revascularization is declared complete if all ischemic myocardial territories are reperfused; areas of old infarction with no viable myocardium are not required to be reperfused. None of the current guidelines set out by the American or European Cardiology societies formally discuss the issue in detail. In a long term (nine-year) follow-up study from the 1985–1986 National Heart, Lung, and Blood Institute PTCA registry, compared to patients who were completely revascularized, incompletely revascularized patients (whether intended, attempted or not achieved) had non-different risks of dying, MI, or repeat revascularization by PTCA or CABG after adjustment for baseline characteristics.[42] Incomplete revascularization remained a significant risk factor for subsequent CABG, and incompletely revascularized patients showed a strong trend towards more recurrent angina, but this risk became weaker after adjustment. Complete revascularization was attempted and achieved in 57% and 46% of patients with two- and three-vessel coronary artery disease.[43] The majority of lesions not amenable to PTCA were total occlusions, and the success rate for attempted occlusions was 54%.

In the more recent ARTS randomized trial, which mandated equivalence of completeness of revascularization, true anatomical completeness of revascularization, as ascertained by experienced independent observers on review of films after completion of the PCI, occurred in 70.5% of patients, higher than in previous studies.[44] Of note, complete revascularization was actually achieved more often in the CABG group over the PCI group, with no mortality difference at one year post-procedure.

As with previous studies, patients who were unable to be completely revascularized had a significantly higher number of diseased segments and vessels. Incompletely revascularized patients also had a 3.6-fold higher incidence of total occlusions compared to completely revascularized patients (19.4% vs. 5.4%, $P < 0.001$). In this study, as with previous studies, stented patients who were incompletely revascularized had a higher requirement for subsequent CABG in the first year of follow-up (10% vs. 2% in those who were completely revascularized, $P < 0.05$), resulting in a lower overall major adverse cardiac and cerebral events (MACCE)-free rate (69.4% vs. 76.6%, $P < 0.05$, Table 12.2 and Figure 12.1).

The ARTS trial was the only one of the three largest randomized trials comparing coronary artery bypass surgery to stenting for multivessel disease to mandate that equivalent revascularization could be achieved by either approach.[7] The SoS trial encouraged but did not mandate equivalent revascularization,[8] while ERACI-2 mandated complete functional revascularization.[9] Consequently, only the ARTS trial has published the one-year outcomes of patients who were completely or incompletely revascularized.[44] In that study, despite the potential for equivalent revascularization, complete revascularization was more frequently achieved in CABG-treated patients (84.1%) as compared to stented patients (70.5%, $P < 0.001$). While no differences in mortality or the combined endpoint of death/stroke/MI were seen in the comparison of the four groups, overall MACCE rates were significantly higher in the incompletely revascularized stented group, driven by an increased need for CABG within the first year of follow-up (Figure 12.1).

The advantages of PCI are that it is performed under local anesthetic, post-procedural morbidity is minimal, and patients endure a short hospital stay. With the current use of drug-eluting stents, long, diffuse stenoses can be effectively treated.

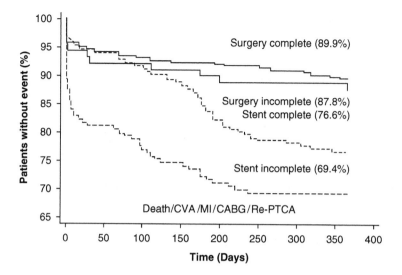

Figure 12.1 Kaplan–Meier curve showing survival free of MACCE at 1-year from the ARTS trial, stratified by treatment and completeness of revascularization. Reprinted with from van den Brand MJ, Rensing BJ, Morel MA et al. The effect of completeness of revascularization on event-free survival at one year in the ARTS trial. J Am Coll Cardiol 2002; 39: 559–64 with permission from American College of Cardiology Foundation.[44]

Despite all the technology that has been described, it however remains restricted by the inability to overcome total occlusions, with varying success rates. Symptomatic failures will eventually require CABG. CABG surgery has the clear advantage of overcoming chronic occlusions, and less repeated revascularizations but is associated with a not-insubstantial postoperative morbidity, longer period of hospitalization and a slower return to normal activities. Multiple, long and diseased coronary segments may be a challenge, with multiple grafts required in small vessels, and longer surgical procedures are associated with higher morbidity.

Hybrid coronary revascularization

The development of hybrid or integrated coronary revascularization in the 1990s to treat multivessel disease by combining percutaneous techniques with minimal access coronary surgery through a mini-thoracotomy has been unsuccessful,[45,46] due to the increased need for repeat revascularization in these patients, driven by incomplete revascularization and in-stent restenosis.[47]

Contrast-induced nephropathy

Patients with renal dysfunction, hypotension and/or diabetes are at increased risk for developing contrast-induced nephropathy (CIN). A risk score has been developed to predict patient outcomes.[48] Importantly, prehydration and the use of N-acetyl cysteine have been shown to be preventive,[49] and the volume of contrast used is an important consideration, as is staging the procedure.

Staged procedures

Treating multivessel disease patients can be particularly challenging and time consuming. Such cases should be performed when the operator is fresh, and possibly with two experienced operators. Staging a procedure, with regard to patient comfort, operator fatigue, radiation dose, and contrast load is an important clinical decision that must be actively considered. In patients with the potential to develop CIN, the second stage should be performed at least one week apart. For other indications no specific recommendations apply.

Treatment of culprit lesion versus total revascularization

In the only study that randomized patients with multivessel disease to either PCI limited to the culprit vessel or PCI of all vessels with ≥50% stenosis, 219 patients were randomized and followed up for 5 years.[50] The culprit vessel was determined by two independent interventional cardiologists based on the clinical evidence available. PCI for an acute MI was an exclusion criterion. This study demonstrated that at long-term follow-up of 4.6 years, the completely revascularized group as compared to the culprit-vessel-treated group had similar target lesion revascularization rates (17.3% vs. 12.0%, $P=0.3$), and not surprisingly, a lower overall need for repeat PCI (21.2% vs. 31.2%, $P=0.06$). The overall long-term death, myocardial infarction or repeat revascularization (MACE) rates were similar between groups (34.6% vs. 40.4% respectively, $P=0.4$, as were estimated costs ($P=0.8$). Despite the low use of stents (only 55% of the cohort was initially treated with stents), this study suggests that the treatment of other non-culprit lesions at the index procedure (i.e. complete revascularization) is associated with less morbidity due to the lower need for a repeat PCI procedure at long-term follow-up.

The importance of this trial was that patients were actively randomized to the treatment groups, and there were patients who were intentionally left untreated, if randomized to the culprit vessel treatment arm alone. This contrasts with previous trials, where patients were incompletely revascularized due to a 'failure' of initial revascularization (intended or otherwise), thus were highly selected and underwent CABG as the second option for revascularization; this was classified as a subsequent CABG. Thus, from a societal perspective while estimated costs were similar, from an individual perspective, complete revascularization was beneficial with less repeat intervention later on.

Bifurcation stenting

In the ARTS 2 trial, bifurcation lesions requiring double wiring were present in 34% of patients. An operator attempting multivessel stenting must be competent with the various types and techniques of bifurcation treatments available. To date, there have been no specific devices developed successfully for bifurcation stenting.

COST-EFFECTIVENESS AND QUALITY OF LIFE

Economic impact of revascularization strategies

The ARTS trial showed that PCI for multivessel disease was associated with lower procedural costs and shorter, less intensive, initial hospitalization; but that

PCI was associated with higher follow-up costs due to the need for repeat revascularizations.[7] Cost savings of €4212 at the end of the procedure had decreased to €2779 after 1 year (in favor of PCI), and after three years further decreased to €1798 (still in favor of PCI).[51] Times have changed as although the price of bare-metal stents used in previous studies has decreased dramatically, higher-priced DES have been introduced with better results in terms of the need for repeat revascularizations. In addition, new less-invasive treatment modalities for multi-vessel disease have been adopted by the surgical community and may be as effec-tive and less costly. Hence, the balance between costs and effects in the treatment of three-vessel disease and/or left main stem disease has changed and requires re-evaluation.

Revascularization strategies on quality of life

In the ARTS trial, PCI was associated with a better quality of life, and patients were able to return to work earlier than the CABG patients.[7] However, these benefits had equalized after 6 months. Patients after PCI had more angina and required more anti-anginal medication. The use of DES is expected to have beneficial effects on quality of life based on the expected decrease in repeat revascularizations. An updated assessment is needed to inform both patients and clinicians about the impact of the recent advances in revascularization strategies in this new era.

THE FUTURE (TABLE 12.4)

SYNTAX

The SYNTAX trial is a multicenter, randomized trial with separate nested registries surrounding the randomized arm, led by Professors Patrick Serruys and Frederick Mohr.[27] The overall goal is to assess the optimum revascularization treatment for patients with *de novo* three-vessel disease and/or left main branch disease (either isolated or with one-, two-, or three-vessel disease) by randomizing patients to either PCI with paclitaxel-eluting stents or to CABG. A total of 1800 patients will be randomized from approximately 90 participating centers, comprising 60–70 sites in Europe and 15–20 sites in the US. The primary endpoint is freedom from MACCE at one year. As with the ARTS trial, patients must have the potential for complete and equivalent revascularization before they may be considered for enrolment. As an 'all-comers' trial, consecutive patients will be enroled, and non-randomizable patients will be entered into the preference registries which will follow patients who cannot be treated by either CABG or PCI because of technical reasons, physician and/or patient preferences or comorbidities. Enrolment began in April 2005. Randomized patients are stratified at each site based on the presence or absence of left main stem disease and medically treated diabetes mellitus (requiring oral medications or insulin).

In addition, the CABG registry data could be used to define the population where drug-eluting stenting is considered unsuitable for treatment of complex, high-risk subsets. Conversely, the PCI registry data using any interventional tech-niques or devices with or without the use of DES establishes the patients where CABG is considered inappropriate. In this trial, CTOs are not an exclusion criteria, and the outcomes of their treatment will be specifically monitored throughout the

Table 12.4   Upcoming randomized trials comparing stenting to coronary artery bypass surgery for multivessel disease

	SYNTAX[27]	FREEDOM	CARDia[52]
Principal Investigator(s)	Patrick W. Serruys and Frederick Mohr	Valentin Fuster	Kevin Beatt and Akhil Kapur
Trial design	Randomized with nested registries	Randomized with nested registries	Randomized with associated registries
Vessels	Three-vessel disease or left main stem disease	Two- or three-vessel disease	Complex one-, two-, or three-vessel disease
Population	All comers	Diabetics	Diabetics
Sample size	1500	2400	600
Number of sites	90	110	21
Geographic location	Europe and USA	USA and Europe	UK and Ireland
Study stent	Taxus paclitaxel-eluting stent	Food and Drug Administration-approved drug-eluting stent: currently Cypher sirolimus-eluting stent and Taxus paclitaxel-eluting stent	Bare-metal stent, or Cypher sirolimus-eluting stent
Trial assumption	Non-inferiority	Non-inferiority	Non-inferiority
Primary endpoint	Freedom from MACCE at 1 year	Mortality at 5 years	Composite of death, non-fatal myocardial infarction, or non-fatal stroke at 1 year
Trial sponsor	Boston Scientific Corporation	National Institutes of Health	Combination of various industry and institutional sponsors

MACCE, composite of death, non-fatal myocardial infarction, non-fatal stroke, or any repeat revascularization.

conduct of the trial. Hence, it is expected that with the new devices not previously available at the time of the previous trials (some of which are described in this article), a substantial proportion of patients enroled will have CTOs, and be treated by CABG and PCI. *Post hoc* analyses of this study, looking at completeness of revascularization, and success of CTO recanalization, within and between groups will provide some useful answers to the current practice of revascularization for multivessel disease. This trial will provide answers in the contemporary treatment of three-vessel and left main stem disease.

FREEDOM

In view of the new results emerging with DES, the multicenter North American and European FREEDOM trial will randomize 2400 diabetic patients with multi (two or three)-vessel disease to either CABG or PCI with DES. The Principal investigator of this government sponsored National Institutes of Health (NIH) study is Dr Valentin Fuster. Device companies with commercialized DES (currently Cordis Johnson and Johnson and Boston Scientific Corporation) will contribute stents for free to the study. The primary endpoint is mortality at 5 years. There will also be nested registries to capture patients treated with either PCI or CABG only.

CARDia (Coronary Artery Revascularisation in Diabetes)

This 21-center, UK and Ireland-based trial currently in progress will randomize 600 diabetic patients with either complex one-vessel disease or multivessel disease to CABG or PCI.[52] A small proportion of the population has received bare stents, and following a protocol amendment the majority will receive sirolimus-eluting stents. The primary endpoint is the composite incidence of death, non-fatal MI, or non-fatal stroke at one year.

COMBAT

The COMparison of Bypass surgery and AngioplasTy using sirolimus-eluting stents in patients with left main coronary disease (COMBAT) randomized trial will randomize 1776 patients to bypass surgery or left main stenting. A further 1000 patients will be entered into registries for PCI, CABG, or medical therapy. The primary endpoint of the trial is the composite of death, MI, or stroke at two years. Key secondary endpoints include MACCE, and ischemia-driven target lesion revascularizaion. Dr Seung-Jung Park is the principal investigator, and Dr Martin Leon will be the co-principal investigator. In addition to the SYNTAX trial, this study should help determine the place of left main stenting in the treatment of coronary disease.

LIMITATIONS

The remaining limitation to multivessel stenting is stent thrombosis, which may be divided up into either early (within the first 30 days after stent implantation) or late (greater than 30 days). Early stent thrombosis is most commonly due to a mechanical reason (underexpansion, unrecognized intimal dissection), while late stent thrombosis is thought to be due to an abnormality with re-endothelialization post-stenting. Early stent thrombosis appears to have similar incidences with DES and BMS in randomized trials and in real-world use, approximating 1%.[53] Concern has evolved with late angiographic stent thrombosis (LAST), given the potent effects of DES on the cell cycle and therefore on endothelial cells, and of hypersensitivity reactions involving the polymer.[54] Comparative studies between BMS and DES are lacking, but the incidence in DES is probably below 1%,[55,56] similar to that reported with BMS,[57,58] but note that the durations of antiplatelet therapy differ between groups (1 month in BMS vs. 3–6 months with DES). More investigation is required to elicit the true etiology of LAST. It is thus imperative that all patients treated with DES remain fully compliant with their long-term dual antiplatelet therapy.

CONCLUSION

Multivessel disease remains the final frontier for interventional cardiology. The randomized trials comparing stenting with bypass surgery have confirmed the similar medium- and long-term mortality; the only difference between the two groups was an excess of restenosis with bare stents. The development of DES may overcome this limitation, and ARTS 2 provided a promising insight. The future results of SYNTAX and FREEDOM will provide the definitive solution to this as-yet unresolved debate.

REFERENCES

1. Favaloro RG. Saphenous vein autograft replacement of severe segmental coronary artery occlusion: operative technique. Ann Thorac Surg 1968; 5: 334–9.
2. Murphy ML, Hultgren HN, Detre K, Thomsen J, Takaro T. Treatment of chronic stable angina. A preliminary report of survival data of the randomized Veterans Administration cooperative study. N Engl J Med 1977; 297: 621–7.
3. Long-term results of prospective randomised study of coronary artery bypass surgery in stable angina pectoris. European Coronary Surgery Study Group. Lancet 1982; 2: 1173–80.
4. Gruntzig AR, Senning A, Siegenthaler WE. Nonoperative dilatation of coronary-artery stenosis: percutaneous transluminal coronary angioplasty. N Engl J Med 1979; 301: 61–8.
5. Serruys PW, de Jaegere P, Kiemeneij F et al, for the Benestent Study Group. A comparison of balloon-expandable-stent implantation with balloon angioplasty in patients with coronary artery disease. N Engl J Med 1994; 331: 489–95.
6. Fischman DL, Leon MB, Baim DS et al, for the Stent Restenosis Study Investigators. A randomized comparison of coronary-stent placement and balloon angioplasty in the treatment of coronary artery disease. N Engl J Med. 1994; 331: 496–501.
7. Serruys PW, Unger F, Sousa JE et al. Comparison of coronary-artery bypass surgery and stenting for the treatment of multivessel disease. N Engl J Med 2001; 344: 1117–24.
8. SoS Investigators. Coronary artery bypass surgery versus percutaneous coronary intervention with stent implantation in patients with multivessel coronary artery disease (the Stent or Surgery trial): a randomised controlled trial. Lancet 2002; 360: 965–70.
9. Rodriguez A, Bernardi V, Navia J et al. Argentine Randomized Study: Coronary Angioplasty with Stenting versus Coronary Bypass Surgery in patients with Multiple-Vessel Disease (ERACI II): 30-day and one-year follow-up results. ERACI II Investigators. J Am Coll Cardiol 2001; 37: 51–8.
10. Morrison DA, Sethi G, Sacks J et al. Percutaneous coronary intervention versus coronary artery bypass graft surgery for patients with medically refractory myocardial ischemia and risk factors for adverse outcomes with bypass: a multicenter, randomized trial. Investigators of the Department of Veterans Affairs Cooperative Study #385, the Angina With Extremely Serious Operative Mortality Evaluation (AWESOME). J Am Coll Cardiol 2001; 38: 143–9.
11. Mercado N, Wijns W, Serruys P et al. One-year outcomes of coronary artery bypass graft surgery versus percutaneous coronary intervention with multiple stenting for multisystem disease: a meta-analysis of individual patient data from randomized clinical trials. J Thorac Cardiovasc Surg 2005; 130: 512–19.
12. Serruys PW, Ong AT, Morice MC et al, on behalf of the ARTS Investigators. Arterial Revascularisation Therapies Study Part II – sirolimus-eluting stents for the treatment of patients with multivessel de novo coronary artery lesions. EuroIntervention 2005; 1: 147–156.
13. Hoffman SN, TenBrook JA, Wolf MP et al. A meta-analysis of randomized controlled trials comparing coronary artery bypass graft with percutaneous transluminal coronary angioplasty: one- to eight-year outcomes. J Am Coll Cardiol 2003; 41: 1293–304.
14. Morice MC, Serruys PW, Sousa JE et al. A randomized comparison of a sirolimus-eluting stent with a standard stent for coronary revascularization. N Engl J Med 2002; 346: 1773–80.

15. Grube E, Silber S, Hauptmann KE et al. TAXUS I: six- and twelve-month results from a randomized, double-blind trial on a slow-release paclitaxel-eluting stent for de novo coronary lesions. Circulation 2003; 107: 38–42.
16. Babapulle MN, Joseph L, Belisle P, Brophy JM, Eisenberg MJ. A hierarchical Bayesian meta-analysis of randomised clinical trials of drug-eluting stents. Lancet 2004; 364: 583–91.
17. Arampatzis CA, Hoye A, Lemos PA et al. Elective sirolimus-eluting stent implantation for multivessel disease involving significant LAD stenosis: one-year clinical outcomes of 99 consecutive patients—the Rotterdam experience. Catheter Cardiovasc Interv 2004; 63: 57–60.
18. Orlic D, Bonizzoni E, Stankovic G et al. Treatment of multivessel coronary artery disease with sirolimus-eluting stent implantation: immediate and mid-term results. J Am Coll Cardiol 2004; 43: 1154–60.
19. Lemos PA, Serruys PW, van Domburg RT et al. Unrestricted utilization of sirolimus-eluting stents compared with conventional bare stent implantation in the 'real world': the Rapamycin-Eluting Stent Evaluated At Rotterdam Cardiology Hospital (RESEARCH) registry. Circulation 2004; 109: 190–5.
20. Ong AT, Serruys PW, Aoki J et al. The unrestricted use of paclitaxel versus sirolimus-eluting stents for coronary artery disease in an unselected population – One Year Results of The Taxus-Stent Evaluated At Rotterdam Cardiology Hospital (T-SEARCH) Registry. J Am Coll Cardiol 2005; 45: 1135–41.
21. Serruys PW, Lemos PA, van Hout BA. Sirolimus eluting stent implantation for patients with multivessel disease: rationale for the Arterial Revascularisation Therapies Study part II (ARTS II). Heart 2004; 90: 995–8.
22. Park SJ, Park SW, Hong MK et al. Stenting of unprotected left main coronary artery stenoses: immediate and late outcomes. J Am Coll Cardiol 1998; 31: 37–42.
23. Arampatzis CA, Lemos PA, Tanabe K et al. Effectiveness of sirolimus-eluting stent for treatment of left main coronary artery disease. Am J Cardiol 2003; 92: 327–9.
24. Valgimigli M, van Mieghem CA, Ong AT et al. Short- and long-term clinical outcome after drug-eluting stent implantation for the percutaneous treatment of left main coronary artery disease: insights from the Rapamycin-Eluting and Taxus Stent Evaluated At Rotterdam Cardiology Hospital registries (RESEARCH and T-SEARCH). Circulation 2005; 111: 1383–9.
25. Chieffo A, Stankovic G, Bonizzoni E et al. Early and mid-term results of drug-eluting stent implantation in unprotected left main. Circulation 2005; 111: 791–5.
26. Park SJ, Kim YH, Lee BK et al. Sirolimus-eluting stent implantation for unprotected left main coronary artery stenosis: comparison with bare-metal stent implantation. J Am Coll Cardiol 2005; 45: 351–6.
27. Ong AT, Serruys PW, Mohr FW et al. The SYNergy between Percutaneous Coronary Intervention with TAXus™ and Cardiac Surgery (SYNTAX) Study: design, rationale and run-in phase. Am Heart J 2006; 151: 1194–204.
28. Moussa I, Leon MB, Baim DS et al. Impact of sirolimus-eluting stents on outcome in diabetic patients: a SIRIUS (SIRolImUS-coated Bx Velocity balloon-expandable stent in the treatment of patients with de novo coronary artery lesions) substudy. Circulation 2004; 109: 2273–8.
29. Ong AT, Aoki J, van Mieghem CA et al. Comparison of short- (one month) and long- (twelve months) term outcomes of sirolimus- versus paclitaxel-eluting stents in 293 consecutive patients with diabetes mellitus (from the RESEARCH and T-SEARCH registries). Am J Cardiol 2005; 96: 358–62.
30. Hoye A, Tanabe K, Lemos PA et al. Significant reduction in restenosis after the use of sirolimus-eluting stents in the treatment of chronic total occlusions. J Am Coll Cardiol 2004; 43: 1954–8.
31. Mollet NR, Hoye A, Lemos PA et al. Value of preprocedure multislice computed tomographic coronary angiography to predict the outcome of percutaneous recanalization of chronic total occlusions. Am J Cardiol 2005; 95: 240–3.

32. Serruys PW, Hamburger JN, Koolen JJ et al. Total occlusion trial with angioplasty by using laser guidewire. The TOTAL trial. Eur Heart J 2000; 21: 1797–805.
33. Abbas AE, Bewington SD, Dixon SR et al. Intracoconary fibrin-specific thrombolytic infusion facilitates percutaneous recanalization of chronic total occlusion. J Am Coll Cardiol 2005; 46: 793–8.
34. Yang YM, Mehran R, Dangas G et al. Successful use of the frontrunner catheter in the treatment of in-stent coronary chronic total occlusions. Catheter Cardiovasc Interv 2004; 63: 462–8.
35. Tsuchikane E, Katoh O, Shimogami M et al. First clinical experience of a novel penetration catheter for patients with severe coronary artery stenosis. Catheter Cardiovasc Interv 2005; 65: 368–73.
36. Hoye A, Onderwater E, Cummins P, Sianos G, Serruys PW. Improved recanalization of chronic total coronary occlusions using an optical coherence reflectometry-guided guidewire. Catheter Cardiovasc Interv 2004; 63: 158–63.
37. Baim DS, Braden G, Heuser R et al. Utility of the Safe-Cross-guided radiofrequency total occlusion crossing system in chronic coronary total occlusions (results from the Guided Radio Frequency Energy Ablation of Total Occlusions Registry Study). Am J Cardiol 2004; 94: 853–8.
38. Colombo A, Mikhail GW, Michev I et al. Treating chronic total occlusions using subintimal tracking and reentry: The STAR Technique. Catheter Cardiovasc Interv 2005; 64: 407–11.
39. Werner GS, Krack A, Schwarz G et al. Prevention of lesion recurrence in chronic total coronary occlusions by paclitaxel-eluting stents. J Am Coll Cardiol 2004; 44: 2301–6.
40. Ge L, Iakovou I, Cosgrave J et al. Immediate and mid-term outcomes of sirolimus-eluting stent implantation for chronic total occlusions. Eur Heart J 2005; 26: 1056–62.
41. Garcia-Garcia HM, Valgimigli M, Lotan C. Beyond crossing a chronic total occlusion Are the drug-eluting stents the solution for this old problem? EuroIntervention 2005; 1: 129–31.
42. Bourassa MG, Yeh W, Holubkov R, Sopko G, Detre KM. Long-term outcome of patients with incomplete vs complete revascularization after multivessel PTCA. A report from the NHLBI PTCA Registry. Eur Heart J 1998; 19: 103–11.
43. Bourassa MG, Holubkov R, Yeh W, Detre KM. Strategy of complete revascularization in patients with multivessel coronary artery disease (a report from the 1985–1986 NHLBI PTCA Registry). Am J Cardiol 1992; 70: 174–8.
44. van den Brand MJ, Rensing BJ, Morel MA et al. The effect of completeness of revascularization on event-free survival at one year in the ARTS trial. J Am Coll Cardiol 2002; 39: 559–64.
45. Angelini GD, Wilde P, Salerno TA, Bosco G, Calafiore AM. Integrated left small thoracotomy and angioplasty for multivessel coronary artery revascularisation. Lancet 1996; 347: 757–8.
46. Cohen HA, Zenati M, Smith AJ et al. Feasibility of combined percutaneous transluminal angioplasty and minimally invasive direct coronary artery bypass in patients with multivessel coronary artery disease. Circulation 1998; 98: 1048–50.
47. Murphy GJ, Bryan AJ, Angelini GD. Hybrid coronary revascularization in the era of drug-eluting stents. Ann Thorac Surg 2004; 78: 1861–7.
48. Mehran R, Aymong ED, Nikolsky E et al. A simple risk score for prediction of contrast-induced nephropathy after percutaneous coronary intervention: development and initial validation. J Am Coll Cardiol 2004; 44: 1393–9.
49. Tepel M, van der Giet M, Schwarzfeld C, Laufer U, Liermann D, Zidek W. Prevention of radiographic-contrast-agent-induced reductions in renal function by acetylcysteine. N Engl J Med 2000; 343: 180–4.
50. Ijsselmuiden AJ, Ezechiels J, Westendorp IC et al. Complete versus culprit vessel percutaneous coronary intervention in multivessel disease: a randomized comparison. Am Heart J 2004; 148: 467–74.
51. Legrand VM, Serruys PW, Unger F et al. Three-year outcome after coronary stenting versus bypass surgery for the treatment of multivessel disease. Circulation 2004; 109: 1114–20.

52. Kapur A, Malik IS, Bagger JP et al. The Coronary Artery Revascularisation in Diabetes (CARDia) trial: background, aims, and design. Am Heart J 2005; 149: 13–19.
53. Ong AT, Hoye A, Aoki J et al. Thirty-day incidence and six-month clinical outcome of thrombotic stent occlusion following bare-metal, sirolimus or paclitaxel stent implantation. J Am Coll Cardiol 2005; 45: 947–53.
54. Virmani R, Guagliumi G, Farb A et al. Localized hypersensitivity and late coronary thrombosis secondary to a sirolimus-eluting stent: should we be cautious? Circulation 2004; 109: 701–5.
55. Ong AT, Mc Fadden EP, Regar E et al. Late angiographic stent thrombosis (LAST) events with drug-eluting stents. J Am Coll Cardiol 2005; 45: 2088–92.
56. Iakovou I, Schmidt T, Bonizzoni E et al. Incidence, predictors, and outcome of thrombosis after successful implantation of drug-eluting stents. JAMA 2005; 293: 2126–30.
57. Wang F, Stouffer GA, Waxman S, Uretsky BF. Late coronary stent thrombosis: early vs. late stent thrombosis in the stent era. Catheter Cardiovasc Interv 2002; 55: 142–7.
58. Wenaweser P, Rey C, Eberli FR et al. Stent thrombosis following bare-metal stent implantation: success of emergency percutaneous coronary intervention and predictors of adverse outcome. Eur Heart J 2005; 26: 1180–7.

13

Highly complex anatomical morphologies: percutaneous intervention versus bypass surgery

Leonardo C Clavijo and Augusto Pichard

What constitutes a complex coronary intervention? • What constitutes an anatomically complex lesion? • The role of intravascular ultrasound in complex percutaneous intervention • Specific anatomical subsets

WHAT CONSTITUTES A COMPLEX CORONARY INTERVENTION?

Complex coronary interventions are those associated with an increased rate of technical failure, morbidity, and mortality. Factors associated with complex coronary interventions include coronary artery anatomy, lesion-specific characteristic, and patient-related cardiac and non-cardiac characteristics (Table 13.1).[1]

WHAT CONSTITUTES AN ANATOMICALLY COMPLEX LESION?

Unfavorable anatomy refers to coronary artery and specific lesion characteristics that limit the ability to access, cross, dilate, or deliver a stent or device to the lesion. In addition, lesion-specific unfavorable characteristics increase the risk of procedural complications, including: dissection, thrombotic occlusion, non-reflow, side-branch closure, and perforation.[1]

It is essential to balance the immediate procedural risk of a complex percutaneous coronary intervention (PCI) with that of coronary artery bypass grafting (CABG), and medical therapy. It is our practice to defer complex PCIs until a detailed lesion and patient-specific risk–benefit analysis has been performed, discussed with the patient, and all therapeutic alternatives reviewed. In fact, most of our complex coronary interventions are performed as a separate procedure offering the secondary benefits of limiting the amount of contrast use during PCI, and allowing enough time to achieve appropriate platelet inhibition at the time of PCI after an oral clopidogrel bolus.

THE ROLE OF INTRAVASCULAR ULTRASOUND IN COMPLEX PERCUTANEOUS CORONARY INTERVENTION

We performed intravascular ultrasound (IVUS) before and after all complex coronary interventions. In our experience IVUS prior to complex PCIs is a valuable tool to appropriately select devices and formulate a revascularization strategy; IVUS

Table 13.1   Characteristics contributing to percutaneous coronary angioplasty complexity

Type A: Low risk	Lesion type Type B: moderate risk	Type C: high risk
Length <10 mm	Length 10–20 mm	Length >20 mm
Easily accessible	Moderate proximal tortuosity	Excessive proximal tortuosity
<45° of angulation	>45° but <90° of angulation	>90° of angulation
Less than totally occlusive	Total occlusion <3 months	Total occlusion >3 months
No branch involvement	Bifurcation able to protect the side branch	Bifurcation unable to protect the side branch
Smooth contour	Irregular contour	Degenerated vein graft
Mild or no calcification	Moderate to heavy calcification	
Concentric	Eccentric	
No thrombus	Thrombus present	
Not ostial	Ostial location	
Patient characteristics		
cardiac	non-cardiac	
ejection fraction <25%	age	
acute clinical presentation	renal insufficiency	
hemodynamic status	diabetes	
	peripheral arterial disease	
	difficult vascular access	

permits accurate assessment of the degree of calcification, ostial involvement, side branch involvement, and lesion composition, and is very accurate in establishing true vessel size and lesion length,[2,3] If the lesion cannot be crossed with the IVUS catheter due to calcification, we routinely perform rotational atherectomy. After stenting, IVUS helps to determine stent expansion and apposition, full lesion coverage, and minimal cross-sectional area, and helps avoiding gaps in overlapping segments and rule out edge dissections.

SPECIFIC ANATOMICAL SUBSETS

Bifurcations

Despite advancements in drug-eluting stent technology, coronary bifurcations remain some of the most complex and challenging interventions, at least in part due to the inadequacy of current technology to conform to the bifurcating coronary anatomy and appropriately cover the side-branch ostium. Bifurcation lesions are associated with increased risk of side-branch closure due to plaque shifting, side-branch ostial recoil, and/or propagation of dissection.[4] Anatomical features associated with increased risk of side-branch closure include side-branch size, angulation from the main vessel, side-branch ostial involvement, and side-branch ostial composition. We based our approach to intervention in coronary bifurcations on IVUS lesion assessment of both the main vessel and side branch (Figure 13.1). We favor

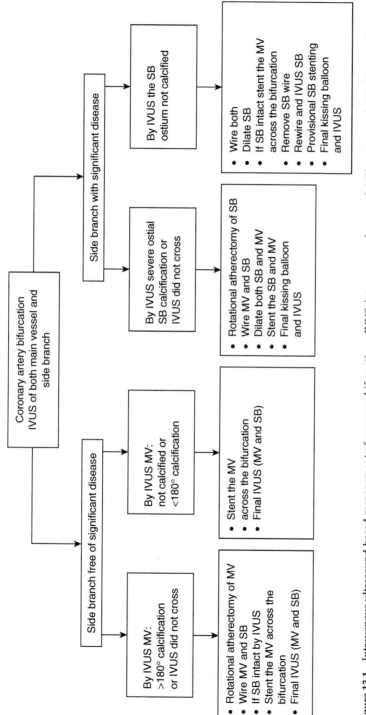

Figure 13.1 Intravenous ultrasound-based management of coronary bifurcations. IVUS, intravenous ultrasound; MV, main vessel; SB, side branch.

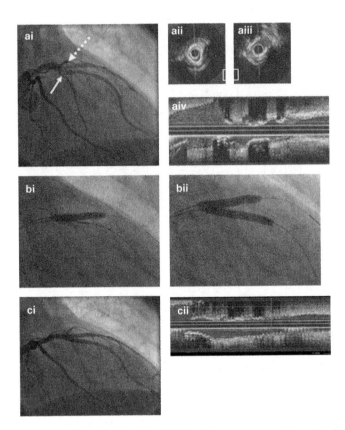

Figure 13.2 Coronary bifurcation stenting. (ai) Baseline coronary angiography demonstrates severe obstructive disease of the left anterior descending artery (LAD) and first diagonal branch (D1) bifurcation; (aii) IVUS cross-section at the ostium of D1 reveals 360° severe calcification; (aiii) and (aiv) IVUS cross-section and long axis views of the LAD reveal tandem severe concentric calcified lesions. Rotational atherectomy of both the LAD and D1 was performed. (bi) Double barrel stenting of the LAD and D1 deploying each stent separately at 20 atmospheres; (bii) kissing balloon at 10 atmospheres. (ci) and (cii) Final angiography and IVUS demonstrate excellent angiographic result, complete stent expansion and apposition, and carina formation

the use of a single stent across the bifurcation when the ostium of the side branch is free of significant disease.[5,6] If the side-branch ostium is diseased but not severely calcified, we first dilate the side branch, stent the main vessel, and reserve side-branch provisional stenting for suboptimal IVUS results. In cases of severe fibrocalcific disease in the ostium of the side branch, or if unable to cross with the IVUS catheter, we perform rotational atherectomy. Rotational atherectomy of the side branch is usually followed by stenting, unless the IVUS and angiographic results are pristine. When two stents are required and the vessels are of large size, main-branch ≥3.0 mm and side branch ≥2.75 mm, we prefer to use the simultaneous kissing stent (double-barrel stenting) technique (Figure 13.2). Even in the absence of ostial side-branch disease we recommend wiring and protecting the side branch if the internal angle of the bifurcation is less than 45° or if the side branch is 2.0–2.5 mm.

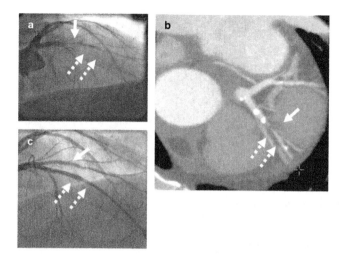

Figure 13.3   Chronic total occlusion percutaneous revascularization. (a) Baseline coronary angiography demonstrates chronic total occlusion of the left anterior descending artery (dotted line), and subtotal occlusion of a large diagonal branch; (b) computed tomography revealed a short segment of moderately calcified occlusion, therefore favorable for a percutaneous approach; (c) final angiographic result after simultaneous kissing stenting with two drug-eluting stents.

Chronic total occlusions

Chronic total occlusions (CTO) are present in approximately 20–40% of patients with angiographic evidence of coronary artery disease (CAD), and represent approximately 10% of PCIs.[7] The rationale for attempting recanalization of a chronically occluded coronary artery includes symptom improvement, normalization of a positive stress test, improvement of left ventricular function, prevention of arrhythmias, and decreased need for CABG surgery.[8] Traditionally, because of high rates of restenosis associated with CTOs, in patients with multivessel CAD the presence of a CTO tilted the balance towards bypass surgery, despite the distribution and characteristics of the other lesions.[9] Nowadays, because of excellent results with drug-eluting stents in CTOs (which decreased restenosis rates from 30–40% with bare-metal stents to <10% with drug-eluting stents),[10,11] and advancements in computerized tomography (CT) scanning resolution, the focus has shifted to achieving complete revascularization by selecting CTOs with a high likelihood of successful revascularization, and considering other associated coronary lesions to accomplish global myocardial perfusion. We now perform CT angiography in patients considered for a CTO revascularization procedure; it not only provides a roadmap during intervention, but is highly predictive of revascularization success (Figure 13.3).[12] Increased length and calcification of a chronic occlusion by CT angiography correlates with low chance of percutaneous coronary revascularization success, and favors coronary artery bypass surgery.

The success rate for recanalization of total occlusions has increased significantly (to 90% in expert hands) thanks to the new wires and techniques.[13]

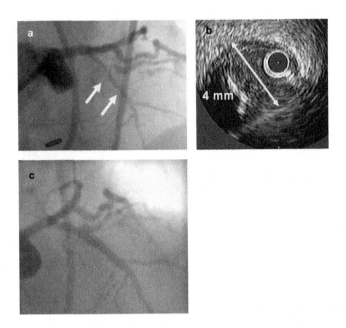

Figure 13.4   Vessel size discrepancy between angiography and intravascular ultrasound. (a) Baseline coronary angiography demonstrates a diffusely diseased left anterior descending artery (arrows), angiographically 2.25–2.5 mm in diameter; (b) intravascular ultrasound reveals a large vessel (4 mm in diameter) with severe diffuse disease; (c) final angiographic result after stenting with a 3.5 mm-diameter drug-eluting stent.

Very small vessels

There is no clear consensus as to what constitutes a small vessel; nevertheless most trials consider small vessels to be those with a diameter of less than 2.5 mm. Vessels of less than 2.25 mm generally perfuse small areas of myocardium and do not required PCI.

Since angiography frequently underestimates vessel size, IVUS is often required to establish true vessel size (Figure 13.4), determine the need of PCI, select devices, and assess postintervention results.[2] The greatest discrepancy between IVUS and coronary angiography in estimating vessel size is found in diabetic patients, angiographically small vessels, and proximal segments. It is important to differentiate large vessels with diffuse disease and small lumen that appear small angiographically, from true small vessels. Bare-metal stents have similar restenosis rates to optimal balloon angioplasty in small vessels,[14] and cutting balloons seem to offer a restenosis benefit over conventional balloon angioplasty.[15] Late lumen loss after stenting is independent of vessel size; therefore the percentage of restenosis is greater as vessel size decreases.[16] The utmost benefit of drug-eluting stents is for the treatment of small vessels. Rates of restenosis and major adverse cardiac events (MACE) correlate with adequate stent expansion and final minimal lumen area (MLA), consequently it is important to perform IVUS post-stenting of small vessels to ensure a minimum stent area >6 mm^2 in bare-metal stents, and >5 mm^2 in drug-eluting stents.[17]

Very long lesions

In the bare-metal stent era, the treatment of long coronary lesions was associated with a poor outcome because of increased rates of restenosis and need for repeat revascularization procedures. Frequently, treatment of long native coronary lesions requires the use of multiple stents. Whether overlapping stents implantation is associated with worse outcomes has been controversial. Lee et al studied patients with long native coronary lesions treated with either one long or two overlapping bare-metal stents.[18] The in-stent restenosis rate at 6 months was found to be equivalently high in both groups (39% vs. 41%). Kastrati et al also showed that lesion length was a significant independent risk factor for restenosis, and that overlapping stenting was an independent risk factor for restenosis.[19]

Nevertheless, in the contemporary drug-eluting stent era, Degertekin and colleagues demonstrated that overlapping sirolimus-eluting stents (SES) implantation is safe and effective for very long coronary lesions.[20] We recently reported our experience with overlapping drug-eluting stents for the treatment of long, native coronary lesions, and found low target lesion revascularization (TLR) rates (3.6% and 5.5% for overlapping paclitaxel- and sirolimus-eluting stents, respectively), but increased rate of periprocedural myonecrosis (23.6% for overlapping drug-eluting stents vs. 7.7% for non-overlapping drug-eluting stents, $P = 0.04$).[21]

Despite previous concern regarding the risk for thrombosis with increased stent length with overlapping stents, we and others have found no evidence of increased acute or subacute thrombosis.[20,21]

Recently, a subgroup analysis of the paclitaxel-eluting stent trial, TAXUS-V, in patients treated with overlapping paclitaxel-eluting stents showed a higher rate of post-procedural myonecrosis as compared to the control patients.[22] We also observed a higher rate of non-Q-wave myocardial infarction in the overlapping drug-eluting stent group.[21] Consistent with the results from TAXUS-V, our main vessel analysis did not show any differences between overlapping and non-overlapping groups regarding no-reflow phenomenon, abrupt closure, dissection, or distal embolization, and thus these factors were not contributory to the higher rate of non-Q-wave myocardial infarction in the overlapping drug-eluting stent. However, the side-branch analysis demonstrated a higher rate of branch Thrombolysis In Myocardial Infarction (TIMI) flow reduction after implantation of the second overlapping stent. Furthermore, the patients with non-Q-wave myocardial infarction had significantly higher rates of branch occlusion, narrowing, and TIMI flow reduction.

In conclusion, implantation of multiple overlapping drug-eluting stents for the treatment of long, native coronary lesions is associated with high technical success and low restenosis rate. The increased rate of periprocedural myonecrosis does not have any adverse impact on late clinical events.

Left main stenosis

The accepted treatment for left main coronary artery (LMCA) disease is CABG. However, the excellent results obtained with drug-eluting stents have renewed interest in the strategy of unprotected left stenting with drug-eluting stents.[23,24] PCI of the unprotected LMCA is feasible and relatively safe with high technical success, but limited by frequent restenosis, most often involving the left circumflex coronary artery ostium. Price et al performed angiographic surveillance of patients who underwent stenting of the LMCA and reported a need for target lesion revascularization of

38%, and a rate of restenosis of 44% over a median follow-up of 9.2 months.[25] In that study, the angiographic follow-up rate was 98%, and 84% of the patients underwent stenting of the LMCA bifurcation. The pattern of stenosis was focal involving the branch ostia in 81% of cases and, uncommonly, the body of the left main branch.

The lack of drug-eluting stents in sizes larger than 3.5 mm limits the ability to match the LMCA vessel size, and imposes the need to perform aggressive overdilation of the drug-eluting stent with the theoretical disadvantage of polymer disruption. The decision to perform LMCA stenting must be individualized, and take into consideration the morbidity and mortality at each institution. In our hospital the mortality of CABG for treatment of LMCA disease is 0.5%, and 1.2% for elective and emergent cases respectively. Therefore, we do not perform routine LMCA stenting, and reserve this option only for patients who are not candidates for surgery after a cardiovascular surgery consultation.

REFERENCES

1. Ryan TJ, Faxon DP, Gunnar RM et al. Guidelines for the percutaneous transluminal angioplasty: a report of the American College of Cardiology/American Heart Association Task Force on Assessment of Diagnostic and Therapeutic Cardiovascular Procedures (Subcommittee of percuatenous TRansluminal Coronary Angioplasty). Circulation. 1993; 88: 2987–3007.
2. Mintz GS, Pichard AD, Kovach JA et al. Impact of preintervention intravascular ultrasound imaging on transcatheter treatment strategies in coronary artery disease. Am J Cardiol 1994; 73: 423–30.
3. Goldberg SL, Colombo A, Nakamura S et al. Benefit of intracoronary ultrasound in the deployment of Palmaz–Schatz stents. J Am Coll Cardiol 1994; 24: 996–1003.
4. Louvard Y, Lefèvre T, Morice M-C. Percutaneous coronary intervention for bifurcation coronary disease. Heart 2004; 90: 713–22.
5. Pan M, de Lezo JS, Medina A et al. Rapamycin-eluting stents for the treatment of bifurcated coronary lesions: a randomized comparison of a simple versus complex strategy. Am Heart J 2004; 148: 857–64.
6. Colombo A, Moses JW, Morice M-C et al. Randomized study to evaluate sirolimus-eluting stents implanted at coronary bifurcation lesions. Circulation 2004; 109: 1244–9.
7. Detre K, Holubkov R, Kelsey S et al. and Co-investigators of the National Heart Lung and Blood Institute's Percutaenous Coronary Angioplasty Registry: percutaneous transluminal coronary angioplasty in 1985–1986 and 1977–1981: The National Heart, Lung, and Blood Institute Registry. N Engl J Med 1988; 318: 265–270.
8 Bell MR, Berger PB, Bresnahan JF et al. Initial and long-term outcome of 354 patients after coronary ballon angioplasty of total coronary artery occlusions. Circulation 1992; 85: 1003–11.
9. Delacrétaz E, Meier B. Therapeutic strategy with total coronary artery occlusions. Am J Cardiol 1997; 79: 185–7.
10. Suttorp M. PRISON II. A prospective randomized trial of sirolimus-eluting and bare-metal stents in patients with chronic total occlusions. TCT 2005; October 16–21, 2005; Washington, DC. (http://www.tct2005.com/index.php?page_id=1525)
11. Werner GS, Krack A, Schwarz G et al. Prevention of lesion recurrence in chronic total occlusions by paclitaxel-eluting stents. J Am Coll Cardiol 2004; 44: 2301–6.
12. Mollet NR, Hoye A, Lemos PA et al. Value of preprocedure multislice computed tomographic coronary angiography to predict the outcome of percutaneous recanalization of chronic total occlusions. Am J Cardiol 2005; 95: 240–3.
13. Nakamura S, Muthusamy TS, Bae JH, Cahyadi YH et al. Impact of sirolimus-eluting stent on the outcome of patients with chronic total occlusions. Am J Cardiol 2005; 95: 161–6.

14. Agostino P, Biondi-Zoccai GL, Gasparini GL et al. Is bare-metal stenting superior to balloon angioplasty for small vessel coronary artery disease? Evidence from a meta-analysis of randomized trials. Eur Heart J 2005; 26: 881–9.
15. Izumi M, Tsuchikane E, Funamoto M et al. Final results of the CAPAS trial. Am Heart J 2001; 142: 782–9.
16. Hoffman R., Mintz GS, Mehran R et al. Intimal hyperplasia thickness is independent of stent size: A serial intravascular ultrasound study. J Am Coll Cardiol 1998; 31: 2 (Suppl): 881–5.
17. Sonoda S, Morino Y, Ako J et al. Impact of final stent dimensions on long-term results following sirolimus-eluting stent implantation. Serial intravascular ultrasound analysis from the SIRIUS trial. J Am Coll Cardiol 2004; 43: 1959–63.
18. Lee SH, Jang Y, Oh SJ et al. Overlapping vs. one long stenting in long coronary lesions. Catheter Cardiovasc Interv 2004; 62: 298–302.
19. Kastrati A, Elezi S, Dirschinger J et al. Influence of lesion length on restenosis after coronary stent placement. Am J Cardiol 1999; 83: 1617–22.
20. Degertekin M, Arampatzis CA, Lemos PA, Saia F et al. Very long sirolimus-eluting stent implantation for de novo coronary lesions. Am J Cardiol 2004; 93: 826–9.
21. Chu WW, Kuchulakanti PK, Torguson R et al. Impact of overlapping drug-eluting stents in patients undergoing percutaneous coronary intervention. Catheter Cardiovasc Interv 2006; 67: 595–9.
22. Stone GW, Ellis SG, Cannon L, et al; TAXUS V Investigators. Comparison of a polymer-based paclitaxel-eluting stent with a bare-metal stent in patients with complex coronary artery disease: a randomized controlled trial. JAMA 2005; 294: 1215–23.
23. Valgimigli M, Malagutti P, Aoki J et al. Sirolimus-eluting stent versus paclitaxel-eluting stent implantation for the percutaneous treatment of left main coronary artery disease. A combined RESEARCH and T-SEARCH long-term analysis. J Am Coll Cardiol 2006; 47: 507–14.
24. Park SJ, Hong MK, Lee CW et al. Elective stenting of unprotected left main coronary artery stenosis: effect of debulking before stenting and intravascular ultrasound guidance. J Am Coll Cardiol 2001; 38: 1054–60.
25. Price MJ, Cristea E, Sawhney N et al. Serial angiographic follow-up of sirolimus-eluting stents for unprotected left main coronary artery revascularization. J Am Coll Cardiol 2006; 47: 871–7.

14

Advanced atherosclerotic diseases in multiple vascular bed sites

Luis A Guzman and Theodore Bass

Atherosclerosis • Associations between the pathogenic process and clinical manifestations • Epidemiology and involvement of multiple vascular beds • Atherosclerosis and renal artery stenosis • Coronary and carotid artery atherosclerosis • Atherosclerosis in the lower extremities • Contrast-induced nephropathy in patients with multiple vascular beds • Conclusions

Atherosclerosis is a complex and systemic disease. Even though the most common clinical presentation of the disease involves the coronary arteries, multiple vascular beds are usually implicated. The involvement of multiple vascular beds appears to be an expression of more advanced process associated with worse prognosis. The understanding of this process is critical for the development of preventive strategies, and institution of appropriate treatment. New imaging modalities have significantly improved our understanding, and provide an opportunity for early detection of the disease process. Technological advances have made possible the utilization of more effective and lower-risk percutaneous revascularization techniques to improve symptoms and decrease morbidity and mortality in the different anatomical territories. In this chapter we will discuss the atherosclerotic process and its manifestations in different territories, the epidemiological and clinical implications of the disease, as well as the global invasive approach to the multiple vascular bed involvement of these patients.

ATHEROSCLEROSIS

Atherosclerosis is a complex systemic disease involving mainly medium and large arteries, including not only the coronary arteries but the aorta, the carotid, the renal, and the lower-extremity arteries. It initially affects the intima of the vessels, and progressively affects the media as well as the adventitia. Recently, the American Heart Association Committee on Vascular Lesion divided the atherosclerotic process into five phases with different plaque components in each phase (Figure 14.1).[1] This description importantly takes into consideration not only the pathological components but also the clinical manifestations of the process. Atherosclerosis is a heterogeneous process, with different proportions of plaque components in different plaques within the same patient and within the same artery, as well as a dynamic process, with different components at different stages of the evolution of the process, with the possibility of returning to a prior stage of the process. From the pathological stand point, atherosclerotic lesions have been classified into seven different types according to the plaque composition.[2] The different lesion types

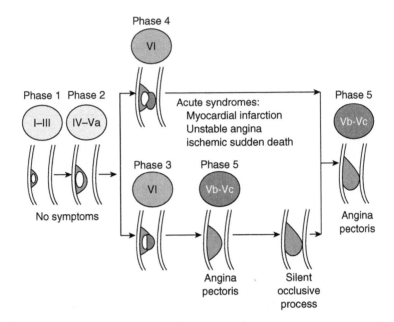

Figure 14.1   Phases of the Atherosclerotic Process. American Heart Association Committee on Vascular Lesion.[1]

develop as a consequence of a complex pathophysiological mechanism at the cellular and molecular level, with participation of multiple pro-inflammatory cytokines, growth factors, matrix metalloproteinase, and coagulation factors. In the early phases, endothelial dysfunction is the main contributor. The exposure to multiple hemodynamic (shear stress, high blood pressure) and biohumoral factors (high cholesterol, high glucose, etc), causes the endothelium to gradually lose its protective function, with the consequent loss of vessel wall homeostasis. Increased permeability to circulating lipoproteins and monocytes creates an intraplaque inflammatory state which will stimulate the proliferation of smooth muscle cells, deposition of extracellular matrix, and development of a prothrombotic environment (phase 1 and lesions type I–III). Continuous exposure of the pro-atherogenic milieu will increase chemotaxis of monocytes and other pro-inflammatory cells, leading to lipid accumulation, necrotic core, and fibrous cap formation, characteristics of the more advanced atherosclerotic process.

ASSOCIATION BETWEEN THE PATHOGENIC PROCESS AND CLINICAL MANIFESTATIONS

Vulnerable plaque and the vulnerable patient

Even though atherosclerosis progresses in subclinical forms, the smaller subset of patients presenting with clinical manifestations usually carry a significant morbidity and mortality risk. The clinical manifestations of the atherosclerotic process are primarily related to the concept of vulnerable plaque, and the presence of thrombotic complications. A significant amount of information has linked the presence of a prothrombotic, *'vulnerable plaque'*, and the incidence of an acute coronary event. Based on pathological studies, plaque rupture is the most common substrate for coronary thrombosis and accounts for 60–70% of the cases. In the remaining 30–40% of cases, coronary thrombosis occurs at the site of erosion without evidence of plaque rupture.[3] Systemic procoagulant activity also plays a role in the development of thrombotic complications of the atherosclerotic process – the *'vulnerable patient'*. Among them, cigarette smoking, changes in lipid metabolism (mainly increases slow-density lipoprotein (LDL)), hyperglycemia, increase in circulating tissue factor, and pro-inflammatory factors (like C-reactive protein (CRP), and CD-40 ligand), are all associated with a systemic prothrombotic state. According to the magnitude of the process, the clinical manifestations vary from an asymptomatic event, a non-ST elevation acute coronary syndrome (ACS), an ST elevation ACS or sudden death.

The demonstration of a vulnerable plaque and its association with clinical events appears very compelling in the coronary arteries. However, the clinical manifestation in other vascular beds and its pathological characteristics are not as well studied. It is the paradigm that ischemic strokes and transient ischemic attacks (TIAs) are frequently the consequence of a cerebral embolism from a thrombotic plaque or thrombosis at the site of the plaque rupture.[4] The recent development in imaging and molecular imaging modalities including intravascular ultrasound, magnetic resonance imaging (MRI), and computer tomography, has significantly improved the understanding of the pathophysiology of the atherosclerotic process in different territories. In the carotid territory, plaque rupture has also been identified as the main contributor of ischemic events. Plaque composition is an important determinant of future rupture; however, a major role is played by the systemic high-energy blood flow.[5-9] Intraplaque hemorrhage as a consequence of rupture of the vasa vasorum has been also significantly associated with clinical events in the carotid territory.[10] Recent studies however, have associated the presence of intraplaque hemorrhages with the classical characteristics of vulnerable or 'high-risk' plaque described for the coronary lesions.[11] Even though still not well demonstrated, the involvement of systemic blood composition and thrombogenicity, the 'vulnerable patient', does not appear to be as significant a player in the carotid territory as it is in the coronary.[12]

In the lower extremities, the atherosclerotic process and its clinical manifestations are less known. Acute embolic events are the consequence of either an abdominal aorta ruptured plaque with subsequent thrombosis and embolization, or from a cardiac source. However, these are less common events and an even less frequent mechanism of progression of the disease. Plaque rupture and similar heterogeneous plaque composition like in other territories has been demonstrated in this territory. Recent studies have shown 'high risk' lesions in the peripheral arteries, with large lipid and necrotic core with thrombus in the lumen similar to those found in the coronaries. However, thrombosis is generally observed on the surface of a frequently fibrotic and severely stenotic lesion. Clinical manifestations appear to be more related with the degree of stenosis. In this territory, systemic thrombogenicity associated with classical risk factors (cigarette smoking, hyperglycemia, etc) appears to play a significant role in progression of the atherothrombotic process.[13-16]

Acute clinical events in multiple vascular beds

The concept of multiple vascular bed involvement within the same diseases process appears more compelling based on recent evidence that patients with acute problems in one vascular territory are at higher risk of developing major acute clinical events in other territories. The evidence supports the concept that plaque instability is not merely a local vascular incident, but occurs at multiple sites in the entire vascular bed. The presence of multiple acute coronary lesions in patients admitted with an ACS has been clearly demonstrated in several reports.[17] In the European Carotid Surgery Study, among 3007 patients with cerebrovascular accident (CVA), patients with irregular angiographic plaques had significantly higher incidence of irregular plaques in the contralateral carotid artery.[18] Importantly, these patients were more prone to develop subsequent coronary events as compared with patients with smooth plaques, and were more likely to have a non-stroke vascular death, mainly coronary, at follow-up (hazard ratio 1.67 (range 1.15–2.44), $P=0.007$). On the other hand, the presence of prior myocardial infarction (MI) was significantly associated with more irregular carotid plaques at the time of presentation with neurological symptoms (hazard ratio 1.82 (range 1.23–2.64), $P<0.001$). Lombardo et al found that patients with ACS had a six-times higher incidence of complex carotid plaque as compared with stable coronary patients (odds ratio (OR) 6.09; 95% confidence interval (CI) 1.01–33).[19] The prevalence of complex carotid plaque was 23% in patients presenting with ACS versus 3.2% in patients with stable coronary syndromes ($P<0.001$).

Thus, significant pathophysiological and, more importantly, clinical links exist among atherosclerosis in different territories. It is likely that a comprehensive evaluation could provide important prognostic information for the global risk stratification. Evaluation of a particular territory provides important diagnostic and prognostic information not only for the evaluated territory, but also for other vascular territories.

EPIDEMIOLOGY AND INVOLVEMENT OF MULTIPLE VASCULAR BEDS

The clinical consequences of atherosclerosis vary according to the territory involved. Mortality is highly related to the coronary involvement. Cardiac death represents 70% of the overall mortality.[20] Cerebrovascular diseases account for approximately 15% of the death in these patients, and an additional 10% mortality is related to aortic aneurysm and visceral infarction. The involvement of lower extremity arteries, peripheral arterial diseases (PAD), is generally not associated with mortality, and represents only 1–3% of the overall mortality in these patients. However, PAD can be considered a high-risk manifestation of the diseases with three-fold increase in mortality due to cardiovascular diseases as compared with an age-matched control subjects.[21,22] The diagnosis of PAD (symptomatic or not) has a 5% per year mortality rate, and is associated with a 50% 10-year mortality due to cardiac and/or cerebrovascular disease. Approximately 60–70% of patients with clinical manifestations of PAD will have associated coronary artery disease.[20,23–25] Therefore, early diagnosis and aggressive preventive actions are mandatory. The clinical outcome and mortality are significantly associated with the number of territories involved.[24,26,27] The involvement of several territories and its prevalence has been clearly demonstrated in several studies. As shown in Figure 14.2, approximately

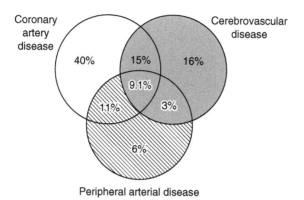

Figure 14.2 Prevalence of atherosclerosis in multiple vascular beds (management of peripheral arterial disease).

30% of patients will have two territories involved, and 98% of patients will have involvement of all three territories.[28]

ATHEROSCLEROSIS AND RENAL ARTERY STENOSIS

Atherosclerotic renal artery stenosis is associated with two common clinical syndromes: renovascular hypertension, and ischemic nephropathy, which often coexist. The presence of renal artery stenosis has been associated with progression to end-stage renal disease, and therefore a potential curable cause of this problem has been suggested. In addition, a high incidence of cardiovascular morbidity and mortality has been associated with the presence of renal artery stenosis. The presence of renal artery stensosis carries a five-fold increase in cardiovascular mortality as compared with an age-matched normal population.[29,30] Importantly, the presence of renal dysfunction played a major role in prognosis in these patients with only a 25–30% five-year survival after renal stenting if the creatinine was >2.5 mg/dl as compared with close to 90% five-year survival if creatinine was normal at the time of the procedure.[31,32] Revascularization, currently the percutaneous approach, is preferred, and has evolved in the last decade, although the clinical impact of this procedure is still controversial. Even though a significant amount of information regarding better blood pressure control and improvement in renal function after renal revascularization in a specific patient population has been demonstrated, prolongation of life after renal revascularization has not been proved. Randomized data comparing percutaneous intervention (balloon or stent) did not show striking differences in favor of revascularization as compared with medical treatment. A modest decrease in blood pressure and modest decreases in the number of blood pressure medications have been reported, with no clear improvement in overall renal function.[33–35] However, major limitations of those trials have been extensively described in order to draw conclusions or make final recommendations (very small sample size, significant cross-over in the medical group, utilization of mainly balloon angioplasty with the high incidence of restenosis, the use of very high-profile and non-dedicated devices, the lack of appropriate definition of treatment effect, etc).[36] Trials currently in progress with larger number of patients, using more advanced technology, with longer follow-up and incorporating clinically meaningful end points (Cardiovascular Outcomes in Renal Atherosclerotic Lesions [CORAL] trial in the USA and the Angioplasty and STent for Renal Artery Lesions [ASTRAL] in the UK), may help to improve our understanding of the role of percutaneous revascularization in this patient population.

Diagnosis of renal artery stenosis in the catheterization lab

The diagnosis of renal artery stenosis has been significantly overlooked. Controversy remains on which patient population and which screening test provides the best balance between accuracy, safety and cost. Non-invasive modalities such as Duplex ultrasound, scintigraphic studies, and more recently computed tomography angiography (CTA) and magnetic resonance angiography (MRA) appear to be the first-line diagnostic tools. Even though the specificity of these new non-invasive imaging modalities appears to be over 90%, the sensitivity has been questioned, falling to 60% and therefore they are not considered gold standards.[37] Digital angiography remains the gold standard. Several clinical features may suggest the presence of renal artery stenosis and the need for further evaluation (Table 14.1). Non-invasive evaluation will be the first approach in these patients. If the study cannot clearly define the presence or degree of stenosis, or it demonstrates the presence of significant stenosis, invasive angiography will be indicated as a confirmatory diagnostic test. Some of the concerns regarding renal angiography were the incidence of complications associated to the procedure. Even though vascular complications represent some of the limitations of the invasive evaluation, the utilization of very low-profile 4F systems has significantly decreased this problem. The most serious complications however, were the incidence of contrast-induced nephropathy and the presence of embolic complications. Non-selective visualization rather than selective renal arteriography, using a pig-tail or a flush catheter, should be the preferred approach. It avoids the risk of serious embolic complications as a consequence of catheter manipulation in a commonly diseased abdominal aorta. Digital subtraction angiography (DSA) should be a mandatory invasive modality for the diagnosis of renal artery stenosis. It provides very accurate images in a single shot with low contrast volume injection. The utilization of both DSA and non-selective visualization significantly decreases the incidence of complications, making this procedure very safe. In a minority of cases this needs to be followed by selective angiography if doubts remain about the significance of a stenosis. Even though not based on validated scientific information, measurement of spontaneous translesion gradient will be recommended in those patients with intermediate stenosis (50–70%), if revascularization is considered. A straight end-hole 4F catheter has been the usual approach; however, measurements using a coronary flow wire have been reported to provide more accurate results. The cut-off limit for considering a lesion hemodynamically significant varies among different studies, with the majority of reports considering gradients above 15–20 mmHg as significant.[38] For the flow wire, the information is less clear. Regardless, the gradient measured with this methodology appears to better correlate with the minimal lumen diameter rather than the percentage of stenosis.[39]

Table 14.1   Clinical features suggestive of atherosclerotic renal artery stenosis
Hypertension or hypertension associated with:

- onset less than 2 years
- onset after age 55 years without family history
- refractory hypertension (HTN) to treatment with ≥ 3 drugs
- increased and refractory HTN in a previously controlled patient
- progressive unexplained renal insufficiency
- abrupt rise in serum creatinine after angiotensin-converting enzyme inhibition treatment
- various atherosclerotic manifestation and/or abdominal aortic aneurysm
- flash pulmonary edema in patient with normal left ventricular and no CAD
- abdominal bruit
- significant discrepancy in size between the two kidneys
- low-grade proteinuria with otherwise unremarkable urinary sediment

Renal angiography in the context of coronary catheterization

Due to the prognostic information as well as the potential percutaneous treatment, routine evaluation of the renal arteries in the setting of a cardiac catheterization has been proposed.[40] However, controversy still remains as to which patient population should be screened in the context of peripheral or coronary catheterization. Prospective and retrospective studies of renal angiography in the setting of cardiac catheterization have shown a prevalence of renal artery stenosis between 11% and 18%.[41-44] Several studies recently have tried to develop predictors of renal artery stenosis in order to further narrow down the group of patients who benefit the most from having an angiographic evaluation in the context of cardiac catheterization. The majority of those studies have found that elderly patients, female sex, the presence of renal dysfunction, the higher number of antihypertension drugs, and the presence of more extensive CAD or of PVD are the major predictors of renal artery stenosis. According to the number of the predictive factors, Cohen et al recently reported a score to predict renal artery stenosis in this context.[44] The prevalence of renal artery stenosis ranged from 0.6% for lower scores, to up to 60% for patients with a score ≥ 18 (Table 14.2). A score ≥ 11 provides the best prediction with a sensitivity 76% and specificity of 71%. Even though based on this or other similar scores one could better define the group with higher prevalence, due to the very low procedural risk, it is still controversial to whether or not lower-risk patients or even all patients undergoing coronary angiography should undergo non-selective renal angiography. The concerns and recommendations mentioned before, regarding contrast utilization, catheter manipulation and the use of DSA will apply to this indication as well.

CORONARY AND CAROTID ARTERY ATHEROSCLEROSIS

A significant number of studies have suggested the association between coronary and carotid artery diseases. Co-existence of both problems has been reported.

Table 14.2   Major predictor factors associated with the presence of renal artery stenosis

Predictor factor	Score
Female sex	2
Age (years)	
>64	0
64–72	2
>73	4
Three-vessel CAD or prior CABG	2
HTN medications	
0–1 drugs	0–1
2 drugs	3
≥3 drugs	4
Creatinine (mg/dl)	
>0.8	0
1.0–1.2	3
1.4–1.6	6
1.8–2.0	9
>2.2	12
Presence of PVD	4

Approximately 15–20% of patients with CAD will have concurrent carotid artery disease.[45] Approximately 40% of patients undergoing coronary bypass (CABG) surgery will have some degree of carotid diseases, and 10% will have associated severe carotid artery stenosis. On the other hand, carotid atherosclerosis significantly correlated with the extension and severity of CAD, evaluated not only by angiography but also by myocardial perfusion.[45,46] Plaque characteristics of the carotid artery significantly correlate with prognosis in patients with CAD. Honda and coworkers evaluated almost 300 mainly stable patients with CAD. The presence of echolucent plaque not only predicted the presence of more complex coronary lesions, but over a 30-month follow-up, patients with echolucent plaques had a 26% incidence of new coronary events versus 4% in patients without echolucent plaques (OR7.0; 95% CI, 2.3–21, $P=0.001$).[47] In the French Aortic Plaque in Stroke Group (FAPS), in which patients were admitted with ischemic strokes, the presence of complex aortic plaques visualized by trans esophageal echocardiogram (TEE) was associated with higher incidence of coronary events during the follow-up.[48] Patients with larger plaque had 4–5 times higher relative risk of cardiovascular events, and large plaque without calcification had 10 times higher relative risk of developing cardiovascular events over a four-year period (relative risk 10.3; 95% CI, 4.2 to 25.2; $P<0.001$). Thus, evidence supports a significant association between ischemic stroke, the presence of carotid artery disease and CAD.

Concurrent carotid disease in patients scheduled for coronary artery bypass surgery

More than 20 years ago Brener and coworkers evaluated 2026 patients undergoing CABG for the presence of carotid artery stenosis.[49] Even though the incidence was low, they found that the incidence of hemispheric neurological deficit following cardiac surgery in the 47 patients with carotid disease was 14.9%, whereas the incidence in patients without carotid disease was 1.9% ($P < 0.001$). Since then, it has remained clear that the presence of carotid artery diseases carries an increased risk for patients undergoing CABG. More contemporary information showed similar findings. Based on several studies, the stroke risk for CABG is <1.8%, with <50% carotid diseases, 3.0% in unilateral asymptomatic 50–99% stenosis, 5.2% if bilateral carotid stenosis is present, and 11.2% in patients with unilateral carotid occlusion.[50–52] On the other hand, carotid endarterectomy carries a 12% combined incidence of death, stroke, and MI in a higher-risk population; in particular, advanced coronary artery disease has been identified as the major risk factor for this procedure.[53,54] Co-existence of carotid and coronary diseases can present significant management challenge, over and above that posed by the respective conditions in isolation. Even though the guidelines by the American Heart Association (AHA)/American College of Cardiology (ACC) state that carotid endarterectomy is probably recommended before CABG or concomitant to CABG in patients with a symptomatic carotid stenosis, or in asymptomatic patients with a unilateral or bilateral internal carotid stenosis of 80% or more (Indication IIa; Level of Evidence: C), significant controversy regarding this recommendation still persists.[55] Even though retrospective studies have clearly demonstrated an increased risk, the presence of carotid artery stenosis by itself was not found to be an independent predictor of adverse clinical events. The etiology of stroke has been considered multifactorial and not only related to carotid artery diseases.[52] Another important consideration in this group of patients is a lack of data regarding whether combined surgery, a staged procedure, or no procedure at all is the indicated treatment approach. In fact, recent systematic review of 97 published studies following 8972 staged or synchronous operations, concluded that in asymptomatic patients, the available data do not support a clear benefit in stroke prevention by performing carotid endarterectomy (either staged or synchronous procedures) in the context of CABG.[52,56] The death and stroke rate was 9.5% (95% CI 7.2–11.8) for combined procedure, and 6.6% (95% CI 4.4–8.8) for staged procedure. Even though no clear information exists and even less data from comparison studies, the incidence of major clinical events appears to be similar to the rate in patients with carotid stenosis undergoing bypass surgery without carotid treatment. This raises two main questions. The first one is whether or not patients scheduled to undergo CABG operation will require a previous evaluation of the status of the carotid arteries, and second, if a stenosis is found what is the treatment approach. The second question does not appear to have a clear-cut answer. The decision to intervene or not will be left to each practice standard, taking into consideration each particular patient. Proposed criteria for higher-risk patients in whom revascularization (concomitant or staged) would be advisable, include: a greater than 80% stenosis in the dominant hemisphere, contralateral occlusion, and >50% stenosis, unilateral symptomatic >70% stenosis, and bilateral stenosis when the addition of both lesions is >150%.[57]

Who should be screened and how?

Due to the increased stroke risk, some surgeons mandate the screening of every patient for the presence of carotid disease prior to bypass surgery. However, this approach is still controversial and not accepted in many centers. Even though the prevalence of the disease is not negligible, the majority of patients will have no significant findings, making screening every patient not cost-effective. Several studies have tried to determine the population at higher risk for concomitant coronary and carotid diseases, focusing the screening to this group of patients. Table 14.3 summarizes the clinical findings associated with higher incidence of carotid stenosis, which helps to select the population in whom the screening will be recommended. This recommendation will be primarily for assessment of the patient surgical risk. Several diagnostic tests are available. The most commonly used with very high sensitivity (99%) and good specificity (84%), is the carotid duplex ultrasound.[58] New imaging modalities such as CTA and MRA are excellent techniques with very high diagnostic accuracy; however, several limitations of these two techniques, including higher cost, equipment availability, the need for large amount of contrast, radiation exposure, etc, make ultrasound the primary screening modality, but either or both techniques can be used for confirmatory indications. Contrast angiography is also a very accurate diagnostic modality; however, limitations of this technique include the fact that it is an invasive procedure and carries a small but not negligible risk of stroke. Therefore angiography should not be considered as part of the screening test. Some investigators, however, have suggested the visualization of the carotid arteries in the context of a diagnostic coronary angiography if, based on the findings, the patient will be considered a candidate for surgical revascularization. There is not a clear recommendation for this approach, and several limitations including increase in contrast utilization, radiation exposure, procedural time, as well as the increase in stroke risk, make the recommendation for all patients not advisable. Even though some of the limitation could be overcome by non-selective aortic arch injection, and by obtaining images with DSA in the catheterization lab suite with larger image intensifier, clear visualization and opening of the carotid bifurcation might not be possible, and selective visualization in multiple projections will be frequently required. Therefore, only the subgroup of patients with the association of high-risk clinical characteristic should be considered candidates for combined coronary and carotid angiography (Table 14.3).

Table 14.3   Carotid artery diseases in the context of coronary artery bypass surgery

Predictors of carotid artery diseases

- Advanced age > 65 years
- Female sex
- Prior cerebrovascular accident or transient ischemic attack
- Smoking habit
- Carotid bruit
- Advanced CAD or LMT
- History of PVD

Predictors of neurological events after coronary artery bypass surgery

- Prior CEA
- Advanced age
- History of PVD
- Symptomatic carotid stenosis
- Stenosis > 50% with contralateral occlusion
- Unilateral carotid stenosis > 80%

CEA, carotid endartherectomy; LMT, left main trunk.

The role of carotid stenting in patients scheduled for coronary artery bypass surgery

Carotid artery stenting has recently emerged as a promising alternative to surgical carotid endarterectomy. Several prospective registries and randomized trials have shown results at least as good as surgical revascularization in high-risk patients, mainly with co-existent coronary artery diseases.[53,59,60] For this reason, and due to the high incidence of complication with the combined or staged coronary and carotid surgical revascularization, carotid stenting prior to CABG surgery appears to be a reasonable alternative. To date, no randomized data are available, and no current trials are addressing the role of carotid stenting in this group of patients. Few small studies based on single-center experience have been reported. Overall, six studies with a total of 242 patients undergoing a staged carotid stenting followed by CABG have been reported. In all the studies, stable patients were included with the majority of the coronary procedures performed several weeks after the carotid intervention. The incidence of clinical events 30 days after bypass surgery, including all events after carotid stenting, were as follows: stroke was 3.6%, mortality 7.4%, and the incidence of death and stroke, 9.5% (Table 14.4).[57,61-65] Importantly, there were only two patients (0.8%) that died during the stent procedure; the majority of the events occurred during bypass surgery, again reinforcing the concept of a higher-risk population independently of solving the carotid problem. Even though this is encouraging information, these numbers represent a very small group of patients in selected centers. In addition, the combined incidence of stroke and mortality is still significantly elevated, and more importantly these events were mainly associated with the bypass surgical procedure (stroke associated with stent, 2.4% and mortality 0.8%; stroke during surgery, 1.2% and mortality 6.6%). More information is required in order to better understand the role of carotid revascularization in the context of CABG surgery in general, and stenting in particular.

Table 14.4   Carotid artery angioplasty/stenting in patients scheduled for coronary artery bypass surgery with concomitant diseases: 30 days event rate

Investigators	Year	*n*	</> Stroke	Death	Death/stroke
Babatasi et al	1996	12	1/0	0	1
Waigand et al[a]	1998	50	1/1	3	4
Lopes et al	2002	49	0/1	4	5
Ziada et al	2005	56	0/1	3	4
Kovacic et al	2006	23	1/0	0	1
Randall et al[b]	2006	52	1/2	8	8
Total		242	4/5 (3.6%)	18 (7.4%)	23 (9.5%)

Results include events from the carotid stent procedure up to 30 days after surgery. >, major stroke; <, minor stroke.
[a]Two deaths were 2 weeks after surgery and not related with neurological problems. The major stroke was fatal and it was related to the stent procedure.
[b]All the strokes were after bypass surgery. One death was related to the carotid stenting procedure, and the remaining seven to the bypass surgical procedure.

ATHEROSCLEROSIS IN THE LOWER EXTREMITIES

Atherosclerosis affecting the lower extremities (PAD) is the most common form of peripheral vascular disease (PVD). The incidence of asymptomatic PAD in the 55–74-year-old age range is about 10%.[66] However, the incidence varies according to age, with 2.5% incidence in those below 60 years, 8.3% between 60–69 years and >19% in those older than 70 years.[67] Individuals with PAD, whether asymptomatic or not, face a risk of progressive limb ischemia. However, only a minority will progress to critical limb ischemia and amputation (1–2%). The symptoms of chronic PAD progress rather slowly over time. Thus, after 5–10 years, more than 70% of patients report either no change or improvement in their symptoms, while 20–30% have progressive symptoms. However, more importantly, the vast majority of these patients with PAD will have a short-term high risk for cardiovascular morbidity and mortality, including MI and stroke (30% prevalence at 5 years). For this reason, the main target treatment in this patient population is the prevention of cardiovascular events. All patients with PAD should achieve risk reduction and treatment targeting blood pressure control, antiplatelet treatment, lipid lowering, and use of angiotensin-converting enzyme inhibitors (ACEI) similarly to patients with coronary artery diseases.[55] Approximately 30% of this population will have symptoms or clinical situations in which revascularization modalities will be considered. It is important to emphasize that at present, no revascularization procedure has been proven to prolong life. The main indication is to improve quality of life and/or to preserve limb viability. The recently published ACC/AHA guidelines give a Class 1 recommendation for revascularization for symptomatic patients. However, they state that patients with symptoms of claudication should have significant functional impairment with a reasonable likelihood of symptomatic improvement with the planned procedure (an absence of other diseases that would limit the exercise ability) before undergoing an evaluation for revascularization.[55]

Prognostic implications of peripheral vascular disease in patients with coronary artery disease

The presence of PAD is a high-risk manifestation for patients with chronic stable coronary diseases, and has been associated with worse outcome in patients admitted with acute coronary syndromes.[68–70] Among 10 281 patients admitted with acute coronary syndromes in the Orbofiban in Patients with Unstable Coronary Syndromes–Thrombolysis In Myocardial Infarction (OPUS-TIMI) 16 trial, 11% had symptoms or history of PAD.[68] The 10-month mortality rate was 8.8% for PAD-positive patients versus 3.9% ($P<0.001$) for PAD-negative patients (OR 1.4; 95% CI 1.1–1.8). The incidence of death and MI was 15.1% versus 8.3%, respectively ($P<0.001$). In patients with chronic stable angina or asymptomatic CAD, the presence of PAD is a strongly associated with a more advance degree of coronary diseases, including three-vessel diseases and higher incidence of significant left main trunk (LMT) stenosis.[71]

The impact of PAD in the in-hospital outcome of patients undergoing coronary revascularization has been emphasized in several studies. Minakata et al found in approximately 600 patients undergoing CABG surgery, that the OR for perioperative MI was 3.4 (95% CI 1.3–8.6), and the OR for in-hospital mortality was 4.3 (95% CI 2.0–9.5).[72] Even though, patients undergoing CABG with history of PAD are generally a sicker population (older age, higher incidence of prior stroke, impaired renal function, etc), several studies have shown that PAD is an independent predictor of very high morbidity and mortality in this setting.[72,73] Similar findings were also reported in the context of percutaneous revascularization. In the Bypass Angioplasty Revascularization Investigation (BARI) trial, patients with PAD had a significant increase in major clinical event, 11.7% versus 7.8% in those without PAD ($P=0.027$).[73] In multivariate analysis, this represented a 50% increase in the odds of having any major complication (multivariate odds ratio, 1.5; $P=0.032$).

Diagnosis of peripheral arterial disease

Based on the epidemiological importance and the possibility for early treatment, diagnosis of PAD has recently been highlighted. Several awareness programs endorsed by different societies have been promoted. The PARTNERS study has clearly demonstrated the high prevalence of the disease, as well as the very large proportion of patients without diagnosis.[74] It also emphasizes the high incidence of asymptomatic patients as well as the very frequent atypical symptoms (Figure 14.3). The most cost-effective, highly specific and sensitive diagnostic screening test for PAD is the ankle/brachial index (ABI). This test can be performed in any physician's office. It provides very valuable diagnostic and prognostic information. Patients with an abnormal ABI (<0.9) have a two-fold increase in cardiovascualr morbidity (MI and stroke) and mortality.[75] In patients with abnormal ABIs and symptoms of limiting claudication or critical limb ischemia, further diagnostic modalities will be indicated if revascularization is considered. Even though angiography remains the goal standard, CTA and MRA are currently widely accepted as the preferred non-invasive imaging modalities for patients with PAD. They provide very accurate images of the aorto-iliac and lower-extremity vascular tree, including below the knee vessels, without the discomfort and risk associated with angiographic invasive study. As stated before, some limitations of these techniques include radiation and contrast exposure, overestimation of the degree of stenosis, availability, etc. These modalities not only provide diagnostic information but are also very helpful in patients with advanced or known PAD, to define access approaches in the context of coronary or peripheral invasive procedures, and difficult anatomies, as well as a treatment approach in the context of percutaneous intervention. Angiography still remains the gold standard, and in case of no clear diagnosis obtained with the non-invasive test or contraindications (claustrophobia, overweight patients, renal dysfunction, permanent pacemaker, etc), angiography will be indicated. In addition, due to the fact that angiography will be the imaging modality to guide a percutaneous intervention, if based on the clinical findings and ABI and/or duplex scan findings, percutaneous intervention will be of high consideration, and angiography would be an appropriate first imaging modality. When performing diagnostic angiography in this particular patient population, certain consideration will be important to highlight. First are vascular access considerations. A thorough clinical history and physical evaluation is mandatory. This is not only to avoid access problems and complications, but also to be able to proceed with revascularization if indicated. If concerns remain regarding access problems, a non-invasive imaging modality might be required before proceeding with the invasive evaluation. History of contrast allergy, renal dysfunction, and recent creatinine should be documented. Many of these patients will have atherosclerotic nephropathy as well as a higher incidence of renal artery stenosis. This information will be important in order to

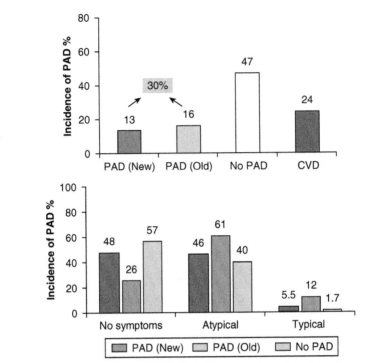

Figure 14.3 Awareness, incidence and clinical presentation of peripheral arterial disease (PAD). The PARTNERS Study.[74] Patients were screened for PAD in primary care offices. (a) Incidence of PAD based on ABI measurement. New, indicates patients newly diagnosed with PAD, and Old indicates patient with history of the diseases; (b) patient's symptom–complaints and its association with the diagnosis or not of PAD.

define the need for additional imaging and the restriction in contrast agent utilization as well as to include prophylaxis for contrast-induce nephropathy. Digital subtraction angiography (DSA) is mandatory in today's practice. It provides significantly higher definition images as well as optimizing contrast utilization. Complete anatomical assessment of the affected vascular territory with significant attention to the *inflow* and *outflow* is very important. Selective and super-selective angiography should be performed in the involved areas, with the use of DSA to improve sensitivity of the procedure as well as to reduce contrast utilization. Invasive angiography also allows defining the hemodynamic significance of an intermediate stenosis and thus increasing the diagnostic capabilities of the test. Pressure gradient across a lesion that is not well defined should be obtained to better define treatment.

Coronary evaluation in the context of lower-extremity angiography and vice versa

In the context of a cardiac catheterization procedure, several groups have suggested the evaluation of PAD during the same procedure. First, since imaging modalities will be indicated 'only' in case revascularization is contemplated, angiography will not be indicated as a screening diagnostic study in this context. The patient is exposed to a longer procedure, with increased radiation exposure, and significant increases in the amount of contrast. For patient with severely symptomatic PAD undergoing coronary angiography, even though not a contraindication, the risk/benefit will be defined on an individual patient basis. The length of the procedure, amount of contrast utilization, and feasibility to perform an appropriate diagnostic study (appropriate catheterization lab suite, with DSA capability, large image intensifier, etc) will need to be considered.

The other scenario is the evaluation of the coronary arteries in the context of a PAD angiographic study. As stated before, CAD is the main morbidity and mortality problem in patients with PAD. The prevalence of CAD in patients with PAD is significantly elevated, up to 70% in the elderly population. The indication for a diagnostic procedure is based on whether or not the additional information will modify the patient's medical management. With that concept in mind, if the angiographic findings are consistent with the need for surgical revascularization, taking into consideration the well-known morbidity and mortality associated with cardiovascular events during vascular surgery, then coronary angiography could be contemplated in the same setting. However, scientific bases for this indication do not exist. Older patients, patients with lower ejection fraction, patients with prior MI, patients with prior CABG surgery, patients with prior stroke, and very obese patients, could be considered a higher-risk group in whom cardiac catheterization in the same setting of PAD evaluation could be advisable. On the other hand, for patients in whom percutaneous revascularization will be indicated, or medical management will be the treatment of choice, there are no data suggesting that the performance of a coronary angiography in the same setting will change the patient's management or prognosis, and therefore it will not be indicated.

Peripheral arterial disease and surgical revascularization: pre-operative cardiovascular risk assessment

Patients with severe claudication and/or critical limb ischemia and who are non-candidates for percutaneous revascularization, will be candidates for surgical revascularization. As previously stated, PAD is significantly associated with the presence of coronary artery disease, with increasing incidence as the population ages.[15,76,77] In addition, patients with PAD have a significantly higher incidence of more advanced degree of CAD. Sukhija and coworkers found that in patients undergoing cardiac catheterization to define CAD, patients with PAD had 18% incidence of LMT compared with 1% in patients without PAD ($P < 0.001$), and 63% had three-vessel CAD compared with only 11% if PAD negative ($P < 0.001$).[71] The presences of other manifestations of vascular diseases further increase the risk of CAD. Patients with PAD and history of CVD have an OR of 2.86 (95% CI 1.3–5.8) of having CAD, compared with patients with PAD and no history of CVD.[78] Patients may have prior history of the disease or may have an asymptomatic covered form. Since in the majority of these patients their functional capacity is significantly impaired, functional status and the presence of symptoms are usually not helpful. Thus, global assessment of the cardiovascular risk will be indicated in all patients who are candidates for non-coronary surgical revascularization. This includes clinical evaluation of the coronary and cerebrovascular status. The modality of evaluation will vary according to the clinical history and presentation, physical examination and electrocardiogram (ECG) findings. Guidelines and recommendations have been reported, but they exceed the focus of this chapter.[79]

CONTRAST-INDUCED NEPHROPATHY IN PATIENTS WITH MULTIPLE VASCULAR BEDS

Even though the subject of contrast-induced nephropathy (CIN; the term used to define the toxic effect to the iodinated contrast agents) is still controversial, with no clear understanding of its pathophysiology or the different possible players involved, this complication during coronary and peripheral diagnostic and interventional procedures is clear. Prevalence varies according to the different populations evaluated. Renal function prior to the procedure is the main predictor of CIN.[80] Patients with clearance >50 ml/min had no CIN, with increasing prevalence as the clearance decreased, reaching 50% if the clearance was <20 ml/min.[81] Even though a small percentage will end up in dialysis (<1%), 15–50% of those requiring dialysis will depend on dialysis permanently.[81,82] The presence of renal failure after a procedure has been strongly associated with worse outcome including increased mortality, both in hospital and during long-term follow-up.[81,83–85] Several predictors have been associated with increased risk of developing CIN, and pre-procedural scores have been developed with the intention of preventing this complication (Table 14.5). Patients with atherosclerotic multivascular bed involvement are at higher risk of developing this complication. The majority of the predictors (Table 14.5) are highly prevalent in this patient population, making them more susceptible to developing the complication. For this reason, appropriate preventive measurements and

Table 14.5   Risk score for acute renal failure after angiography

	Score
Hemodynamic decompensation	5
Use of intra aortic balloon pump (IABP)	5
Age >75 years	4
Hematrocrit <39 male, <36 female	3
Diabetes	3
Contrast	1 per 100 ml
Creatinine >1.5 mg/dl	4
Glomerular filtration rate (GFR) <60 (ml/min/(1.73 m²))	2: 40–60
	4: 20–39
	6: <20
Total risk score for renal failure (increase in creatinine >0.5 mg/dl or >25%)	
<5	7.5%
6–10	14%
11–15	26%
>16	57%

Estimated glomeruar filtration (GFR) = 186 × (creatinine (mg/dl)) − 1.154 × (age (years)) − 0.203 × 0.742 (in females × 1.21).

cautious contrast utilization is critical. The use of DSA in territories other than the coronary vessels, contrast dilution when high iodine content is used, and the use of lower-osmolarity contrast agents will be important considerations when performing diagnostic or interventional procedures in these patients. Proven interventions to decrease CIN in addition to the lowest possible contrast utilization, include good hydration prior to the procedure with 0.9% normal saline intravenous (1 ml/kg/h if there is normal left ventricular function, or 0.75 ml/kg/h if function is depressed), beginning 2–12 h prior to the procedure, followed by 6 h after the procedure.[86] The use of intravenous sodium bicarbonate has been efficient in one randomized study, and therefore further confirmatory studies are needed before there is a generalized recommendation.[87] The use of *N*-acetylcysteine is still controversial. Even though a pool analysis of all randomized trials showed benefit (pooled OR 0.54–0.73), inconsistent results raise some concerns.[88,89]

CONCLUSIONS

As the population ages, and the new advances in preventive measures and treatment of coronary artery disease continues to reduce mortality, healthcare providers will increasingly face the problem of concomitant 'non-coronary' arterial diseases. Invasive cardiologists today are facing a new paradigm with the chance to impact the diagnosis and treatment and improve prognosis of patients with different manifestations of atherosclerotic disease. Multivascular therapeutic approaches are needed because atherosclerosis has a common systemic pathogenesis and simultaneously affects multiple circulations, but more importantly, because clinical links exist among different territories. The achievement of health, without amputation, stroke, end-stage renal disease, or MI will require clinical wisdom. Defining the risk/benefit as well as the cost/benefit of this multicirculatory intervention is very complex, and will probably need to be tailored to the individual at risk. In general these patients currently seek consultation and care from multiple specialists, with poor interaction among them. A team approach with an integrated management of these patients will be the main challenge for the future.

REFERENCES

1. Stary H, Chandler A, Dinsmore R et al. A definition of advanced types of atherosclerotic lesions and a histological classification of atherosclerosis. A report from the Committee on Vascular Lesions of the Council on Arteriosclerosis, American Heart Association. Arterioscler Thromb Vasc Biol 1995; 15: 1512–31.
2. Virmani R, Kolodgie F, Burke A, Farb A, Schwartz S. Lessons from sudden coronary death: a comprehensive morphological classification scheme for atherosclerotic lesions. Arterioscler Thromb Vasc Biol 2000; 20: 1262–75.
3. Farb A, Burke A, Tang A et al. Coronary plaque erosion without rupture into a lipid core. A frequent cause of coronary thrombosis in sudden coronary death. Circulation 1996; 93: 1354–63.
4. Bamford J, Sandercock P, Dennis M, Burn J, Warlow C. Classification and natural history of clinically identifiable subtypes of cerebral infarction. Lancet 1991; 337: 1521–6.
5. Fisher M, Paganini-Hill A, Martin A, Cosgrove M, Toole J, Barnett H, Norris J. Carotid plaque pathology: thrombosis, ulceration, and stroke pathogenesis. Stroke 2005; 36: 253–7.
6. Rothwell P, Villagra R, Gibson R, Donders R, Warlow C. Evidence of a chronic systemic cause of instability of atherosclerotic plaques. Lancet 2000; 355: 19–24.

7. Sitzer M, Muller W, Siebler M et al. Plaque ulceration and lumen thrombus are the main sources of cerebral microemboli in high-grade internal carotid artery stenosis. Stroke 1995; 26: 1231–3.
8. Rothwell P, Gutnikov S, Warlow C, Collaboration ECSTs. Reanalysis of the final results of the European Carotid Surgery Trial. Stroke 2003; 34: 514–23.
9. Shaalan W, Cheng H, Gewertz B et al. Degree of carotid plaque calcification in relation to symptomatic outcome and plaque inflammation. J Vasc Surg 2004; 40: 262–9.
10. Imparato A, Riles T, Mintzer R, Baumann F. The importance of hemorrhage in the relationship between gross morphologic characteristics and cerebral symptoms in 376 carotid artery plaques. Ann Surg 1983; 197: 195–203.
11. Montauban van Swijndregt A, Elbers H, Moll F, de Letter J, Ackerstaff R. Cerebral ischemic disease and morphometric analyses of carotid plaques. Ann Vasc Surg 1999; 13: 468–74.
12. Fuster V, Moreno P, Fayad Z, Corti R, Badimon J. Atherothrombosis and high-risk plaque: part I: evolving concepts. J Am Coll Cardiol 2005; 46: 937–54.
13. Ouriel K. Peripheral arterial disease. Lancet 2001; 358: 1257–64.
14. Schmieder F, Comerota A. Intermittent claudication: magnitude of the problem, patient evaluation, and therapeutic strategies. Am J Cardiol 2001; 87: 3D–13D.
15. Dieter R, Chu W, Pacanowski JJ, McBride P, Tanke T. The significance of lower extremity peripheral arterial disease. Clin Cardiol 2002; 25: 3–10.
16. Faxon D, Fuster V, Libby P et al. American Heart Association. Atherosclerotic Vascular Disease Conference: Writing Group III: pathophysiology. Circulation 2004; 109: 2617–25.
17. Goldstein J, Demetriou D, Grines C et al. Multiple complex coronary plaques in patients with acute myocardial infarction. N Engl J Med 2000; 343: 915–22.
18. Jander S, Sitzer M, Schumann R et al. Inflammation in high-grade carotid stenosis: a possible role for macrophages and T cells in plaque destabilization. Stroke 1998; 29: 1625–30.
19. Lombardo A, Biasucci L, Lanza G et al. Inflammation as a possible link between coronary and carotid plaque instability. Circulation 2004; 109: 3158–63.
20. Fowkes F, Housley E, Cawood E et al. Edinburgh Artery Study: prevalence of asymptomatic and symptomatic peripheral arterial disease in the general population. Int J Epidemiol 1991; 20: 384–92.
21. Jackson M, Clagett G. Antithrombotic therapy in peripheral arterial occlusive disease. Chest 2001; 119: 283S–299S.
22. Ogren M, Hedblad B, Isacsson S et al. Non-invasively detected carotid stenosis and ischaemic heart disease in men with leg arteriosclerosis. Lancet 1993; 342: 1138–41.
23. Criqui M, Denenberg J, Langer R, Fronek A. The epidemiology of peripheral arterial disease: importance of identifying the population at risk. Vasc Med 1997; 2: 221–6.
24. Leng G, Fowkes F, Lee A et al. Use of ankle brachial pressure index to predict cardiovascular events and death: a cohort study. BMJ 1996; 313: 1440–4.
25. Zheng Z, Sharrett A, Chambless L et al. Associations of ankle-brachial index with clinical coronary heart disease, stroke and preclinical carotid and popliteal atherosclerosis: the Atherosclerosis Risk in Communities (ARIC) Study. Atherosclerosis 1997; 131: 115–25.
26. Eagle K, Rihal C, Foster E, Mickel M, Gersh B. Long-term survival in patients with coronary artery disease: importance of peripheral vascular disease. The Coronary Artery Surgery Study (CASS) Investigators. J Am Coll Cardiol 1994; 23: 1091–5.
27. Sutton-Tyrrell K, Rihal C, Sellers M et al. Long-term prognostic value of clinically evident noncoronary vascular disease in patients undergoing coronary revascularization in the Bypass Angioplasty Revascularization Investigation (BARI). Am J Cardiol 1998; 81: 375–81.
28. No author listed. TransAtlantic Inter-Society Consensus (TASC). Eur J Vasc Endovasc Surg 2000; 19 (Suppl A): S1–S250.
29. Johansson M, Herlitz H, Jensen G, Rundqvist B, Friberg P. Increased cardiovascular mortality in hypertensive patients with renal artery stenosis. Relation to sympathetic activation, renal function and treatment regimens. J Hypertens 1999; 17: 1743–50.
30. Conlon P, Little M, Pieper K, Mark D. Severity of renal vascular disease predicts mortality in patients undergoing coronary angiography. Kidney Int 2001; 60: 1490–7.

31. Zeller T, Muller C, Frank U et al. Survival after stenting of severe atherosclerotic ostial renal artery stenoses. J Endovasc Ther 2003; 10: 539–45.
32. Dorros G, Jaff M, Mathiak L et al. Four-year follow-up of Palmaz–Schatz stent revascularization as treatment for atherosclerotic renal artery stenosis. Circulation 1998; 98: 642–7.
33. Plouin P, Chatellier G, Darne B, Raynaud A. Blood pressure outcome of angioplasty in atherosclerotic renal artery stenosis: a randomized trial. Essai Multicentrique Medicaments vs Angioplastie (EMMA) Study Group. Hypertension 1998; 31: 823–9.
34. Webster J, Marshall F, Abdalla M et al. Randomised comparison of percutaneous angioplasty vs continued medical therapy for hypertensive patients with atheromatous renal artery stenosis. Scottish and Newcastle Renal Artery Stenosis Collaborative Group. J Hum Hypertens 1998; 12: 329–35.
35. van Jaarsveld B, Krijnen P, Pieterman H et al. The effect of balloon angioplasty on hypertension in atherosclerotic renal-artery stenosis. Dutch Renal Artery Stenosis Intervention Cooperative Study Group. N Engl J Med 2000; 342: 1007–14.
36. Safian R, Textor S. Renal-artery stenosis. N Engl J Med 2001; 344: 431–42.
37. Qanadli S, Soulez G, Therasse E et al. Detection of renal artery stenosis: prospective comparison of captopril-enhanced Doppler sonography, captopril-enhanced scintigraphy, and MR angiography. AJR Am J Roentgenol 2001; 177: 1123–9.
38. Rocha-Singh K. Aortorenal artery translesion pressure gradients in renovascular hypertension: In search of clinical significance. Catheter Cardiovasc Interv 2003; 59: 378–9.
39. Colyer WJ, Cooper C, Burket M, Thomas W. Utility of a 0.014″ pressure-sensing guidewire to assess renal artery translesional systolic pressure gradients. Catheter Cardiovasc Interv 2003; 59: 372–7.
40. Rigatelli G, Rigatelli G. Routine screening angiography of extra-cardiac arteries during cardiac catheterization: angiographer's delirium or common sense? Am J Med 2004; 117: 443–4.
41. Harding M, Smith L, Himmelstein S et al. Renal artery stenosis: prevalence and associated risk factors in patients undergoing routine cardiac catheterization. J Am Soc Nephrol 1992; 2: 1608–16.
42. Khosla S, Kunjummen B, Manda R et al. Prevalence of renal artery stenosis requiring revascularization in patients initially referred for coronary angiography. Catheter Cardiovasc Interv 2003; 58: 400–3.
43. Buller C, Nogareda J, Ramanathan K et al. The profile of cardiac patients with renal artery stenosis. J Am Coll Cardiol 2004; 43: 1606–13.
44. Cohen M, Pascua J, Garcia-Ben M et al. A simple prediction rule for significant renal artery stenosis in patients undergoing cardiac catheterization. Am Heart J 2005; 150: 1204–11.
45. Tanimoto S, Ikari Y, Tanabe K et al. Prevalence of carotid artery stenosis in patients with coronary artery disease in Japanese population. Stroke Epub 2005; 36: 2094–8.
46. Hallerstam S, Larsson P, Zuber E, Rosfors S. Carotid atherosclerosis is correlated with extent and severity of coronary artery disease evaluated by myocardial perfusion scintigraphy. Angiology 2004; 55: 281–8.
47. Honda O, Sugiyama S, Kugiyama K et al. Echolucent carotid plaques predict future coronary events in patients with coronary artery disease. J Am Coll Cardiol 2004; 43: 1177–84.
48. Cohen A, Tzourio C, Bertrand B et al. Aortic plaque morphology and vascular events: a follow-up study in patients with ischemic stroke. FAPS Investigators. French Study of Aortic Plaques in Stroke. Circulation 1997; 96: 3838–41.
49. Brener B, Brief D, Alpert J et al. A four-year experience with preoperative noninvasive carotid evaluation of two thousand twenty-six patients undergoing cardiac surgery. J Vasc Surg 1984; 1: 326–38.
50. Brener B, Brief D, Alpert J, Goldenkranz R, Parsonnet V. The risk of stroke in patients with asymptomatic carotid stenosis undergoing cardiac surgery: a follow-up study. J Vasc Surg 1987; 5: 269–79.

51. Naylor A, Mehta Z, Rothwell P, Bell P. Carotid artery disease and stroke during coronary artery bypass: a critical review of the literature. Eur J Vasc Endovasc Surg 2002; 23: 283–94.
52. Naylor A, Cuffe R, Rothwell P, Bell P. A systematic review of outcomes following staged and synchronous carotid endarterectomy and coronary artery bypass. Eur J Vasc Endovasc Surg 2003; 25: 380–9.
53. Yadav J, Wholey M, Kuntz R et al, Stenting and Angioplasty with Protection in Patients at High Risk for Endarterectomy Investigators. Protected carotid-artery stenting versus endarterectomy in high-risk patients. N Engl J Med 2004; 351: 1493–501.
54. Winslow C, Solomon D, Chassin M et al. The appropriateness of carotid endarterectomy. N Engl J Med 1988; 318: 721–7.
55. No authors listed. ACC/AHA 2005 Practice Guidelines for the Management of Patients With Peripheral Arterial Disease (Lower Extremity, Renal, Mesenteric, and Abdominal Aortic). Circulation 2006; 113: 1474–1547.
56. Naylor A, Cuffe R, Rothwell P, Bell P. A systematic review of outcomes following staged and synchronous carotid endarterectomy and coronary artery bypass: Influence of surgical and patient variables. Eur J Vasc Endovasc Surg 2003; 26: 230–41.
57. Randall M, McKevitt F, Cleveland T, Gaines P, Venables G. Is there any benefit from staged carotid and coronary revascularization using carotid stents? A single-center experience highlights the need for a randomized controlled trial. Stroke 2006; 37: 435–9.
58. Roederer G, Langlois Y, Chan A. Ultrasonic duplex scanning of extracranial carotid arteries. J Cardiovasc Ultrasound 1982; 4; 373–80.
59. CAVATAS I. Endovascular versus surgical treatment in patients with carotid stenosis in the Carotid and Vertebral Artery Transluminal Angioplasty Study (CAVATAS): a randomised trial. Lancet 2001; 357: 1729–37.
60. Gray W. Endovascular treatment of extra-cranial carotid artery bifurcation disease. Minerva Cardioangiol 2005; 53; 69–77.
61. Kovacic J, Roy P, Baron D, Muller D. Staged carotid artery stenting and coronary artery bypass graft surgery: Initial results from a single center. Catheter Cardiovasc Interv 2006; 67: 142–8.
62. Babatasi G, Theron J, Massetti M et al. Associated carotid and coronary lesions: carotid endoluminal angioplasty before coronary surgery. Presse Med 1996; 25: 1623–6.
63. Lopes D, Mericle R, Lanzino G et al. Stent placement for the treatment of occlusive atherosclerotic carotid artery disease in patients with concomitant coronary artery disease. J Neurosurg 2002; 96: 490–6.
64. Waigand J, Gross C, Uhlich F et al. Elective stenting of carotid artery stenosis in patients with severe coronary artery disease. Eur Heart J 1998; 19: 1365–70.
65. Ziada K, Yadav J, Mukherjee D et al. Comparison of results of carotid stenting followed by open heart surgery versus combined carotid endarterectomy and open heart surgery (coronary bypass with or without another procedure). Am J Cardiol 2005; 96: 519–23.
66. Weitz J, Byrne J, Clagett G et al. Diagnosis and treatment of chronic arterial insufficiency of the lower extremities: a critical review. Circulation 1996; 94: 3026–49.
67. Criqui M, Fronek A, Barrett-Connor E et al. The prevalence of peripheral arterial disease in a defined population. Circulation 1985; 71: 510–15.
68. Cotter G, Cannon C, McCabe C et al, Investigators O-T. Prior peripheral arterial disease and cerebrovascular disease are independent predictors of adverse outcome in patients with acute coronary syndromes: are we doing enough? Results from the Orbofiban in Patients with Unstable Coronary Syndromes–Thrombolysis In Myocardial Infarction (OPUS-TIMI) 16 study. Am Heart J 2003; 145: 622–7.
69. Smith G, Shipley M, Rose G. Intermittent claudication, heart disease risk factors, and mortality. The Whitehall Study. Circulation 1990; 82: 1925–31.
70. Aronow W, Ahn C, Mercando A, Epstein S. Prognostic significance of silent ischemia in elderly patients with peripheral arterial disease with and without previous myocardial infarction. Am J Cardiol 1992; 69: 137–9.
71. Sukhija R, Yalamanchili K, Aronow W. Prevalence of left main coronary artery disease, of three- or four-vessel coronary artery disease, and of obstructive coronary artery disease in

patients with and without peripheral arterial disease undergoing coronary angiography for suspected coronary artery disease. Am J Cardiol 2003; 92: 304–5.

72. Minakata K, Konishi Y, Matsumoto M et al. Influence of peripheral vascular occlusive disease on the morbidity and mortality of coronary artery bypass grafting. Jpn Circ J 2000; 64: 905–8.

73. Rihal C, Sutton-Tyrrell K, Guo P et al. Increased incidence of periprocedural complications among patients with peripheral vascular disease undergoing myocardial revascularization in the bypass angioplasty revascularization investigation. Circulation 1999; 100: 171–7.

74. Hirsch A, Criqui M, Treat-Jacobson D et al. Peripheral arterial disease detection, awareness, and treatment in primary care. JAMA 2001; 286: 1317–24.

75. Newman A, Siscovick D, Manolio T et al. Ankle-arm index as a marker of atherosclerosis in the Cardiovascular Health Study. Cardiovascular Heart Study (CHS) Collaborative Research Group. Circulation 1993; 88: 837–45.

76. Aronow W, Ahn C. Prevalence of coexistence of coronary artery disease, peripheral arterial disease, and atherothrombotic brain infarction in men and women >or=62 years of age. Am J Cardiol 1994; 74: 64–5.

77. Ness J, Aronow W. Prevalence of coronary artery disease, ischemic stroke, peripheral arterial disease, and coronary revascularization in older African-Americans, Asians, Hispanics, whites, men, and women. Am J Cardiol 1999; 84 : 932–3.

78. Kawarada O, Yokoi Y, Morioka N et al. Carotid stenosis and peripheral artery disease in Japanese patients with coronary artery disease undergoing coronary artery bypass grafting. Circ J 2003; 67: 1003–6.

79. Eagle K, Berger P, Calkins H et al. ACC/AHA guideline update for perioperative cardiovascular evaluation for noncardiac surgery – executive summary a report of the American College of Cardiology/American Heart Association Task Force on Practice Guidelines. Circulation 2002; 105: 1257–67.

80. Rudnick M, Goldfarb S, Wexler L et al. Nephrotoxicity of ionic and nonionic contrast media in 1196 patients: a randomized trial. The Iohexol Cooperative Study. Kidney Int 1995; 47: 254–61.

81. McCullough P, Wolyn R, Rocher L, Levin R, O'Neill W. Acute renal failure after coronary intervention: incidence, risk factors, and relationship to mortality. Am J Med 1997; 103: 368–75.

82. Gruberg L, Mintz G, Mehran R et al. The prognostic implications of further renal function deterioration within 48 h of interventional coronary procedures in patients with pre-existent chronic renal insufficiency. J Am Coll Cardiol 2000; 36: 1542–8.

83. Rihal C, Textor S, Grill D et al. Incidence and prognostic importance of acute renal failure after percutaneous coronary intervention. Circulation 2002; 105: 2259–64.

84. Bartholomew B, Harjai K, Dukkipati S et al. Impact of nephropathy after percutaneous coronary intervention and a method for risk stratification. Am J Cardiol 2004; 93: 1515–19.

85. Dangas G, Iakovou I, Nikolsky E et al. Contrast-induced nephropathy after percutaneous coronary interventions in relation to chronic kidney disease and hemodynamic variables. Am J Cardiol 2005; 95: 13–19.

86. Barrett B, Parfrey P. Clinical practice. Preventing nephropathy induced by contrast medium. N Engl J Med 2006; 26: 379–86.

87. Merten G, Burgess W, Gray L et al. Prevention of contrast-induced nephropathy with sodium bicarbonate: a randomized controlled trial. JAMA 2004; 291: 2328–34.

88. Kshirsagar A, Poole C, Mottl A et al. N-acetylcysteine for the prevention of radiocontrast induced nephropathy: a meta-analysis of prospective controlled trials. J Am Soc Nephrol 2004; 15: 761–9.

89. Nallamothu B, Shojania K, Saint S et al. Is acetylcysteine effective in preventing contrast-related nephropathy? A meta-analysis. Am J Med 2004; 117: 938–47.

15

The intermediate coronary lesion

Pedro A Lemos and Patrick W Serruys

Clinical impact of intermediate lesions • Diagnostic evaluation of intermediate lesions

Coronary angiography is currently the gold standard for the diagnosis of atherosclerotic heart disease. Nevertheless, it is well known that conventional angiography has several important limitations. Although angiography is a reliable tool to evaluate the luminal dimensions of a coronary segment, its ability to estimate the flow-limiting significance of lesions classified as 'intermediate' (commonly defined as a diameter stenosis between 40% and 70%) is suboptimum. Angiographic analysis of intermediate lesions is well known to have a poor correlation with the induction of myocardial ischemia or with patients' complaints. Unfortunately, intermediate or ambiguous lesions are frequently found in the daily practice of any catheterization laboratory, and often pose a diagnostic dilemma. In this chapter we discuss the advantages and disadvantages of invasive and non-invasive strategies currently available for the evaluation of intermediate lesions.

CLINICAL IMPACT OF INTERMEDIATE LESIONS

Angiography is known to only weakly predict the presence of myocardial ischemia, even when aided by quantitative analysis with either edge detection algorithms, or densitometric techniques.[1-4] The angiographic severity of lesions treated with percutaneous coronary intervention was analyzed in a recent metanalysis including 3812 patients from 14 studies.[5] Curiously, it was observed that approximately 6% of the cases enrolled in these trials had a lesion with <50% diameter stenosis at quantitative angiography. It should be noted that all such patients had documented ischemia and/or chest pain, clearly indicating a mismatch between angiographic and clinical findings.

Intermediate coronary lesions are frequently found in daily practice. Between June 1994 and June 2004, a total of 70721 diagnostic coronary angiographies were performed at the Heart Institute of the University of Sao Paulo, Brazil. Of these, 20107 (28%) had at least one lesion with a stenosis ≥50% and <70% by visual analysis. It is therefore easy to see that the evaluation of an angiographic intermediate lesion is a challenging clinical dilemma that is commonly posed to both the angiographer and the referring physician.

Patients with suspected or diagnosed coronary heart disease commonly (if not always) undergo cardiac catheterization only after a comprehensive clinical and non-invasive evaluation, with the invasive procedure habitually being considered the last diagnostic step. In this context, finding intermediate lesions at angiography may be a frustrating result, since the flow-limiting nature of intermediate lesions cannot be assessed with certainty using angiography alone. In this context, two main strategies are possible for the evaluation of an intermediate lesion found at a coronary angiography: (1) lesion-specific invasive testing at the time of the procedure; or (2) non-invasive ischemia testing after the catheterization. Table 15.1 shows the advantages and disadvantages of invasive and non-invasive testing.

DIAGNOSTIC EVALUATION OF INTERMEDIATE LESIONS

Angiographic techniques

A number of angiographic techniques have been described aiming to improve the diagnostic accuracy of the method. Computerized systems have been developed to (semi-) automate the measurements of coronary dimensions, so-called quantitative coronary angiography. The determination of coronary diameters using computer-based edge detection or videodensitometric algorithms has been proven to greatly minimize inter- and intra-observer variability, compared to visual estimation. Because of its good reproducibility, quantitative coronary angiography is established as the basis for most clinical trials with angiographic endpoints. However, although improving the variability of the measurements, quantitative angiographic parameters have shown conflicting results in their ability to predict the functional significance of

Table 15.1   Advantages and limitations of non-invasive or invasive testing for intermediate lesions[a]

Non-invasive testing	Invasive testing
Advantages	
Evaluation of myocardial ischemia in all territories	Permits differentiation between epicardial and microvascular components
Evaluation of global and segmental left ventricular function	Time saving if performed at the time of the initial catheterization
Evaluation of myocardial viability	Lesion specific: differentiates the significance of distinct lesions even if located in the same vessel
Evaluation of the amount of jeopardized myocardium	Possibly more accurate than non-invasive testing to assess the flow-limiting nature of a specific epicardial lesion
	May be performed without pharmacological stress or without systemic administration of drugs
Limitations	
Delay in final clinical decision	Needs intracoronary manipulation
Needs physical exercise or systemic pharmacological stress	Needs anticoagulation
	May induce myocardial ischemia
	Does not allow global evaluation of the entire coronary bed

[a]The advantages and disadvantages listed reflect an overall evaluation of all current available invasive and non-invasive methods and may apply to a specific method.

a coronary lesion.[3,6-12] It is important to note that studies showing a good correlation between quantitative coronary angiography and functional testing included only angiograms acquired under optimal settings, a scenario that is rarely found in daily practice. Many series have found a significant relationship between quantitative coronary angiography and functional parameters, but with a large variability.

Several factors may potentially decrease the ability of angiography to reflect the true significance of a lesion. Angiography is in fact a two-dimensional projected 'lumenography', which is not ideal to fully assess complex three-dimensional coronary anatomy. The angiographic representation of the coronaries is frequently impaired by (1) foreshortening of the target segment; (2) overlap with other branches; (3) origin of a side branch close to the target lesion; (4) diffuse disease; (5) pre- or post-stenotic ectatic segments; (6) target lesion at ostial location; (7) luminal irregularities; (8) intimal dissection; (9) intraluminal filling defects; and (10) lesions with local flow disturbances. It is important to note that edge detection and videodensitometry, the most widely used methods for quantitative angiography, are greatly impaired by the factors above. Most certainly, the wide range of results precludes the use of angiography to evaluate the significance of an intermediate lesion in an individual patient.

Coronary flow can theoretically be assessed by means of the Thrombolysis in Myocardial Infarction (TIMI) frame count method,[13] which evaluates the number of cine frames between the beginning of contrast filling until the opacification reaches predefined anatomical landmarks.[14] Previous studies have analyzed the 'angiographic coronary flow reserve', comparing the results of TIMI frame count at baseline and after pharmacological hyperemic stimulus.[15-17] However, when compared to intracoronary Doppler wire-derived flow reserve, the results of the abovementioned angiographic index were not consistent across the studies, suggesting that the method needs to be better validated before more conclusive recommendations can be made.

Overall, angiography does not seem to be an appropriate tool to evaluate the significance of intermediate coronary lesions in an individual patient. Although advanced approaches are potentially able to improve its accuracy, angiography still remains a limited modality for the analysis of ambiguous lesions.

Intravascular ultrasound

Intravascular ultrasound has the unique capacity to visualize and measure the luminal and transmural coronary dimensions, *in vivo*, online, and with a high spatial resolution. Intravascular ultrasound examination accurately provides measurements of luminal areas and diameters at the obstruction site and at the references. Also, the outer limits of the vessel and the atherosclerotic plaque can be easily assessed at the lesion and at the reference segments. Moreover, intravascular ultrasound provides planar (cross-sectional) as well as longitudinal (three-dimensional) imaging of the coronary vessel.[18,19] Because of its higher accuracy for detecting atherosclerosis and quantifying the luminal obstruction, intravascular ultrasound appears to be a potential tool for evaluating ambiguous coronary lesions at angiography.

The intravascular ultrasound minimum cross-sectional area at the lesion site has been demonstrated to significantly correlate with the coronary flow reserve ($r = 0.831$, $P < 0.0001$ for lesions tested before coronary intervention).[20] Also, it has been shown that the ratio of minimum luminal area to lesion length (both measured by intravascular ultrasound) was independently associated with the fractional flow reserve.[21] A previous study identified subsequent intravascular ultrasound figures as the best cutoff values to predict myocardial ischemia, according to a fractional flow reserve <0.75: (1) percentage area stenosis at the lesion site >70% (sensitivity 100%, specificity 68%); (2) minimum luminal diameter ≤1.8 mm (sensitivity 100%, specificity 66%); (3) minimum luminal area ≤4.0 mm^2 (sensitivity 92%, specificity 56%); and (4) lesion length >10 mm (sensitivity 41%, specificity 80%).[22] Combining percentage area of stenosis and minimum luminal diameter increased the specificity of intravascular ultrasound to predict a fractional flow reserve <0.75 (sensitivity 100%, specificity 76%). In another study, the minimum luminal area showed a positive correlation ($r^2=0.62$, $P<0.01$) with the percentage area of stenosis, and an inverse correlation with the fractional flow reserve ($r^2=0.60$, $P<0.01$).[23] The best cutoff values to detect a fractional flow reserve <0.75 were minimum luminal area <3.0 mm^2 (sensitivity 83%, specificity 92%), and area of stenosis >60% (sensitivity 92%, specificity 89%) – all lesions, without exception, with a minimal luminal area <3.0 mm^2 and a percentage area of stenosis <60% had a fractional flow reserve <0.75.[23]

Intravascular ultrasound has been used to indicate, or defer, invasive treatment for patients with intermediate lesions. An observational study included 300 patients (357 intermediate lesions) in whom percutaneous intervention was deferred based on intravascular ultrasound, according to a 'general' criterion of a minimum lumen area ≥4.0 mm^2, or a minimum lumen diameter ≥2.0 mm.[24] During a mean follow-up period of 13 months, the need for lesion-related revascularization was 6%. In particular, for patients with a minimum lumen area ≥4.0 mm^2, the target lesion revascularization was only 2.8%.[24] Importantly, no angiographic parameter had the ability to differentiate patients with an increased probability of adverse events.[24]

The severity of lesions located in the left main coronary is frequently difficult to interpret with angiography alone. Intravascular ultrasound was compared to fractional flow reserve in 55 patients with an angiographically ambiguous left main stenosis.[25] A minimal luminal diameter <2.8 mm had the highest sensitivity and specificity (93% and 98%, respectively) for predicting the significance of the lesion (fractional flow reserve <0.75), followed by a minimal luminal area <5.9 mm^2 (93% and 95%, respectively).[25] In another study, intravascular ultrasound imaging was obtained in 121 patients with an angiographically normal left main coronary trunck.[26] This cohort was used to determine the lower normal limit for minimum luminal area (defined as the mean minus two standard deviations), which was found to be 7.5 mm^2. In a subsequent phase, revascularization or medical treatment was recommended for 214 patients with ambiguous left main arteries who had a minimal luminal area below or above 7.5 mm^2 respectively. After 3.3±2.0 years, no significant difference in the incidence of adverse events was observed between patients with a minimum luminal area <7.5 mm^2 (who underwent revascularization), and those with a minimum luminal area ≥7.5 mm^2 (in whom revascularization was deferred). The authors concluded that deferring revascularization for patients with an indeterminate left main lesion with a minimum lumen area ≥7.5 mm^2 appeared to be a safe strategy.[26]

Intravascular ultrasound techniques have been recently developed with the aim to characterize the atherosclerotic plaque, in an attempt to identify features of plaque 'vulnerability'.[27,28] Such methods will potentially add to morphological measurements currently obtained with quantitative intravascular ultrasound, and will provide more insightful information for the clinical decision making relating to intermediate lesions. At the moment, however, the value of vulnerable plaque imaging has not been established for prognosis assessment, and cannot be incorporated as a routine tool for the evaluation of patients with intermediate lesions.

Intravascular ultrasound is frequently employed to examine ambiguous lesions in many catheterization laboratories, providing useful additional information in determining whether the stenosis is clinically significant or not. However, it is important to note that intravascular ultrasound has several limitations for this application. For instance, evaluation of intermediate lesions with intravascular ultrasound has not been sufficiently studied in small vessels, diffuse disease, saphenous grafts, ectatic segments, or patients with acute coronary syndromes. Most importantly, it must be emphasized that intravascular ultrasound does not provide physiological information *per se*.[18]

Coronary flow measurements

Intracoronary blood flow velocity can be measured distal to an intermediate lesion by a 0.014 inch Doppler guidewire inserted under fluoroscopic guidance. Alternatively, a thermodilution technique has been more recently introduced to measure blood flow using a regular 0.014 inch pressure wire.[29–32] Because of their thin diameter, both wires can be advanced through the lesion without significantly impeding blood flow.

A previous study has evaluated the prognostic value of intracoronary Doppler-derived coronary flow velocity reserve, compared to myocardial perfusion scintigraphy for intermediate lesions in 191 patients with stable angina.[33] Coronary flow reserve was defined as the ratio between maximum (drug-induced) and baseline flow velocities. Percutaneous intervention of the intermediate lesion was deferred when coronary flow reserve was ≥ 2.0, or scintigraphy was negative. At one-year follow-up, coronary flow velocity reserve was a more accurate predictor of cardiac events than scintigraphy (relative risk: coronary flow reserve 3.9, $P < 0.05$; scintigraphy 0.5, $P = $ non-significant). Patients with a coronary flow reserve ≥ 2.0 had an event rate of 6% during the first year.[33]

Even though intracoronary flow (velocity) measurements are helpful in identifying better candidates for revascularization, these methods have several important limitations for the evaluation of intermediate lesions, namely: (1) flow measurements are not stenosis specific, and are strongly influenced by the microvascular circulation; (2) flow measurements are highly sensitive to hemodynamic conditions; (3) baseline myocardial flow (measured for the calculation of coronary flow reserve) have a high inter- and intra-individual variability; and (4) as a consequence normal and cut-off values are not sharply defined, which limits the use of flow measurement indexes as an optimum tool to be used in daily practice.

Fractional flow reserve

The concept of fractional flow reserve (FFR) is illustrated in Figure 15.1. Briefly, the FFR measures the ratio of myocardial blood flow at maximum hyperemia in the presence of a luminal stenosis, in relation to the flow that would exist if no stenosis was present (hyperemic myocardial flow in the presence of stenosis ÷ hyperemic myocardial flow in the absence of stenosis). The driving pressure in a stenotic vessel is calculated by the pressure distal to the lesion minus the venous pressure

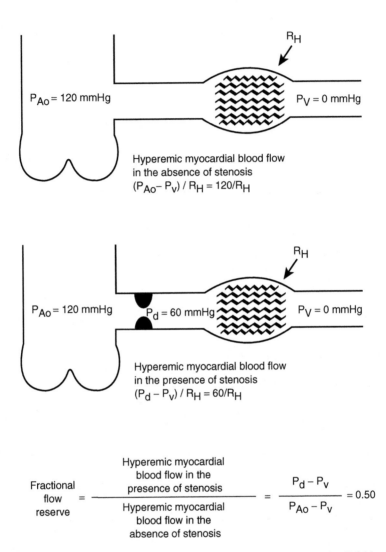

$$\text{Fractional flow reserve} = \frac{\text{Hyperemic myocardial blood flow in the presence of stenosis}}{\text{Hyperemic myocardial blood flow in the absence of stenosis}} = \frac{P_d - P_V}{P_{Ao} - P_V} = 0.50$$

Figure 15.1 Calculation of fractional flow reserve. The hyperemic myocardial blood flow (induced by a microvascular vasodilator such as adenosine) is directly proportional to the perfusion pressure (inflow pressure minus outflow pressure [right atrial pressure, P_V]) and inversely proportional to the hyperemic myocardial resistance (R_H). In the absence of coronary stenosis (upper panel), the inflow pressure is equal to the aortic pressure (P_{Ao}), while in the presence of a coronary stenosis (lower panel), the inflow pressure is represented by the intra-coronary pressure distal to the stenosis (P_d). The fractional flow reserve is calculated as the ratio between the hyperemic myocardial blood flow in the presence of stenosis (calculated using the P_d) and the theoretical hyperemic myocardial blood flow in case the stenosis would not be present (calculated using the P_{Ao}). The final formula for calculation of the fractional flow reserve is $(P_d - P_V) \div (P_{Ao} - P_V)$. For practical reasons, the right atrial pressure (P_V) is frequently ignored for the calculation of the fractional flow reserve due to its low values in comparison to the arterial pressures. Therefore, a simplified formula would be $P_d \div P_{Ao}$ (this simplified approach has the advantage of avoiding the need for right heart catheterization, but may be a source of error, which can be a limitation when dealing with fractional flow reserves very close to the ischemic threshold).

0 mmHg – 0 mmHg in Figure 15.1). The theoretical driving pressure if no stenosis is present is calculated with the aortic pressure, since no pressure drop is expected to occur in the trajectory of normal epicardial coronary arteries (120 mmHg – 0 mHg in Figure 15.1). It is easy to see that FFR represents the fraction of maximum normal flow that is still maintained in the presence of a stenosis. In the example of Figure 15.1, the luminal stenosis limits the maximum flow to only half (fractional flow reserve = 0.50) of what the expected normal hyperemic myocardial flow would be.

In a validation study, FFR was compared to a sophisticated gold standard index that combined the results of exercise testing, thallium scintigraphy, dobutamine stress echocardiography, quantitative coronary arteriography, and the follow-up findings after revascularization.[34] Every patient was evaluated with all non-invasive methods before intracoronary pressure measurement. Patients with a FFR < 0.75 detected during catheterization underwent revascularization. In these patients, all non-invasive tests that had yielded positive results were subsequently repeated within 6 weeks post-procedure. FFR was compared to a composite gold standard that used the following criteria for the definition of the presence or absence of a significant lesion: (1) important stenoses were present only if one or more non-invasive tests were clearly positive and reverted to normal after successful revascularization; (2) significant stenoses were absent only if all non-invasive tests were negative. The authors observed that in all 21 patients with a FFR < 0.75, unequivocal reversible myocardial ischemia was demonstrated in at least one non-invasive test (after coronary angioplasty or bypass surgery all positive test results reverted to normal). Moreover, 21 of the 24 patients with FFR ≥ 0.75 had negative findings in all non-invasive tests. Therefore, the sensitivity of FFR in detecting reversible ischemia according to this composite gold standard was 88%, and the specificity 100%.[34]

FFR is the most extensively tested method for the evaluation of angiographically intermediate coronary lesions. A randomized clinical trial included 325 patients with scheduled angioplasty, who did not have documented ischemia.[35] If FFR was ≥ 0.75, patients were randomly allocated to deferral (deferral group) or performance (performance group) of percutaneous intervention. If FFR was < 0.75, angioplasty was undertaken as planned (reference group). At 24-month follow-up, event-free survival was similar between the deferral and performance groups (89% vs. 83%), but was significantly lower in the reference group (78%). These findings strongly indicate that patients with an intermediate lesion and a FFR above the cut-off value (≥ 0.75) should be maintained on medical therapy, since revascularization did not add any benefit to this subset.[35]

The clinical value of FFR for the evaluation of angiographically ambiguous lesions has been reported for several subgroups, including patients with previous myocardial infarction,[36,37] acute coronary syndromes,[38] multivessel disease,[39-42] left main coronary disease,[25,43,44] and ostial lesions.[45] Importantly, FFR translates the resistance to flow of the epicardial vessel and is mostly not affected by the microcirculatory function. Also, FFR is minimally or not influenced by hemodynamic or load conditions.[46] Interestingly, the results of FFR are poorly predicted by the angiographic aspect of the lesions, even when analyzed by experienced operators.[4,47]

A recent prospective registry detected that a policy of encouraging the routine use of FFR for all ambiguous lesions led to the utilization of the technique in approximately 6% of all coronary angiographies.[48] On the basis of FFR, two-thirds of patients with intermediate lesions were not revascularized. The event-free survival after one year was comparable in patients with versus without revascularization (94% vs. 93%, respectively).[48]

Taken together, these characteristics make FFR an attractive diagnostic tool for investigating intermediate lesions in daily practice.

Non-invasive myocardial ischemia testing

The functional significance of intermediate lesions can be assessed by several modalities of non-invasive ischemia testing, including exercise stress test, nuclear medicine, stress echocardiography, and magnetic resonance imaging. Each of these methods has advantages and limitations for the evaluation of coronary lesions. A detailed technical description of these methods is beyond the scope of this chapter.

A recent report compared single photon emission computer tomography with FFR for intermediate coronary lesions.[49] Final analysis identified a regional summed difference score ≥1, and a regional summed stress score ≥3 as the best cut-off values to predict a FFR <0.75. The sensitivity and specificity of regional summed difference score were 80% and 76% for patients without prior myocardial infarction, and 57% and 50% for patients with prior myocardial infarction, respectively. Regional summed stress score had a sensitivity and specificity of 70% and 93% for patients without prior myocardial infarction, and 100% and 50% for patients with prior myocardial infarction respectively.[49]

In another study, dobutamine stress echocardiography and single photon emission computer tomography were compared to intracoronary FFR measurements for the evaluation of angiographically intermediate lesions.[50] The sensitivity and specificity for the detection of a FFR <0.75 was 67% and 77% for echocardiography, and 69% and 87% for scintigraphy respectively. Importantly, the sensitivity of both non-invasive methods was significantly reduced for a target lesion located distally. In addition, stress echocardiography had poor results for lesions in the left circumflex artery as well as for patients with previous myocardial infarction.[50]

The best choice of the non-invasive imaging modality for the evaluation of intermediate lesions is controversial. It should be noted that agreement among the different methods is frequently less than perfect. A previous study comparing contrast-enhanced transthoracic Doppler echocardiography with thallium-201 scintigraphy for intermediate lesions showed that the agreement between the methods was only moderate, at best (agreement=59%, kappa=0.28, P <0.05).[51] The selection of the non-invasive test should be guided by local availability and expertise, particularly for methods that are highly dependent on operator experience.

Invasive versus non-invasive testing for intermediate lesions: practical recommendations

Patients undergoing cardiac catheterization in whom an intermediate lesion has been identified may fall into one of the following categories: (1) without non-invasive testing obtained before the angiography; (2) inconclusive non-invasive testing obtained before the angiography; or (3) conclusive non-invasive testing obtained before angiography. The strategy to further evaluate an angiographically intermediate lesion in a particular patient will vary among the groups above. Overall, patients without precatheterization testing, or with inconclusive ischemia testing will benefit from invasive lesion-directed evaluation during the invasive procedure. Patients with a good-quality non-invasive testing obtained before the angiography should have their intermediate lesion evaluated in light of those results.

Additional invasive evaluation should be performed in these latter patients if the findings of the non-invasive testing do not fit with the clinical scenario, and false-positive or false-negative results are suspected.

Non-invasive imaging for intermediate lesions is an adequate option if a more global evaluation of left ventricle perfusion is needed, such as in patients with multiple coronary lesions. Nevertheless, it should be noted that invasive testing (particularly pressure-derived FFR) has been extensively validated as a reliable method for evaluating patients with multivessel coronary disease.[33,39–41]

If the assessment of viable myocardium is clinically indicated when evaluating patients with intermediate lesions, coupled ischemia and viability with non-invasive methods should be strongly considered. However, it is important to note that the accuracy of non-invasive methods to analyze the flow-limiting nature of an intermediate lesion is greatly reduced in patients with previous myocardial infarction.[49,50] Conversely, intracoronary measurement of FFR has been demonstrated to be an accurate diagnostic option for patients with prior infarction.[36]

Non-invasive testing to assess the functional significance of an intermediate lesion after initial coronary angiography has the potential to increase the length of hospitalization or to prolong the time until a final therapeutic decision is taken, when compared to invasive evaluation undertaken at the time of the first catheterization (Table 15.1). On the other hand, invasive testing of intermediate lesions potentially increases initial costs and may be associated with an augmented risk of procedural complications. To evaluate this issue, the costs and benefits of FFR versus stress perfusion scintigraphy were analyzed in a randomized trial that included 70 patients with intermediate lesions admitted with acute coronary syndrome. Patients with negative nuclear testing or with a fractional flow reserve ≥ 0.75 were discharged; patients with a positive scintigraphy or with a FFR <0.75 underwent percutaneous intervention. Patients randomized to FFR had a significantly reduced duration and cost of hospitalization compared with those randomized to scintigraphy (11 h vs. 49 h, $P < 0.001$; and US\$1329 vs. US\$2113, respectively, $P < 0.05$). There were no significant differences in adverse event rates during one-year follow-up.[38] In another study, a decision model was developed to compare the cost-effectiveness profile of three strategies: (1) nuclear stress testing after the coronary angiography to evaluate the appropriateness of further treatment; (2) FFR at the time of angiography to guide the therapeutic decision; and (3) stenting of all intermediate lesions.[52] It was estimated that 40% of intermediate lesions would be associated with ischemia. The cost of FFR was set at US\$761, the cost of nuclear test at US\$1093, and the cost of medical treatment for angina at US\$1775 per year. The extra cost of splitting the angiogram and angioplasty with the nuclear imaging strategy was US\$3886. The FFR was found to save US\$1795 per patient compared with the nuclear strategy, and US\$3830 compared with the unrestricted stenting strategy.[52] This evidence strongly suggests that invasive evaluation of intermediate coronary lesions (especially with FFR) is an attractive approach from a clinical and a resource utilization standpoint, compared to both non-invasive testing (with nuclear medicine) or no additional testing.

REFERENCES

1. Di Carli M, Czernin J, Hoh CK et al. Relation among stenosis severity, myocardial blood flow, and flow reserve in patients with coronary artery disease. Circulation 1995; 91: 1944–51.

2. Uren NG, Melin JA, De Bruyne B et al. Relation between myocardial blood flow and the severity of coronary-artery stenosis. N Engl J Med 1994; 330: 1782–8.
3. Zijlstra F, Fioretti P, Reiber JH, Serruys PW. Which cineangiographically assessed anatomic variable correlates best with functional measurements of stenosis severity? A comparison of quantitative analysis of the coronary cineangiogram with measured coronary flow reserve and exercise/redistribution thallium-201 scintigraphy. J Am Coll Cardiol 1988; 12: 686–91.
4. Fischer JJ, Samady H, McPherson JA et al. Comparison between visual assessment and quantitative angiography versus fractional flow reserve for native coronary narrowings of moderate severity. Am J Cardiol 2002; 90: 210–15.
5. Mercado N, Maier W, Boersma E et al. Clinical and angiographic outcome of patients with mild coronary lesions treated with balloon angioplasty or coronary stenting. Implications for mechanical plaque sealing. Eur Heart J 2003; 24: 541–51.
6. Hadjimiltiades S, Watson R, Hakki AH, Heo J, Iskandrian AS. Relation between myocardial thallium-201 kinetics during exercise and quantitative coronary angiography in patients with one vessel coronary artery disease. J Am Coll Cardiol 1989; 13: 1301–8.
7. Baptista J, Arnese M, Roelandt JR et al. Quantitative coronary angiography in the estimation of the functional significance of coronary stenosis: correlations with dobutamine-atropine stress test. J Am Coll Cardiol 1994; 23: 1434–9.
8. Folland ED, Vogel RA, Hartigan P et al. Relation between coronary artery stenosis assessed by visual, caliper, and computer methods and exercise capacity in patients with single-vessel coronary artery disease. The Veterans Affairs ACME Investigators. Circulation 1994; 89: 2005–14.
9. Tron C, Kern MJ, Donohue TJ et al. Comparison of quantitative angiographically derived and measured translesion pressure and flow velocity in coronary artery disease. Am J Cardiol 1995; 75: 111–17.
10. Piek JJ, Boersma E, di Mario C et al. Angiographical and Doppler flow-derived parameters for assessment of coronary lesion severity and its relation to the result of exercise electrocardiography. DEBATE study group. Doppler Endpoints Balloon Angioplasty Trial Europe. Eur Heart J 2000; 21: 466–74.
11. Wilson RF, Marcus ML, White CW. Prediction of the physiologic significance of coronary arterial lesions by quantitative lesion geometry in patients with limited coronary artery disease. Circulation 1987; 75: 723–32.
12. Zijlstra F, van Ommeren J, Reiber JH, Serruys PW. Does the quantitative assessment of coronary artery dimensions predict the physiologic significance of a coronary stenosis? Circulation 1987; 75: 1154–61.
13. Tanedo JS, Kelly RF, Marquez M et al. Assessing coronary blood flow dynamics with the TIMI frame count method: comparison with simultaneous intracoronary Doppler and ultrasound. Catheter Cardiovasc Interv 2001; 53: 459–63.
14. Gibson CM, Cannon CP, Daley WL et al. TIMI frame count: a quantitative method of assessing coronary artery flow. Circulation 1996; 93: 879–88.
15. Manginas A, Gatzov P, Chasikidis C et al. Estimation of coronary flow reserve using the Thrombolysis In Myocardial Infarction (TIMI) frame count method. Am J Cardiol 1999; 83: 1562–5, A7.
16. Stoel MG, Zijlstra F, Visser CA. Frame count reserve. Circulation 2003; 107: 3034–9.
17. Chugh SK, Koppel J, Scott M et al. Coronary flow velocity reserve does not correlate with TIMI frame count in patients undergoing non-emergency percutaneous coronary intervention. J Am Coll Cardiol 2004; 44: 778–82.
18. Mintz GS, Nissen SE, Anderson WD et al. American College of Cardiology Clinical Expert Consensus Document on Standards for Acquisition, Measurement and Reporting of Intravascular Ultrasound Studies (IVUS). A report of the American College of Cardiology Task Force on Clinical Expert Consensus Documents. J Am Coll Cardiol 2001; 37: 1478–92.
19. De Winter SA, Hamers R, Degertekin M et al. Retrospective image-based gating of intracoronary ultrasound images for improved quantitative analysis: the intelligate method. Catheter Cardiovasc Interv 2004; 61: 84–94.

20. Abizaid A, Mintz GS, Pichard AD et al. Clinical, intravascular ultrasound, and quantitative angiographic determinants of the coronary flow reserve before and after percutaneous transluminal coronary angioplasty. Am J Cardiol 1998; 82: 423–8.

21. Takayama T, Hodgson JM. Prediction of the physiologic severity of coronary lesions using 3D IVUS: validation by direct coronary pressure measurements. Catheter Cardiovasc Interv 2001; 53: 48–55.

22. Briguori C, Anzuini A, Airoldi F et al. Intravascular ultrasound criteria for the assessment of the functional significance of intermediate coronary artery stenoses and comparison with fractional flow reserve. Am J Cardiol 2001; 87: 136–41.

23. Takagi A, Tsurumi Y, Ishii Y et al. Clinical potential of intravascular ultrasound for physiological assessment of coronary stenosis: relationship between quantitative ultrasound tomography and pressure-derived fractional flow reserve. Circulation 1999; 100: 250–5.

24. Abizaid AS, Mintz GS, Mehran R et al. Long-term follow-up after percutaneous transluminal coronary angioplasty was not performed based on intravascular ultrasound findings: importance of lumen dimensions. Circulation 1999; 100: 256–61.

25. Jasti V, Ivan E, Yalamanchili V, Wongpraparut N, Leesar MA. Correlations between fractional flow reserve and intravascular ultrasound in patients with an ambiguous left main coronary artery stenosis. Circulation 2004; 110: 2831–6.

26. Fassa AA, Wagatsuma K, Higano ST et al. Intravascular ultrasound-guided treatment for angiographically indeterminate left main coronary artery disease: a long-term follow-up study. J Am Coll Cardiol 2005; 45: 204–11.

27. Schaar JA, Regar E, Mastik F et al. Incidence of high-strain patterns in human coronary arteries: assessment with three-dimensional intravascular palpography and correlation with clinical presentation. Circulation 2004; 109: 2716–19.

28. Rodriguez-Granillo GA, Garcia-Garcia HM, Mc Fadden EP et al. In vivo intravascular ultrasound-derived thin-cap fibroatheroma detection using ultrasound radiofrequency data analysis. J Am Coll Cardiol 2005; 46: 2038–42.

29. Pijls NH, De Bruyne B, Smith L et al. Coronary thermodilution to assess flow reserve: validation in humans. Circulation 2002; 105: 2482–6.

30. De Bruyne B, Pijls NH, Smith L, Wievegg M, Heyndrickx GR. Coronary thermodilution to assess flow reserve: experimental validation. Circulation 2001; 104: 2003–6.

31. Fearon WF, Farouque HM, Balsam LB et al. Comparison of coronary thermodilution and Doppler velocity for assessing coronary flow reserve. Circulation 2003; 108: 2198–200.

32. Barbato E, Aarnoudse W, Aengevaeren WR et al. Validation of coronary flow reserve measurements by thermodilution in clinical practice. Eur Heart J 2004; 25: 219–23.

33. Chamuleau SA, Tio RA, de Cock CC et al. Prognostic value of coronary blood flow velocity and myocardial perfusion in intermediate coronary narrowings and multivessel disease. J Am Coll Cardiol 2002; 39: 852–8.

34. Pijls NH, De Bruyne B, Peels K et al. Measurement of fractional flow reserve to assess the functional severity of coronary-artery stenoses. N Engl J Med 1996; 334: 1703–8.

35. Bech GJ, De Bruyne B, Pijls NH et al. Fractional flow reserve to determine the appropriateness of angioplasty in moderate coronary stenosis: a randomized trial. Circulation 2001; 103: 2928–34.

36. De Bruyne B, Pijls NH, Bartunek J et al. Fractional flow reserve in patients with prior myocardial infarction. Circulation 2001; 104: 157–62.

37. Usui Y, Chikamori T, Yanagisawa H et al. Reliability of pressure-derived myocardial fractional flow reserve in assessing coronary artery stenosis in patients with previous myocardial infarction. Am J Cardiol 2003; 92: 699–702.

38. Leesar MA, Abdul-Baki T, Akkus NI et al. Use of fractional flow reserve versus stress perfusion scintigraphy after unstable angina. Effect on duration of hospitalization, cost, procedural characteristics, and clinical outcome. J Am Coll Cardiol 2003; 41: 1115–21.

39. Wongpraparut N, Yalamanchili V, Pasnoori V et al. Thirty-month outcome after fractional flow reserve-guided versus conventional multivessel percutaneous coronary intervention. Am J Cardiol 2005; 96: 877–84.

40. Chamuleau SA, Meuwissen M, Koch KT et al. Usefulness of fractional flow reserve for risk stratification of patients with multivessel coronary artery disease and an intermediate stenosis. Am J Cardiol 2002; 89: 377–80.
41. Berger A, Botman KJ, MacCarthy PA et al. Long-term clinical outcome after fractional flow reserve-guided percutaneous coronary intervention in patients with multivessel disease. J Am Coll Cardiol 2005; 46: 438–42.
42. Botman KJ, Pijls NH, Bech JW et al. Percutaneous coronary intervention or bypass surgery in multivessel disease? A tailored approach based on coronary pressure measurement. Catheter Cardiovasc Interv 2004; 63: 184–91.
43. Bech GJ, Droste H, Pijls NH et al. Value of fractional flow reserve in making decisions about bypass surgery for equivocal left main coronary artery disease. Heart 2001; 86: 547–52.
44. Jimenez-Navarro M, Hernandez-Garcia JM, Alonso-Briales JH et al. Should we treat patients with moderately severe stenosis of the left main coronary artery and negative FFR results? J Invasive Cardiol 2004; 16: 398–400.
45. Ziaee A, Parham WA, Herrmann SC et al. Lack of relation between imaging and physiology in ostial coronary artery narrowings. Am J Cardiol 2004; 93: 1404–7, A9.
46. Pijls NH, de Bruyne B. Independence of fractional flow reserve of hemodynamic loading conditions. In: Pijls NH, de Bruyne B, eds. Coronary Pressure. Dordrecht, The Netherlands: Kluwer Academic Publishers, 1997: 157–78.
47. Brueren BR, ten Berg JM, Suttorp MJ et al. How good are experienced cardiologists at predicting the hemodynamic severity of coronary stenoses when taking fractional flow reserve as the gold standard. Int J Cardiovasc Imaging 2002; 18: 73–6.
48. Legalery P, Schiele F, Seronde MF et al. One-year outcome of patients submitted to routine fractional flow reserve assessment to determine the need for angioplasty. Eur Heart J 2005; 26: 2623–9.
49. Hacker M, Rieber J, Schmid R et al. Comparison of Tc-99m sestamibi SPECT with fractional flow reserve in patients with intermediate coronary artery stenoses. J Nucl Cardiol 2005; 12: 645–54.
50. Rieber J, Jung P, Erhard I et al. Comparison of pressure measurement, dobutamine contrast stress echocardiography and SPECT for the evaluation of intermediate coronary stenoses. The COMPRESS trial. Int J Cardiovasc Intervent 2004; 6: 142–7.
51. Okayama H, Sumimoto T, Hiasa G et al. Assessment of intermediate stenosis in the left anterior descending coronary artery with contrast-enhanced transthoracic Doppler echocardiography. Coron Artery Dis 2003; 14: 247–54.
52. Fearon WF, Yeung AC, Lee DP, Yock PG, Heidenreich PA. Cost-effectiveness of measuring fractional flow reserve to guide coronary interventions. Am Heart J 2003; 145: 882–7.

16

Percutaneous coronary intervention in the treatment of cardiogenic shock complicating acute myocardial infarction

Expedito Ribeiro, Pedro E Horta,
Marcus N da Gama, and Eulógio E Martinez

Cardiogenic shock constitutes a dreadful complication of acute coronary syndromes, occurring predominantly after an acute myocardial infarction with ST elevation (STEMI) but also among patients with non-ST elevation acute syndromes. When occuring in the acute phase of a myocardial infarction (MI), it is usually consequent to severe left ventricular dysfunction. Cardiogenic shock may also be due to mechanical complications, represented by acute mitral valve regurgitation, and acute ventricular septal rupture. These events constitute relatively late complications of acute myocardial infarction (AMI), usually occurring more than two days after the onset of symptoms, and requiring prompt echocardiographic confirmation of diagnosis and urgent surgical correction. In large series of patients, cardiogenic shock is observed in 6–7% of AMI, with mortality rates still very high, ranging from 56% to 74% in several publications.[1–6] The mortality rate in patients in cardiogenic shock in GUSTO-IIb (Global Utilization of Streptokinase and t-PA in Occluded Coronary Arteries) was similar in those with an STEMI or a non-ST elevation acute coronary syndrome.[4]

Left ventricular failure in patients with post-AMI cardiogenic shock is usually due to large areas of ischemia in consequence to extensive coronary disease. Accordingly, in the SHOCK (Should we emergently revascularize Occluded Coronaries for cardiogenic shock) trial registry, 53% of patients had obstructive lesions in three major coronary vessels, and 16% had significant left main disease.[5] In this registry, prognosis was better for patients with Thrombosis in Myocardial Infarction (TIMI) grade 3 flow in the culprit vessel (in-hospital mortality was 26% for TIMI 3 versus 47% for TIMI grade 0/1), emphasizing the importance of coronary reperfusion for the improvement in survival.

Percutaneous revascularization was proven to be efficacious in the treatment of AMI, and is the preferential treatment for cardiogenic shock complicating AMI.[6–15]

Ideally, patients with AMI complicated by cardiogenic shock and treated by primary percutaneous coronary intervention (PCI) should have support started before coronary angiography. Use of intra aortic balloon pump (IABP) is important not only during the procedure, but also post-intervention, particularly in patients without immediate hemodynamic improvement following coronary reperfusion.

Guidelines published by the American College of Cardiology (ACC)/American Heart Association (AHA) in 2004 gave a class I recommendation for the use of IABP as a stabilizing measure in acute MI in patients with cardiogenic shock not quickly reversed with pharmacological therapy or with acute mitral regurgitation (MR), or ventricular septal defect.

There are no randomized controlled trials to test the efficacy of IIb/IIIa glycoprotein inhibitors as an adjunct pharmacological agent during primary PCI in patients with cardiogenic shock. However, there is evidence that use of IIb/IIIa glycoprotein inhibitors may be beneficial. Giri et al recently reported a non-randomized study that involved 113 patients with post-infarction cardiogenic shock, of whom 54 were given abciximab.[16] Patients who received abciximab had a significantly higher rate of TIMI 3 flow (87% vs. 58% without abciximab), and a lower rate of the no-reflow phenomenon (9% vs. 37%).

A patent infarct-related artery is a strong determinant of survival in patients with cardiogenic shock. Accordingly, among 200 patients treated at Duke University the in-hospital mortality was 33% in patients with a patent infarct-related artery, compared to 75% in patients with closed arteries.[17] Similarly, in the SHOCK trial registry,[6] in-hospital mortality was lower in patients with TIMI grade 3 flow compared to TIMI grade 0/1 (26% vs. 47%, respectively).

In the SHOCK trial, 302 patients with confirmed cardiogenic shock developing within 36 h of an AMI were randomly assigned within 12 h of the diagnosis of shock to emergency revascularization (coronary artery bypass graft (CABG) in 40%, and PCI in 60%) within 6 h, or to initial medical stabilization.[14] Late revascularization was performed in 25% of patients in the medical stabilization arm at a minimum of 54 h after randomization. Intra-aortic balloon counterpulsation was utilized in 86% of patients in both groups. At 30 days, there was no significant difference in mortality comparing the two strategies (47% for emergency revascularization, and 56% for initial medical stabilization). However, the mortality benefit with emergency revascularization increased over time, the reduction in mortality compared to medical stabilization becoming significant at six months and one year (50% vs. 63%, and 53% vs. 66%, respectively).

A review from the National Registry of Myocardial Infarction (NRMI) of 25 311 patients with cardiogenic shock seen between 1995 and 2004, documented significant in-hospital mortality benefit for patients who underwent primary PCI (odds ratio 0.46, 95% confidence interval (CI) 0.40–0.53); in hospitals with catheterization and cardiac surgery facilities there was a progressive increase in the rate of primary PCI over the time period of the study, from 27% to 54% of patients, without concomitant increase in the rate of immediate CABG (2.1% to 3.2%).[18] The increase in use of primary PCI was associated with a significant reduction in in-hospital mortality from 60% in 1995 to 48% in 2004.

Traditionally, after recanalization of the infarct-related artery, patients with multivessel disease undergo staged percutaneous revascularization or surgical bypass grafting of the non-culprit lesions. In modern times, with the use of stents and potent antiplatelet agents, multivessel angioplasties are performed with high rates of success.[19,20] It is then reasonable to admit that simultaneous percutaneous revascularization of non-culprit arteries during primary PCI may be an alternative strategy for AMI patients found to have multiple lesions during acute angiography. Multivessel coronary disease occurs in between 40% and 65% of patients with AMI at presentation.[21-23] Among patients with non-complicated AMI, primary PCI is usually performed exclusively on the infarct-related artery. Treatment of non-culprit lesions is traditionally deferred and indicated after demonstration of ischemia.

Theoretically, treatment of non-culprit lesions in patients with AMI and multivessel disease should be avoided for two main reasons:

1. In the acute phase of a MI, there is an enhancement in the systemic thrombotic state, together with a generalized inflammatory reaction.[24-29] We can predict that in this setting there is a high risk for acute and post-procedural complications if multiple areas of vascular injury are created by multiple vessel interventions.
2. The severity of non-culprit lesions is often exaggerated in coronary angiograms of patients with AMI.[30] Many factors possibly contribute to this phenomenon, including vasoconstriction induced by increased levels of circulating cate-cholamines, serotonin, endothelin, angiotensin, and thromboxane, together with oxidative stress-induced attenuation of the vasodilatory activity of nitric oxide, adenosine, and prostacyclin.

Additionally, treatment of non-culprit lesions increases the utilization of contrast medium and the duration of the procedure.

Recently, the outcomes of 820 consecutive primary PCIs performed at the Middle America Heart Institute of Kansas were reported by Corpus et al.[31] Patients were treated between 1998 and 2002 and classified into two groups: patients with single-vessel disease (SVD) and patients with multiple-vessel disease (MVD), defined by the finding of $\geq 70\%$ stenosis of ≥ 2 coronary arteries. Patients with MVD were subdivided into three groups on the basis of the revascularization strategy: (1) patients undergoing PCI of the infarct-related artery (IRA) only; (2) patients undergoing PCI of both the IRA and non-IRA(s) during the initial procedure; and (3) patients undergoing PCI of the IRA followed by staged, in-hospital PCI of the non-IRA(s).

At 1 year, compared with patients with SVD, patients with MVD had a higher incidence of re-infarction (5.9% vs 1.6%, $P=0.003$), revascularization (18% vs. 9.6%, $P<0.001$), mortality (12% vs. 3.2%, $P<0.001$), and major adverse cardiac events (MACEs; 31% vs. 13%, $P<0.001$). In patients with MVD, compared with PCI restricted to the IRA only, multivessel PCI was associated with higher rates of re-infarction (13.0% vs. 2.8%, $P<0.001$), revascularization (25% vs. 15%, $P=0.007$), and MACEs (40% vs. 28%, $P=0.006$). Multivessel PCI was an independent predictor of MACEs at 1 year (odds ratio = 1.67, $P=0.01$).

Based on their findings the authors suggested that in patients with MVD, PCI should be directed at the IRA only. In their view, decisions about PCI of non-culprit lesions should be guided by objective evidence of residual ischemia at late follow-up. However, among their 506 patients with MVD, only 3.4% had Killip class IV on admission.

Similar findings were reported by Roe et al, in an analysis of a series of primary PCI in 79 patients with multivessel coronary disease.[32] Compared with patients undergoing culprit artery PCI, patients undergoing simultaneous multivessel PCI had a higher risk of death (25% vs. 16.4%), re-infarction (8.8% vs. 1.6%), CABG (4.4% vs. 0%), and stroke (10.3% vs. 0%).[15] Again, in this small series of patients less than one-third of those with multivessel disease presented with Killip class IV on admission. Thus, in order to limit procedural and in-hospital complications, primary PCI has traditionally been restricted to the IRA.

Recently, however, Katayama et al reported a series of 56 Japanese patients with AMI in hemodynamic subset 4 of Forrester's classification at hospitalization.[33] Patients underwent primary PCI within 12h (6.1±3.4h) of the onset of AMI. All patients had significant MVD. In 36 patients, PCI was performed exclusively in the culprit lesion; 20 patients also underwent PCI for non-culprit vessel lesions. Although the rates of all in-hospital deaths were not different when the two strategies were compared, the rate of cardiac deaths was higher in the group of patients in whom PCI was exclusively performed in the culprit lesion when compared with patients undergoing PCI of multiple lesions (42% vs. 15%, $P<0.05$). MACEs occurred more often among patients undergoing PCI of the culprit lesion only, than in patients treated also by PCI of non-culprit lesions (58% vs. 25%, $P<0.05$). Multivariate logistic regression analysis showed that complete revascularization (odds ratio 0.11, 95% CI 0.02–0.95, $P<0.05$) and duration from onset of AMI to PCI <6h (odds ratio 0.25, 95% CI 0.06–0.98, $P<0.05$) were negative predictors of in-hospital cardiac death, and prior MI (odds ratio 4.97, 95% CI 1.09–22.67, $P<0.05$) was a positive predictor.

According to the ACC and AHA, primary PCI or emergent surgical revascularization should be performed in patients who develop circulatory shock within 36h of an AMI, and can be treated within 18h of the onset of shock. An IABP should be inserted in patients with cardiogenic shock that is not quickly reversed with pharmacological therapy. Primary PCI is preferred to CABG for patients with one- or two-vessel coronary disease and technically suitable lesions. Immediate CABG is the preferred treatment for left main or severe three-vessel disease. If CABG cannot be performed, single-vessel or multivessel PCI may be attempted. Patients admitted within three hours of symptom onset to hospitals without facilities for revascularization, and scheduled to be transferred for a tertiary care center, may benefit from thrombolytic therapy prior to transfer.

We believe that when shock persists after recanalization of the IRA, simultaneous interventions on non-culprit lesions may be life saving. This strategy should only be followed by interventionalists with large experience in the treatment of acute coronary syndromes, considering that the consequences of any procedural complication when treating these additional lesions may be catastrophic. Meticulous analysis of coronary anatomy and lesion characteristics is fundamental for patient selection. In our view, acute simultaneous intervention in non-culprit lesions should be avoided in the presence of a visible thrombus, in severely calcified and/or tortuous vessels, in bifurcations, and when the non-culprit lesion is located in the left main coronary artery and/or in a saphenous vein graft.

REFERENCES

1. Goldberg RJ, Gore JM, Thompson CA, Gurwitz JH. Recent magnitude of and temporal trends (1994–1997) in the incidence and hospital death rates of cardiogenic shock complicating acute myocardial infarction: The second National Registry of Myocardial Infarction. Am Heart J 2001; 141: 65–72.
2. Holmes DR Jr, Bates ER, Kleinman NS et al. Contemporary reperfusion therapy for cardiogenic shock: The GUSTO-I trial experience. Global Utilization of Streptokinase and Tissue Plasminogen Activator for Occluded Coronary Arteries. J Am Coll Cardiol 1995; 26: 668–74.
3. Goldberg RJ, Samad NA, Yarzebski J et al. Temporal trends in cardiogenic shock complicating acute myocardial infarction. N Engl J Med 1999; 340: 1162–8.

4. Holmes DR Jr, Berger PB, Hochman JS et al. Cardiogenic shock in patients with acute ischemic syndromes with and without ST-segment elevation. Circulation 1999; 100: 2067–73.
5. Hochman JS, Boland J, Sleeper LA et al and the SHOCK Registry Investigators. Current spectrum of cardiogenic shock and effect of early revascularization on mortality: Results of an international registry. Circulation 1995; 91: 873–81.
6. Wong SC, Sanborn T, Sleeper LA et al. Angiographic findings and clinical correlates in patients with cardiogenic shock complicating acute myocardial infarction: a report from the SHOCK Trial Registry. SHould we emergently revascularize Occluded Coronaries for cardiogenic shocK? J Am Coll Cardiol 2000; 36: 1077–83.
7. O'Neill WW, Brodie BR, Ivanhoe R et al., Primary coronary angioplasty for acute myocardial infarction (the Primary Angioplasty Registry). Am J Cardiol 1994; 73: 627–34.
8. Keeley EC, Boura JA, Grines CL. Primary angioplasty or thrombolysis for acute myocardial infarction? Lancet 2003; 361: 967–8.
9. Grines CL, Browne KF, Marco J et al. A comparison of immediate angioplasty with thrombolytic therapy for acute myocardial infarction. The Primary Angioplasty in Myocardial Infarction Study Group. N Engl J Med 1993; 328: 673–9.
10. O'Neill WW. Angioplasty therapy of cardiogenic shock: Are randomized trials necessary? J Am Coll Cardiol 1992; 19: 915–17.
11. Bates E, Topol E. Limitations of thrombolytic therapy for acute myocardial infarction complicated by congestive heart failure and cardiogenic shock. J Am Coll Cardiol 1991; 18: 1077–84.
12. Antoniucci D, Valenti R, Santoro GM et al. Systematic direct angioplasty and stent-supported direct angioplasty therapy for cardiogenic shock complicating acute myocardial infarction: in-hospital and long-term survival. J Am Coll Cardiol 1998; 31: 294–300.
13. Berger PB, Holmes DR, Stebbins AL et al., for the GUSTO-I Investigators. Impact of an aggressive invasive catheterization and revascularization strategy on mortality in patients with cardiogenic shock in the Global Utilization of Streptokinase and Tissue Plasminogen Activator for Occluded Coronary Arteries (GUSTO-I) trial. Circulation 1997; 96: 122–7.
14. Hochman, JS, Sleeper, LA, Webb, JG et al, for the SHOCK Investigators. Early revascularization in acute myocardial infarction complicated by cardiogenic shock. N Engl J Med 1999; 341: 625–34.
15. Hochman JS. One-year survival following early revascularization for cardiogenic shock. JAMA 2001; 285: 190–2.
16. Giri S, Mitchel J, Azar RR et al. Results of primary percutaneous transluminal coronary angioplasty plus abciximab with or without stenting for acute myocardial infarction complicated by cardiogenic shock. Am J Cardiol 2002; 89: 126–31.
17. Bengtson JR, Kaplan AJ, Pieper KS et al. Prognosis of cardiogenic shock after acute myocardial infarction in the interventional era. J Am Coll Cardiol 1992; 20: 1482–9.
18. Babaev A, Frederick PD, Pasta DJ et al. Trends in management and outcomes of patients with acute myocardial infarction complicated by cardiogenic shock. JAMA 2005; 294: 448–54.
19. Kornowski R, Mehran R, Satler LF et al. Procedural results and late clinical outcomes following multivessel coronary stenting. J Am Coll Cardiol 1999; 33: 420–6.
20. Moussa I, Reimers B, Moses J et al. Long-term angiographic and clinical outcome of patients undergoing multivessel coronary stenting. Circulation 1997; 96: 3873–9.
21. Muller DW, Topol EJ, Ellis SG et al. Multivessel coronary artery disease: a key predictor of short-term prognosis after reperfusion therapy for acute myocardial infarction. Thrombolysis and Angioplasty in Myocardial Infarction (TAMI) Study Group. Am Heart J 1991; 121: 1042–9.
22. Jaski BE, Cohen JD, Trausch J et al. Outcome of urgent percutaneous transluminal coronary angioplasty in acute myocardial infarction: comparison of single-vessel versus multivessel coronary artery disease. Am Heart J 1992; 124: 1427–33.
23. Kahn JK, Rutherford BD, McConahay DR et al. Results of primary angioplasty for acute myocardial infarction in patients with multivessel coronary artery disease. J Am Coll Cardiol 1990; 16: 1089–96.

24. Shah PK, Forrester JS. Pathophysiology of acute coronary syndromes. Am J Cardiol 1991; 68: 16–23C.
25. Ambrose JA, and M. Weinrauch M. Thrombosis in ischemic heart disease. Arch Intern Med 1996; 156: 1382–94.
26. Dangas G, Colombo A. Platelet glycoprotein IIb/IIIa antagonists in percutaneous coronary revascularization. Am Heart J 1999; 138: S16–23.
27. Fuster V. Understanding the coronary disease process and the potential for prevention: a summary. Prev Med 1999; 29: S9–10.
28. Chierchia SL. Inflammation and acute coronary syndromes [in Spanish]. Rev Esp Cardiol 2001; 54: 1135–40.
29. Barrett TD, Hennan JK, Marks RM et al. C-reactive-protein-associated increase in myocardial infarct size after ischemia/reperfusion. J Pharmacol Exp Ther 2002; 303: 1007–13.
30. Hanratty CG, Koyama Y, Rasmussen HH et al. Exaggeration of nonculprit stenosis severity during acute myocardial infarction: implications for immediate multivessel revascularization. J Am Coll Cardiol 2002; 40: 911–16.
31. Corpus RA, House JA, Marso SP et al. Multivessel percutaneous coronary intervention in patients with multivessel disease and acute myocardial infarction. Am Heart J 2004; 148: 493–500.
32. Roe MT, Cura FA, Joski PS et al. Initial experience with multivessel percutaneous coronary intervention during mechanical reperfusion for acute myocardial infarction. Am J Cardiol 2001; 88: 170–3.
33. Katayama N, Horiuchi K, Nakao K, Kasanuki H, Honda T. Does percutaneous coronary intervention in non-culprit vessels improve the prognosis of acute myocardial infarction complicated by pump failure? J Cardiol 2005; 46: 1–8.

17

The hypotensive patient after angioplasty: occult life-threatening percutaneous coronary intervention-related complications

Eulógio E Martinez, Marco A Perin, and Luiz J Kajita

Dehydration • Vasovagal reactions • Arrhythmias • Retroperitoneal hematoma • Cardiac tamponade • Treatment of coronary perforation

Hypotension during or after percutaneous coronary intervention (PCI) may be due to a variety of causes that include dehydration, vasovagal reaction, cardiac arrhythmias, myocardial ischaemia, anaphylaxis, access site bleeding, retroperitoneal haematoma, and cardiac tamponade.

DEHYDRATION

Due to prolonged fasting before the procedure some degree of dehydration is common, particularly among patients on diuretic therapy. Routine pre-procedural administration of sublingual nitrates to these patients may precipitate severe hypotension; for that reason, in our view, sublingual nitrates should be replaced by intracoronary nitrates (200 µg of nitroglycerin, for example), particularly in patients with systolic blood pressure below 120 mmHg at the beginning of the intervention. Rapid intravenous infusion of a 0.9% sodium chloride solution will usually normalize blood pressure when hypotension is due to dehydration.

VASOVAGAL REACTIONS

Reflex reactions to arterial manipulation – vasovagal reactions – may cause severe bradycardia and hypotension and are seen in up to 3% of cardiac catheterizations. The usual treatment consists of volume administration and atropine 0.5–1.0 mg intravenously. Rapid reversion of hypotension may be mandatory in cases of hemodynamic deterioration caused by vagally mediated hypotension, particularly in patients with critical coronary or valvular disease. Of course myocardial ischemia must be excluded as a cause of vasovagal reaction, and in most cases the 12-lead electrocardiogram (ECG) can be used to assess this. The absence of ST deviation particularly in the inferior leads should exclude this possibility.

ARRHYTHMIAS

Atrial and ventricular arrhythmias frequently occur during cardiac catheterization. Cardiac arrhythmias leading to hemodynamic compromise require urgent treament that may include pharmacological agents, electrical cardioversion, or pacemaker stimulation. There are specific chapters in the book dealing with anaphylaxis and with management of patients with severe ischaemic ventricular dysfunction.

The two most serious occult life-threatening complications causing hypotension are represented by retroperitoneal hematoma (RPH) and cardiac tamponade.

RETROPERITONIAL HEMATOMA

Retroperitoneal hematoma is a life-threatening complication of access site injury when PCI is performed by the femoral route.[1-6] According to several studies the incidence of RPH is low, ranging from 0.15% to 0.44%.[7] The real incidence could possibly be higher, as milder cases may go undetected and fatal cases may not be diagnosed.

The absolute number of reported cases of RPH is significant, considering that approximately one million percutaneous coronary interventions per year are currently performed in the US alone. A large volume of blood can silently accumulate in the retroperitoneum before signs and symptoms of hypovolemia are manifested, with consequent delayed diagnosis, high morbidity and potential mortality. The access to the femoral artery can be guided by direct palpation, as well as anatomical and radiographic landmarks.[8,9] The ideal access site for the common femoral artery is located at the junction between the middle and the lower third of the femoral head. This approach is specially useful for obese patients and patients with weak pulses, such as those in cardiogenic shock.

Retroperitoneal extension of a hematoma originating from the femoral access site is more likely to occur when the arterial puncture is done above the inguinal ligament. When the puncture site is located above the inguinal ligament, the artery is accessed in the retroperitoneal space, and is called the external iliac artery.[9] On the other hand, if the puncture site is too low, below the distal common femoral bifurcation, access site complications are also increased, due to lack of support from the femoral head during mechanical compression.[8,9]

The predictors of retroperitoneal hematoma as a femoral access site complication were examined in two recent articles.[10,11] Farouque et al reported a retrospective analysis of 26 cases of RPH out of 3508 consecutive patients undergoing PCI between January 2000 and January 2004 at Stanford University.[10] Twenty-five patients had computed tomographic scan documentation, and one patient had autopsy confirmation of RPH. Cases were compared with a randomly selected sample of 50 control subjects without RPH. During the procedures, aspirin and unfractionated heparin were used as antithrombotic agents. Administration of glycoprotein IIb/IIIa inhibitors and use of coronary stents were decided by the operator. A thienopyridine was administered to patients receiving a stent. Use and choice of the type of vascular closure devices were based on operator decision. Sheaths left *in situ* after the procedure were removed when the activated clotting time was < 180 s, and compression was applied to achieve hemostasis. Interestingly, as a routine, femoral artery angiograms were obtained after sheath introduction by hand injection of radiographic contrast through the side arm of the femoral sheath. Images were taken in a shallow (±20°) right or left anterior oblique projection without cranial or caudal angulation. Using the femoral head as a landmark, the puncture site position was arbitrarily divided into two categories: high, when located in the proximal third of the femoral head or above, and low, when in the middle third of the femoral head or below. When compared to the control group, RPH patients had a greater fall in hematocrit percentage points from baseline (11.5 ± 5.1 vs. 2.3 ± 3.3; $P<0.0001$). Blood transfusions to correct severe anemia were given to 92% of RPH patients (mean 2.7 ± 3.3 units (range 1–18 units)). Three patients (12%) required vascular surgical intervention due to persistent hypotension. Two of these patients had punctures in the distal external iliac artery, and one patient had an anterior wall common femoral artery puncture that was inadequately sealed by a suture-mediated closure device, despite the appearance of external hemostasis. These patients had successful vascular repair and recovered uneventfully. One patient (4%) with RPH died from complications of retroperitoneal blood loss. Mean time from the end of the procedure until occurrence of first clinical feature was approximately 2.5 h. Forty-two per cent of the patients had the first clinical manifestation of RPH within the first 90 min, and 73% within the first 3 h after the end of the procedure. Only 4% had the first clinical manifestation later than 6 h after the procedure. Physical signs included blood loss anemia in all patients, hypotension in 92%, abdominal tenderness in 69%, bradycardia in 31%, and external groin hematoma in 31%. Clinical symptoms consisted of diaphoresis in 58%, groin pain in 46%, lower abdominal pain in 42%, and back pain in 23%. Female gender (odds ratio (OR) 5.4), body surface area <1.73 m^2 (OR 7.1), and a higher femoral puncture site (OR 5.3) were identified as independent predictors of RPH. Use of glycoprotein IIb/IIIa inhibitor and vascular closure device was not predictive of RPH. However, patients receiving a higher weight-adjusted heparin dose and those with smaller-caliber femoral arteries had a tendency to develop RPH, of borderline statistical significance. The study of Farouque et al yields several important lessons regarding clinical manisfestations and risk factors for the occurrence of RPH.[10] Clinically, it is noteworthy that the diagnosis is usually made only after significant blood loss has occurred. Additionally, back pain, often regarded as a common feature of RPH, occurred in only 23% of the patients, being less frequent than the complaints of groin pain and lower abdominal pain. Thus, one should not wait for 'typical' clinical manifestations before taking measures to diagnose and treat this potentially fatal complication. The frequent finding of abdominal tenderness (present in 69% of the cases) illustrates the importance of physical examination of the abdomen in cases of suspected RPH. Curiously, 92% of the patients were hypotensive, and bradycardia was detected in only 31%. This unexpected finding may be consequent to powerful vagal stimulation triggered by the hematoma in the retroperitoneal space, blunting the reflex tachycardia that would be expected in response to a fall in blood pressure. According to this finding, we believe that the association of hypotension and bradycardia after a PCI should raise the suspicion of RPH. A higher femoral arterial puncture site, defined as above the middle third of the femoral head on fluoroscopy, was the only procedure-related risk factor for RPH that can be at least partially prevented by the operator. However, in 45% of patients with RPH the arterial puncture site was low (in the middle third of the femoral head or below). In these cases, blood can reach the retroperitonium through the space alongside the femoral sheath. For this reason, the authors advocated applying manual compression to the femoral area at an early stage of all cases of presumed RPH until stabilization of the patient is achieved and the diagnosis confirmed.[10]

The relationship between the angiographic arteriotomy location and the subsequent development of retroperitoneal bleeding was also reported by Sherev et al.[11] Between October 2002 and September 2003, among 1631 left heart catheterization procedures, 1570 (96%) were performed with femoral access, 868 purely diagnostic and 702 PCIs. Through the femoral sheath, angiograms were obtained in 20–30° ipsilateral oblique view with no cranial or caudal angulations. Medial tension to the side arm of the femoral sheath was applied to confirm the arteriotomy location. The authors used anatomical markers of the inferior epigastric artery to classify femoral arteriotomy location. The inferior epigastric artery was used as a surrogate angiographic marker for the inguinal ligament and the retroperitonium, since that it is the last major branch of the external iliac artery before it traverses through the inguinal ligament.[12]

The following criteria were used for patient classification, according to the location of the arterial sheath):

- group 1 or low arteriotomy group: arterial sheath at or below the bifurcation of the common femoral artery into the superficial femoral artery and the profunda femoral artery
- group 2 or middle arteriotomy group: arterial sheath above the femoral bifurcation and below the most inferior border of the inferior epigastric artery (IEA)
- group 3 or high middle arteriotomy group: arterial sheath at or above the most inferior border of the IEA and below the origin of the IEA
- group 4 or high arteriotomy group: arterial sheath at or above the origin of the IEA.

Patients undergoing percutaneous coronary intervention received either 60 u/kg heparin bolus and IIb/IIIa inhibitor or bilivarudin. The femoral sheaths were removed immediately after diagnostic procedures. The artery was sealed by a femoral closure device or manual compression. For PCI patients, the sheaths were removed immediately at the end of the procedure if a closure device was used or there was evidence of an expanding hematoma. Among the 1570 patients undergoing femoral artery catheterization, there were 33 (2%) vascular complications, including 6 (0.4%) retroperitoneal hemorrhages. Blood transfusion ranging from 6 to 8 units of packed red blood cells was required in all retroperitoneal hemorrhages. All patients with RPH survived. Retroperitoneal hemorrhage only occurred in patients undergoing PCI (0.9% of PCI patients). A very important finding was that RPH were exclusively observed among patients with a high and high middle arteriotomy location (5 in group 3, and 1 in group 4). The authors recommend a femoral angiogram to risk-stratify patients after sheath insertion and, if clinically appropriate, advocate the deferral of PCI when arteriotomy is shown to be too high. However, in the article there is no mention of cases in which PCI was deferred due to inappropriately high femoral arteriotomy location. In our view, the importance of these two studies is the teaching that a proper arteriotomy location is the most relevant factor for the prevention of RPH. The inguinal ligament, and the femoral head (by radiographic visualization) should be used as anatomical landmarks to guide all femoral arteriotomies. We believe that if these landmarks are meticulously used, retroperitoneal hemorrhages should become even less common. In our laboratory we have no experience with routine femoral angiograms after sheath insertion. Furthermore, there are no data that closure devices reduce the risk of RPH, and in fact access site bleeding may be higher with their use. New promising antithrombotic regimens are now available. In patients with low-to-moderate-risk for PCI, bivalirudin with provisional glycoprotein IIb/IIIa blockade was associated with fewer major bleeding events as compared with unfractionated heparin and planned glycoprotein IIb/IIIa blockade. Additionally, the incidence of RPH was reduced by 60%, without significant changes in ischemic end points.[13]

CARDIAC TAMPONADE

Cardiac tamponade is usually due to coronary perforation and less frequently to tight ventricular perforation by temporary pacemaker wires. Coronary perforation is a rare but potentially serious complication of PCI, associated with urgent revascularization surgery in over 50% of cases, and high hospital mortality.[14-16] According to the Ellis classification, perforations are considered as class 1: presence of an extraluminal crater without extravasation, in the absence of signs of coronary dissection; class 2: pericardial or myocardial blush without contrast jet extravasation; class 3: extravasation through a clearly identifiable perforation. In a recent analysis of 16298 PCI procedures performed at the Mayo Clinic, 95 (0.58%) coronary perforations were identified, of which 12 patients (12.6%) sustained an acute myocardial infarction (MI), cardiac tamponade developed in 11 patients (11.6%), and eight patients (10%) died.[16] Predictors of mortality among patients with coronary perforation were age and cardiac tamponade. The following variables were tested for the association with perforation: age, sex, body mass index, diabetes, hypertension, renal failure, prior coronary artery bypass graft (CABG), left ventricular ejection fraction, lesion type (American College of Cardiology (ACC)/American Heart Association (AHA) classification), ostial lesion location, calcified lesion, calcium in the treated artery, proximal angulation, lesion on a bend, presence of thrombus, and use of an atheroablative device. Interventions were performed between January 1990 and December 2001. Significant multivariable correlates of coronary perforation were: use of an atheroablative device (OR 2.68), female sex (OR 2.38), ACC/AHA type C lesion classification (OR 2.28), and history of prior CABG (OR 1.70). Death was most common in patients with Ellis class 3 perforations. The incidence of coronary perforation varied with time, probably as a consequence of variations in the frequency of use of atheroablative devices. Clinical outcomes represented by cardiac tamponade, MI, and death were similar for patients who had and had not received a glycoprotein IIb/IIIa inhibitor. However, more patients receiving IIb/IIIa inhibitors required placement of a covered stent or emergency surgery (33.3% vs. 3.2%). In our experience, we have the impression that the use of newer hydrophilic guidewires in conjunction with IIb/IIIa inhibitors is associated with an increased risk of distal wire perforation.

Curiously, although the use of atheroablative devices has decreased, the odds of coronary perforation have not changed. It is reasonable to suppose that, due to great improvements in the technique and in equipment, cases considered too dangerous to be attempted in the past are now routinely attempted, with a higher rate of complication in comparison with simpler cases. Among 30746 PCIs performed between 1990 and 1999 at the Washington Hospital Center, there was an incidence of coronary perforations of 0.29%, among which 10% died.[17] Similarly with the findings from the Mayo Clinic, age and cardiac tamponade were independent predictors of mortality. The incidence, management and clinical outcome of coronary perforations in 39 of 12658 patients (0.3%) from the Massachusets General Hospital were recently reported by Witzke et al.[18] Perforations were more frequent when atheroablative devices were used compared to angioplasty and stent techniques (1% vs 0.2%, $P < 0.001$). Frequencies of class 1, class 2 and class 3 perforations were respectively 20.5%,

38.5% and 41%. Curiously, 51% of coronary perforations were guidewire related. Incidences of major clinical events were much higher in patients who experienced class 3 perforations. There was one death (2.6%), two emergency surgeries (5.2%), and no Q-wave MIs. Among the 39 perforations, pericardial effusions were detected in 18 patients (46.2%), with cardiac tamponade occurring in seven patients.

In an analysis of 7443 procedures performed between 1992 and 1996 reported by Fukotomi et al, the incidence of coronary perforation was 0.93% without in-hospital deaths.[19] However, 74% were Ellis class 1, and no class 3 perforations were observed.

TREATMENT OF CORONARY PERFORATION

Immediately after identification of a class 3 coronary perforation, occlusion of coronary vessel extravasation through deployment of a covered stent or a prolonged balloon inflation (preferentially with a perfusion balloon) should be attempted; other urgent measures are reversal of heparin anticoagulation with protamine, administration of inotropic agents if there is hemodynamic compromise, urgent pericardiocentesis in cases of large pericardial bleeding, and platelet transfusion in those patients treated with abciximab. In cases of pericardiocentesis it has been our practice to re-inject the blood through the side arm of the arterial introducer, particularly in cases of massive pericardial blood accumulation. The efficacy of polytetrafluoroethylene (PTFE)-covered stent in coronary perforations was recently reported by Ly et al.[20] Data related to all consecutive coronary perforations from databases of the Montreal Heart Institute were included in the study. At the operator's discretion, alternatives to seal perforations included deployment of a PTFE-covered stent as first-line strategy, or prolonged balloon inflation with or without bare-metal stenting. If a PTFE-covered stent was deployed, aspirin and clopidogrel were given for ≥3 months. Six-month clinical follow-up was scheduled. Procedural success was defined as successful delivery and deployment of the PTFE-covered or bare-metal stent to the perforation site, complete cessation of dye extravasation at the end of the procedure (after stenting or after prolonged balloon inflation), and postprocedural Thrombolysis in Myocardial Infarction (TIMI) 3 flow. Between April 1999 and June 2003, among 9382 PCI patients there were 25 diagnosed coronary perforations (0.3%). In 14 of these 25 patients, use of the PTFE-covered stent was attempted. There were no differences in baseline clinical (including age, sex and reasons for PCI) and angiographic characteristics between the group of patients treated with prolonged balloon inflation (with or without bare-metal stenting) and the group in which a PTFE-covered stent was used. A very important finding was that most perforations resulted from balloon or stent oversizing (11 of 14 patients in the PTFE group, and 8 of 11 patients in the bare-metal group). Mean balloon-to-artery ratio among the 25 patients with perforations was 1.37 ± 0.09. Other causes of perforations were guidewire damage to the vessel wall in five cases, and rotational atherectomy in one single case. Procedural success was higher in patients treated with PTFE-covered stents (10 of 14 patients, 71.4%, vs. 3 of 11 patients, 27.3%, $P=0.047$); postprocedural mean percentage diameter of stenoses was smaller in the PTFE group (12.7% vs. 35.4%, $P=0.002$). Reasons for failure of PTFE-covered stent were persistence of dye extravasation despite successful stent deployment in one patient, and inability to deliver the stent to the perforation site in three patients. Cardiac tamponade occurred in one patient in the PTFE arm, compared with four patients in the standard measure group ($P=$not significant). Although final TIMI 3 flow rates were comparable in the two treatment groups, persistence of postprocedural dye extravasation was more common in the standard management arm. Also, postprocedural increase in cardiac enzymes occurred in 1 patient among the 14 treated with PTFE-covered stents, and in 6 of the 11 patients treated by the standard strategy. At 6-month follow-up, 13 of 14 patients in the PTFE group remained asymptomatic or had mild angina on exertion, and 1 patient underwent clinically driven target site revascularization for restenosis. In contrast, 3 of 10 survivors in the standard management group were readmitted for acute coronary syndromes. In summary, PTFE-covered stents were significantly better than bare-metal stents at sealing coronary perforations, with greater procedural success, more frequent cessation of dye extravasation, larger postprocedural minimal lumen diameter, and favorable in-hospital and 6-month clinical outcomes. Similar results were reported by Briguori et al: 100% success rate among 11 patients with coronary perforations treated with PTFE-covered stents, compared with 40% success rate in 17 patients in which bare-metal stents were deployed to seal coronary perforations refractory to prolonged balloon inflation and anticoagulation reversal.[21] The sharp reduction in utilization of atheroablative devices was associated with a marked reduction in coronary perforations. However, new devices like distal protection filters, thrombectomy catheters, and stiff wires to facilitate crossing of chronic total occlusions may lead to new increases in the incidence of this serious complication. Special care should be taken in the selection of appropriate equipment, in the avoidance of balloon/stent oversizing, and in the handling of wires and of the abovementioned new devices. We believe that PTFE-covered stents of different sizes should be readily available to be used in cases of perforations with dye extravasation.

Cardiac tamponade can occur acutely, during the procedure, or can be diagnosed as a late event after PCI. The diagnosis of cardiac tamponade is suspected in cases of drop in blood pressure during or following PCI in the absence of causes of hypotension like vasovagal reaction, access site hemorrhage, retroperitoneal bleeding, myocardial ischemia, or anaphylaxis. It is usually heralded by hypotension and bradycardia due to potent vagal reaction triggered by blood in the pericardium. Cardiac tamponade is a consequence of perforation or frank rupture of coronary arteries, occurring in 0.2–0.6% of coronary angioplasties, the incidence being higher when atherectomy devices are utilized.[22-25] As mentioned before, a less frequent cause of tamponade related to cardiac catheterization is represented by right ventricular perforation due to temporary pacing wire. Treatment consists of reversal of heparin with protamine sulfate, attempts to stop the bleeding with prolonged inflation with either an angioplasty balloon or perfusion catheter, placement of a covered stent, pericardiocentesis, or emergency bypass surgery. Surgery is indicated in cases of continued bleeding or hemodynamic compromise unresponsive to pericardiocentesis.[17] The diagnosis can be confirmed by an urgent echocardiogram performed in the catheterization laboratory. However, treatment should be started immediately after the diagnosis is made from other evidence, like the documentation of free coronary perforation (free contrast extravasion) and/or fluoroscopic evidence of contrast medium in the pericardial space. In a recently published analysis of a prospective single center database, Feika et al reported 31 patients who developed cardiac tamponade among over 25 000 PCIs performed at the William Beaumont Hospital.[26]

Similarly to what has been reported in many publications, cardiac tamponade was twice as frequent after use of atheroablative devices compared with coronary angioplasty and stenting (0.26% vs. 0. 11%, $P < 0.05\%$). Interestingly, the incidence of tamponade was similar among patients treated with and without glycoprotein IIb/IIIa inhibitors. The diagnosis of cardiac tamponade was made in the catheterization lab, during the procedure, in 17 of the 31 patients (55%), and late after the intervention in 14 patients (45%) with a mean time of 4.4 h from the end of the intervention to the diagnosis, ranging from 2 to 15 h. The most frequent manifestation was progressive hypotension. Coronary free perforation was detected in all patients with early tamponade, whereas 10 of the 14 patients with late-onset diagnosis had no identifiable cause. Treatment consisted of intravenous volume expanders and inotropic support for all patients. Anticoagulation was reversed (mainly with protamine) in 17 patients (12 early and 5 late). Four patients were receiving a glycoprotein receptor inhibitor when cardiac tamponade developed; in all cases therapy was discontinued upon diagnosis. There was no definite association between use of a glycoprotein IIb/IIIa inhibitor and cardiac tamponade (cardiac tamponade in 4 (0.10%) of 3956 with vs. 27 (0.12%) of 21 741 without glycoprotein IIb/IIIa). A prolonged balloon inflation or perfusion balloon was used in all cases of coronary perforation, but sealing of the perforation was successful in only two patients. However, 'cover stents' were not available during the study period. In this series, cardiac tamponade was associated with a very high global mortality rate of 42% (13 of 31 patients). Mortality was particularly high for patients who developed cardiac tamponade in the cardiac catheterization laboratory (59% for early diagnosis vs. 21% for late diagnosis, $P < 0.05$). Twenty-nine of the 31 cases were due to coronary perforations by interventional devices, and only two were due to right ventricular perforations caused by temporary pacing wires. The poor prognosis observed in this study[26] differs from the study published by Von Sohsten et al, in which in a series of almost 7000 percutaneous coronary interventions, 15 patients developed cardiac tamponade and all survived the index hospitalization.[24] However, half of the cases were consequent to right ventricular rather than coronary artery perforation. It is then very likely that the cause of tamponade and rate of fluid accumulation in the pericardial space may be important determinants of clinical outcome, as suggested by Fejka et al.[26] Although the diagnosis of cardiac tamponade is usually easy when it occurs during the intervention, it may be less obvious in cases of late tamponade, manifested by hypotension after the patient has left the catheterization lab. Except for cases in which the cause of hypotension is easily identifiable, like access site bleeding, severe dehydration, or cardiac arrhythmias, an echocardiogram should be urgently recorded to either rule out or confirm the diagnosis of tamponade. Cases of cardiac tamponade diagnosed late after the procedure are frequently due to small coronary perforations, which are often treatable by percutaneous techniques. We believe coronary angiography is indicated in all cases to define the underlying cause for tamponade. Distal perforations may be managed by placement of embolization coils, or other materials, sacrificing patency of the perfurated branch.[27,28]

It has been our practice to re-infuse the blood removed by pericardiocentesis through the side arm of the arterial sheath. We usually try to drain the pericardium prior to the administration of protamine, because blood in the pericardium may 'gel' upon reversal of anticoagulation.[29]

REFERENCES

1. Steinhubl SR, Berger PB, Mann JT III et al. Early and sustained dual oral antiplatelet therapy following percutaneous coronary intervention: the CREDO trial. JAMA 2003; 288: 2411–20.

2. Lincoff MA, Bittl JA, Harrington RA et al. Bivalirudin and provisional glycoprotein IIb/IIIa blockade compared with heparin and planned glycoprotein IIb/IIa blocade during percutaneous coronary intervention: Replace-2 trial. JAMA 2003; 289: 853–63.
3. EPIC investigators. Use of a monoclonal antibody directed against the platelet glycoprotein IIb/IIIa receptor in high-risk coronary angioplasty. N Engl J Med 1994; 330: 956–61.
4. Van De Werf F, Armstrong PW, Granger C, Wallentin L et al. Efficacy and safety of tencteplase in combination with enoxaparin, abxicimab, or unfractinated heparin: the ASSENT-3 randomized trial in acute myocardial infarction. Lancet 2001; 358: 605–13.
5. Levine GN, Kern MJ, Berger PB et al. Management of patients undergoing percutaneous coronary interventions. Ann Intern Med 2003; 139: 123–36.
6. Jackson JE, Allison DJ, Hemingway AP. Principles, techniques and complications of angiography. In: Grainger RG, Allison D, Adams A, Dixon A, eds. Grainger and Allison's Diagnostic Radiology: a textbook of medical imaging, 4th ed. New York: Churchill Livingston, 2001: 149–59.
7. Nasser TK, Mohler ER 3rd, Wilensky RL, Hathaway DR. Peripheral vascular complications following coronary interventional procedures. Clin Cardiol 1995; 18: 609–14.
8. Safian RD, Freed MS. Coronary intervention preparation, equipment and technique. In: Safian RD, Freed MS, eds. The Manual of Interventional Cardiology, 3rd edn. Royal Oak, IL: Physicians' Press, 2001: 1–32.
9. Baim DS, Grossman W. Complications of cardiac catheterization. In: Baim DS, Grossman W, eds. Grossman's Cardiac Catheterization, Angiography, and Intervention, 6th edn. Philadelphia: Lippincott Williams and Wilkins, 2000: 35–65.
10. Farouque HM, Tremmel JA, Shabari FR et al. Risk factors for the development of retroperitoneal hematoma after percutaneous coronary intervention in the era of glycoprotein IIb/IIIa inhibitors and vascular closure devices. J Am Coll Cardiol 2005; 45: 363–8.
11. Sherev DA, Shaw RE, Brent BN. Angiographic predictors of femoral access site complications: Implication for planned percutaneous coronary intervention. Catheter Cardiovasc Interv 2005; 65: 196–202.
12. Bannister LH, Berry MM, Collins P et al. Common iliac arteries. In: Bannister LH, Berry MM, Collins P et al, eds. Gray's Anatomy: the anatomic basis of medicine and surgery, 38th edn. New York: Pearson Professional, 1995: 1558–68.
13. Lincoff MA, Bittl JA, Harrington RA et al. Bivalirudin and provisional glycoprotein IIb/IIIa blockade compared with heparin and planned glycoprotein IIb/IIa blockade during percutaneous coronary intervention: Replace-2 trial. JAMA 2003; 289: 853–63.
14. Stankovic G, Orlic D, Corvaja N et al. Incidence, predictors, in-hospital, and late outcomes of coronary artery perforations. Am J Cardiol 2004; 93: 213–16.
15. Gunning MG, Williams IL, Jewitt DE et al. Coronary artery perforation during percutaneous intervention: incidence and outcome. Heart 2002; 88: 495–8.
16. Fasseas P, Orford JL, Panetta CJ et al. Incidence, correlates, management, and clinical outcome of coronary perforation: analysis of 16298 procedures. Am Heart J 2004; 147: 140–5.
17. Gruberg L, Pinnow E, Flood R et al. Incidence, management, and outcome of coronary artery perforation during percutaneous coronary interventions. Am J Cardiol 2000; 86: 680–2.
18. Witzke CF, Martin Herrero F, Clarke SC, Pomerantzev E, Palacios IF. The changing pattern of coronary perforation during percutaneous coronary intervention in the new era. J Invasive Cardiol 2004; 16: 257–301.
19. Fukutomi T, Suzuki T, Popma JJ et al. Early and late clinical outcomes following coronary perforation in patients undergoing percutaneous coronary intervention. Circ J 2002; 66: 349–56.
20. Ly H, Awaida JS, Lesperance J, Bilodeau L. Angiographic and clinical outcomes of polytetrafluoroethylene-covered stent use in significant coronary perforations. Am J Cardiol 2005; 95: 244–6.
21. Briguori C, Nishida T, Anzuini A et al. Emergency polytetrafluoroethylene-covered stent implantation to treat coronary ruptures. Circulation 2000; 102: 3028–31.

22. Ellis SG, Ajluni SC, Arnold AZ, Popma JJ, Bittl JA et al. Increased coronary perforation in the new device era. Incidence, classification, management, and outcome. Circulation 1994; 90: 2725–30.
23. Dippel EJ, Kereiakes DJ, Tramuta DA et al. Coronary perforations during percutaneous coronary intervention in the era of abciximab platelet glycoprotein IIb/IIa blockade: an algorithm for percutaneous management. Cathet Cardiovasc Interven 2001; 52: 279–86.
24. Von Sohsten R, Kopistansky C, Cohen M, Kussmaul WG. Cardiac tamponade in the 'new era': evaluation of 6999 consecutive percutaneous coronary interventions. Am Heart J 2000; 140: 279–83.
25. King SB, Yeh W, Holubkov R et al. Balloon angioplasty versus new device intervention: clinical outcomes. A comparison of the NHLBI PTCA and NACI registries. J Am Coll Cardiol 1988; 31: 558–66.
26. Fejka M, Dixon SR, Safian RD et al. Diagnosis, management, and clinical outcome of cardiac tamponade complicating percutaneous coronary intervention. Am J Cardiol 2002; 90: 1183–6.
27. Dixon SR, Webster MW, Ormiston JA, Wattie WJ, Hammett CJ. Gelfoam embolization of a distal coronary artery guidewire perforation. Cathet Cardiovasc Intervent 2000; 49: 214–17.
28. Gaxiola E, Browne KF. Coronary artery perforation using microcoil embolization. Cathet Cardiovasc Diagn 1998; 43: 474–6.
29. Baim DS, Grossman W. Complications of cardiac catheterization. In: Baim DS, Grossman W, eds. Cardiac Catheterization, Angiography and Intervention. Baltimore: Williams & Wilkins, Baltimore, 1996, 17.

18

Percutaneous treatment options for patients with end-stage aortic valve disease

Aamer H Jamali and Raj R Makkar

Case presentation • Percutaneous aortic balloon valvuloplasty • Percutaneous aortic valve replacement • Future directions

CASE PRESENTATION

An 87-year-old female was admitted with recurrent congestive heart failure. She was known to have long-standing severe aortic stenosis (valve area 0.53 cm^2) and coronary artery disease with a left ventricular ejection fraction of 50%. After she was stabilized, the patient was taken to the cardiac catheterization laboratory. Coronary angiography revealed osteal left main coronary stenosis and osteal right coronary stenosis. She refused surgical intervention. High-risk percutaneous coronary intervention was offered. The patient was placed on a TandemHeart percutaneous left ventricular assist device (left atrial to femoral artery bypass), and the left main coronary artery was stented with a Cypher drug-eluting stent (Figure 18.1(a) and (b)). The osteal right coronary artery was then also stented with a Cypher drug-eluting stent (Figure 18.1(c) and (d)). Aortic valvuloplasty was performed using a 20 mm valvuloplasty balloon using the assist device to maintain flow while minimizing balloon movement. The resultant valve area was increased to 0.8 cm^2 The assist device was removed in the catheterization laboratory. At last follow-up (11 months after procedure), the patient was doing well at home without recurrent heart failure symptoms.

Aortic valve stenosis is the most common acquired form of cardiac valvular disease. Though rheumatic etiologies continue to constitute a fair proportion of aortic stenosis, their incidence is declining.[1] Senile calcific aortic valve disease, either stenosis, regurgitation, or mixed disease, represents the most common form of aortic valve disease today, occurring in up to 2.9% of patients over 65 years old.[2]

There is no suitable medical management for calcific aortic stenosis, and the mainstay of treatment remains aortic valve replacement. Over 13 000 aortic valve replacements are performed every year in the US alone.[3] While usually well tolerated, surgical aortic valve replacement can be associated with mortality risks ranging from 4% to 20%, with higher risks associated with left ventricular dysfunction.[3–6]

Traditional percutaneous options have been limited to percutaneous balloon valvuloplasty; however the results of this technique have been very disappointing, largely due to the recoil and restenosis of the aortic valve.[7]

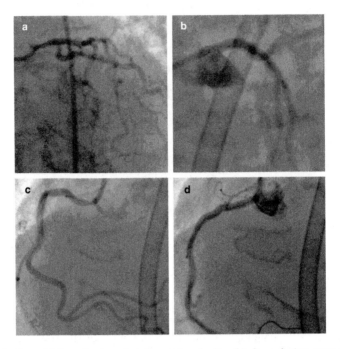

Figure 18.1   Osteal left main stenosis before (a) and after (b) drug-eluting stent placement. Osteal right coronary stenosis before (c) and after (d) drug-eluting stent placement.

Recent advances in interventional techniques have led to the development of what has been termed 'percutaneous aortic valve replacement', a displacement of the native leaflets against the sinuses by a stent-mounted biological valve. Although initial results with this technique and its variations have been promising, it remains a rapidly developing technology which is likely to evolve as it enters the mainstream in the coming years.

PERCUTANEOUS AORTIC BALLOON VALVULOPLASTY

Percutaneous aortic balloon valvuloplasty was first reported approximately 20 years ago.[8,9] Initial enthusiasm was soon tempered, however, by significant concerns regarding the long-term durability of results.[7] While the procedure may still be of particular use in pediatric patients with congenital aortic stenosis, its use in adults is reserved for patients with advanced congestive heart failure who are not surgical candidates. It also may be useful in patients with acute illnesses, as a temporizing measure before aortic valve surgery.

The largest series of patients undergoing percutaneous balloon valvuloplasty was reported by the National Heart Lung and Blood Institute, and consisted of 674 consecutive patients.[10] This series demonstrated relatively modest success of the procedure, with mean gradient reduction from 55 mmHg to 29 mmHg, and an increase in valve area from 0.5 cm^2 to 0.8 cm^2. However, a peri-procedural mortality of 10% was reported, with 8% of patients dying from cardiovascular causes. Though acute

Table 18.1 Summary of major trial experience with aortic valvuloplasty

Investigator	n (total) = 1704	Age (years)	MGr pre	MGr post	CO pre	CO post	AVA pre	AVA post	Clinical outcome
Block and Palacios[13]	90	79	61	30	3.6	3.9	0.4	0.8	72% cumulative survival at 5 months
Lewin et al[14]	125	76	70	30	4.3	4.6	0.6	1.0	62% cumulative survival at 1 year
Kuntz et al[12]	205	78	67	33	4.4	4.8	0.6	0.9	50% event free survival at 1 year
NHLBI[10]	674	78	55	29	4.0	4.1	0.5	0.8	86% cumulative survival at 30 days
O'Neill[15,a]	492		60	29	3.9	4.1	0.51	0.83	43% symptom free survival at 1 year
Letac/ Cribier et al[16]	92	75	75	30	–	–	0.5	0.9	66% cumulative survival at 13 months
Brady et al[17]	26	86	59	31	3.6	3.6	0.5	0.7	68% cumulative survival at 6 months
Weighted mean		78	60	30			0.52	0.84	

AVA, aortic valve area; CO, cardiac output; MGr, mean trans-aortic pressure gradient; pre, pre-valvuloplasty; post, post-valvuloplasty.
[a]Dr O'Neill's analysis is reported in groups of responders versus non-responders. For educational purposes, his numbers are presented as weighted averages between the groups.

clinical improvement was noted in the 86% of patients surviving at least 30 days (75% improved at least one functional class) in this registry, many other studies have shown that the durability of results from balloon valvuloplasty have proven to be quite poor (Table 18.1). The median time to restenosis has been shown to be approximately 6 months,[7] and the median survival after valvuloplasty is approximately 1 year, largely impacted by patient selection.[11,12]

In addition to this concern over 'restenosis' of the aortic valve, valvuloplasty often leaves valve areas of less than 1 cm², compared with the 2 cm² often obtainable with surgery. These issues, combined with the comparable mortality rates of the procedures, have led to a virtual abandonment of balloon valvuloplasty in favor of

Table 18.2   Summary of current experience with percutaneous aortic valve replacement

	Cribier–Edwards[a]	CoreValve[b]
Number of patients to date	68 (presented), >75 total	>27 total
Technology	Balloon-expandable stent	Self-expanding frame
Approach	First anterograde, more recently retrograde	Retrograde
Current delivery cannula	24F	24F
Stabilization	Rapid ventricular pacing	Femoral bypass
Coronary patency	Stent placement below ostea	Incomplete frame apposition to aortic wall in area of coronary ostea

[a]Personal communication Edwards Lifesciences, January 2006.
[b]Personal communication CoreValve Technologies, December 2005.

aortic valve replacement, despite the more invasive nature of the latter. Current indications for balloon valvuloplasty are restricted to non-surgical candidates, and as a temporizing measure in patients awaiting surgery. There has also been increasing consideration of using balloon valvuloplasty as a bridge to percutaneous aortic valve replacement while the latter procedure is being refined.

PERCUTANEOUS AORTIC VALVE REPLACEMENT

The lack of an acceptable alternative to surgical aortic valve replacement, as well as the demand for less invasive strategies for management of cardiovascular disease, have fueled a concerted effort to develop a feasible percutaneous approach to aortic valve replacement.

This effort was brought to fruition in 2002 when Cribier and colleagues described the first case of successful percutaneous orthotopic implantation of an aortic valve in a 57-year-old man with multiple comorbidities and a bicuspid aortic valve.[18] The patient underwent valvuloplasty but continued to decline clinically and had an ejection fraction of 20% with a systolic blood pressure approximately 70 mmHg despite multiple vasopressors. The patient experienced immediate hemodynamic improvement and survived for approximately 17 weeks after the procedure, but succumbed to sepsis after severe peripheral ischemia necessitated an above the knee amputation. Continued refinements since then have led to shorter procedure times, smaller vascular access sites, and, consequently, fewer complications.

Technical considerations

The term 'percutaneous aortic valve replacement' is actually a misnomer, as the native aortic valve tissue is not removed during the procedure. To date, two different systems have been used in humans; although details between the systems vary, both share the same basic technique (Table 18.2). Both consist of a stent or frame deployed within the aortic valve annulus, resulting in compression of the native leaflets against the walls of the sinuses of Valsalva. The interior of the stent contains biological valve tissue in order to maintain the vital physiological functions of an aortic valve.

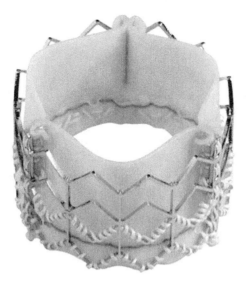

Figure 18.2 The Cribier–Edwards balloon-expandable aortic valve stent. This was the first percutaneously implanted aortic valve used in a human subject.

The Cribier–Edwards Valve (Edwards Lifesciences, Irvine, CA, USA) consists of a balloon-expandable stent, the superior border of which sits below the coronary ostea (Figure 18.2). The CoreValve Revalving system (CoreValve, Irvine, CA, USA) consists of a self-expanding frame spanning the entire sinuses of Valsalva into the ascending aorta (Figure 18.3; note that The CoreValve ReValving System is in the early stages of development and is neither commercially nor investigationally available in the USA).

Positioning

As opposed to the initial experience with pulmonic valve replacement, positioning of the prosthetic aortic valve is made more important by its close proximity to the coronary ostea.

A solution of historical interest is heterotopic aortic valve replacement with placement of the prosthetic aortic valve above the native valve and the coronary ostea in the ascending aorta, or even the descending aorta. Although initially performed by Huffnagel in 1951, this procedure soon fell out of favor thereafter.[19,20] It is only a feasible solution in the relatively small subset of patients with severe aortic insufficiency without significant stenosis. This approach also harbors the potential of changing coronary flow dynamics substantially (in essence ventricularizing the coronary ostea), and potentially precipitating severe coronary ischemia.

One solution is to allow the frame or stent to cross over the coronary ostea. In the CoreValve system, the nitinol framework actually spans across the coronary ostea while not being apposed to them. This allows normal flow through the coronary vessels, as well as catheter access to the ostea through the frame struts, while allowing slightly more flexibility in positioning.

Another solution used in the Cribier–Edwards Valve is to use a shorter stent, and position the superior margin below the coronary ostea. This approach probably

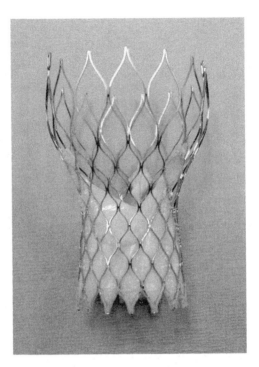

Figure 18.3 CoreValve Technologies ReValving System. Note the three distinct segments: the lower frame which helps position the valve and provides radial strength to prevent paravalvular leak, the middle region which allows access to coronary ostea, and the superior portion used for valve stability.

produces minimal disturbances to coronary flow. However, this limits the length of the stent that can be used, and requires very exact positioning, in turn potentially increasing procedure times. In patients with potentially distorted anatomy, this approach may necessitate the simultaneous use of advanced imaging methods, and both real-time magnetic resonance and intracardiac echocardiography have been looked at in this setting.

Other potentially useful methods of achieving coronary patency that have been investigated include devices that require significant rotational positioning in order to free the ostea or deploy stent grafts into them. However, these have been hampered by significant complexity and correspondingly long procedure times.

Approach

Initial implantations used the antegrade approach in which the aortic valve was accessed through transseptal puncture and subsequent passage of a guidewire through the mitral orifice and left ventricle (Figure 18.4). Concerns quickly arose about damage to the mitral valve as well as the difficulty in maneuvering catheters and wires in the small, hypertrophied ventricular cavities found in most patients with aortic stenosis.[21] For these reasons, the approach has largely been supplanted by the retrograde approach. Though this has obvious concerns of large-caliber arterial access (currently 24F), as well as difficulty in retrograde crossing of the stenotic aortic valve, it is quickly becoming the preferred approach for access for aortic valve stenting. This is likely to continue, as both major valve systems being investigated in humans currently are deployed via the retrograde approach. The adoption of the retrograde approach has been greatly enhanced by the development of deflectable tip catheter systems to facilitate traversing the aortic arch as well as crossing of the stenotic valve. Further advances in catheter-based techniques are likely to improve the issues of arterial cannula size, and devices that can be deployed through catheters as small as 18F are currently in development (personal communication CoreValve Technologies, December 2005).

Stabilization

Stabilization of the device is of prime importance during positioning, as proper positioning is essential to assure normal coronary blood flow, and the margin for error is quite small. This is hampered by the large volume of flow through the left ventricular outflow tract and its tendency to push undeployed prostheses into the ascending aorta. In the cases performed to date, one of the major modes of stabilizing the prosthesis predeployment has been to induce virtual cardiac standstill by rapid ventricular pacing. Cribier and colleagues have shown that they can consistently position the prosthesis during relatively short bursts of ventricular pacing at a rate of 220 beats/min.[22] In addition to reducing blood flow through the outflow tract, however, this method has the disadvantage of reducing vital organ perfusion as well.

Reduction in flow through the left ventricular outflow tract with maintenance of vital organ perfusion would be ideal for these procedures for two reasons. Firstly, by decreasing the blood volume flowing around the device during deployment, device movement is minimized. This is especially true for balloon-expandable systems, which are prone to movement with the balloon inflated in the aortic root. Secondly, the maintenance of vital organ perfusion allows the operator more time to properly position and deploy the device without as much concern for the patient's neurological wellbeing. For these reasons, investigations using the CoreValve system have used femoro-femoral bypass to reduce cardiac output through the aortic valve, while providing uninterrupted cerebral perfusion and hence aiding in positioning. In addition, other percutaneous circulatory assist devices such as the TandemHeart percutaneous LV (left ventricular) assist device may provide a potential means of providing excellent cerebral and vital organ perfusion while reducing flow through the left ventricular outflow tract.

Early human studies

Edwards Lifescience developed the first valve deployed in a human subject in 2002, a balloon-expandable valve which was placed using an anterograde approach through a 24F catheter (Figure 18.4).[18] It consisted of bovine tricuspid valve tissue mounted on a stainless steel stent. CoreValve Technologies has subsequently developed a self-expanding frame designed for a retrograde approach (Figure 18.5). Human trials are ongoing with both.

In 2005, Dr. Cribier presented the results of the first 33 patients to receive the Cribier–Edwards Valve.[23,24] The patients were all deemed to have prohibitive risk for surgery, and had a Parsonett score of greater than 30.[25] The antegrade approach was

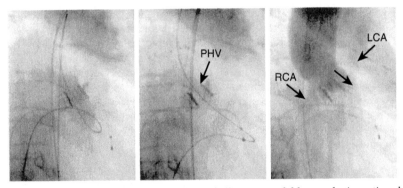

Figure 18.4   From the first in-man report of the balloon expandable prosthetic aortic valve.[18] Left: balloon inflation within the native valve; middle: the prosthetic valve in position (arrow); right: aortic root angiography showing no valvular regurgitation and only mild paravalvular regurgitation (arrow). Note that the valve ends below the coronary ostea. LCA, left coronary artery; PHV, prosthetic heart valve; RCA, right coronary artery.

used in 26 patients, and the retrograde approach in seven patients; however the valve was unable to be crossed retrogradely in three of these seven patients (one patient subsequently underwent antegrade replacement). The mean gradient in all of these patients was reduced from 37 mmHg to 9 mmHg, and the valve area was increased form 0.60 cm^2 to 1.7 cm^2. Most patients ended with some degree of paravalvular leak, though it was not severe in any of them. Though all cases showed immediate and dramatic hemodynamic and clinical improvement, four patients died in the peri-procedural period from procedure-related complications. Overall survival was limited in this study largely by the extremely high risk of the patients enrolled, but the results appear remarkably durable to follow-up as long as 2 years.

The CoreValve Technologies ReValving System consists of a self-expanding nitinol frame deployed through the retrograde approach. This framework houses three different zones – a lower one with excellent radial strength to reduce the risk of para-valvular leak, a middle, contracted segment which theoretically does not occlude coronary blood flow, and an upper segment devoted to providing stable fixation. Currently, feasibility trials are under way in Europe, and over 20 patients have received the device (Table 18.2; personal communication CoreValve Technologies, December 2005).[26] In the initial feasibility trial with a first generation device, six of ten patients were alive at follow-up up to 11 months; one of these patients has subsequently been able to receive a traditional aortic valve replacement. The second-generation device shows nine of ten patients alive, albeit at shorter (up to 5 month) follow-up.

FUTURE DIRECTIONS

Just as coronary stenting has evolved from a treatment for acute vessel closure in non-surgical situations, so too is aortic stent implantation likely to expand in indica-tion and use over the next several years.

Many of the challenges faced by the initial stenting procedures persist for aortic valve stenting, but are amplified by the critical anatomical and physiological role of

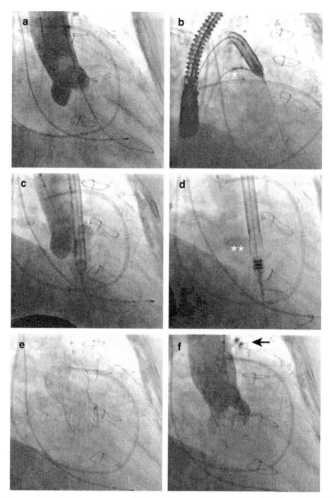

Figure 18.5 From the first in-man report of a self-expanding aortic valve prosthesis.[25] (a) Aortic root angiography pre-intervention; (b) advancing the valve over the aortic arch. A snare (*) is used to facilitate deflection; (c) device positioning; (d) pullback of the outer sheath with deployment of the prosthesis (**); (e) deployed prosthesis; (f) aortic root angiography showing no paravalvular regurgitation. (Reprinted from Grube E, Laborde JC, Zickman B et al. First report on a human percutaneous transluminal implantation of a self-expanding valve prosthesis for interventional treatment of aortic valve stenosis. Catheter Cardiovasc Interv 2005; 66: 465–9, with permission.)

the aortic valve. Issues of coronary patency, mechanical support, device positioning, and vascular access have proved surmountable in early trials, but further refinement of these techniques is necessary.

Currently the greatest challenge facing percutaneous valve implantation is one of patient selection. As initial experience has appropriately focused on critically ill patients with extremely short life expectancy, clinical outcomes following percutaneous techniques have been less impressive than those found with aortic surgery. However, physiological results have been similar. The mean aortic valve area achieved with the Cribier–Edwards Valve was $1.7\,cm^2$, similar to that achieved with traditional surgical aortic prostheses. Thus, to truly understand the impact of this procedure, a fair comparison must be made with surgery. This can only be achieved through randomized clinical trials; such a trial should be delayed, however, until the techniques involved in percutaneous valve replacement reach a higher level of refinement. In the meantime, trials in patients with prohibitive surgical risk are ongoing.

Given the high prevalence of aortic stenosis, the risks and invasiveness of surgical aortic valve replacement, the lack of any alternative treatment for aortic stenosis, and the initial promising results with percutaneous stenting, it is virtually certain that the nascent field of aortic valve stenting will expand dramatically in the near future to change the treatment of heart disease.

REFERENCES

1. Passick CS, Ackermann DM, Pluth JR, Edwards WD. Temporal changes in the causes of aortic stenosis: A surgical pathologic study of 646 cases. Mayo Clin Proc 1987; 62: 119–23.
2. Otto CM, Lind BK, Kitzman DW et al. Association of aortic valve sclerosis with cardiovascular mortality and morbidity in the elderly. N Engl J Med 1999; 341: 142–7.
3. Society for Thoracic Surgeons. Executive Summary 2005. Availble at http:// www.sts.org.
4. Jamieson WRE, Edwards FH, Schwartz M et al. Risk stratification for cardiac valve replacement. National Cardiac Surgery Database. Ann Thoracic Surg 1999; 67: 943–51.
5. Kvidal P, Bergstrom R, Horte L, Stahle E. Observed and relative survival after aortic valve replacement. J Am Coll Cardiol 2000; 35: 747–56.
6. Powell DE, Tunick PA, Rosenzweig BP et al. Aotic valve replacement in patients with aortic stenosis and severe left ventricular dysfunction. Arch Intern Med 2000; 160: 1337–41.
7. Litvack F, Jakubowski AT, Buchbinder NA, Eigler N. Lack of sustained clinical improvement in an elderly population after percutaneous aortic valvuloplasty. Am J Cardiol 1988; 62: 270–5.
8. Cribier A, Saoudi N, Berland J et al. Percutaneous transluminal valvuloplasty of acquired aortic stenosis in elderly patients: an alternative to valve replacement? Lancet 1986; 1: 63–7.
9. McKay RG, Safian RD, Lock JE et al. Balloon dilatation of calcific aortic stenosis in elderly patients: Postmortem, intraoperative, and percutaneous valvuloplasty studies. Circulation 1986; 74: 119–25.
10. NHLBI Balloon Valvuloplasty Registry Participants. Percutaneous balloon aortic valvuloplasty. Circulation 1991; 84: 2383–97.
11. Otto CM, Mickel MC, Kennedy JW et al. Three year outcome after balloon aortic valvuloplasty: Insights into prognosis of valvular aortic stenosis. Circulation 1994; 89: 642–50.
12. Kuntz RE, Tosteson ANA, Berman AD et al. Predictors of event-free survival after balloon aortic valvuloplasty. N Engl J Med 1991; 325: 17–23.
13. Block PC, Palacios IF. Clinical and hemodynamic follow-up after percutaneous aortic valvuloplasty in the elderly. Am J Cardiol 1988; 62: 760–3.
14. Lewin RF, Dorros G, King JF, Mathiak L. Percutaneous transluminal aortic valvuloplasty: acute outcome and follow-up of 125 patients. J Am Coll Cardiol 1989; 14: 1210–17.
15. O'Neill WW. Predictors of long-term survival after percutaneous aortic valvuloplasty: Report of the Mansfield Scientific Balloon Aortic Valvuloplasty Registry. J Am Coll Cardiol 1991; 17: 193–8.
16. Letac B, Cribier A, Koning R, Lefabvre E. Aortic stenosis in elderly patients aged 80 or older. Treatment by percutaneous balloon valvuloplasty in a series of 92 cases. Circulation 1989; 80: 1514–20.
17. Brady ST, Davis CA, Kussmaul WG et al. Percutaneous aortic balloon valvuloplasty in octogenarians: morbidity and mortality. Ann Intern Med 1989; 110: 761–6.
18. Cribier A, Eltchaninoff H, Bash A et al. Percutaneous transcatheter implantation of an aortic valve prosthesis for calcific aortic stenosis. Circulation 2002; 106: 3006–8.

19. Hufnagel CA, Harvey WP. The surgical correction of aortic regurgitation preliminary report. Bull Georgetown Univ Med Ctr 1953; 6: 60–1.
20. Rose JC, Hufnagel CA, Freis ED, Harvey WP, Partenope EA. The hemodynamic alterations produced by a plastic valvular prosthesis for severe aortic insufficiency in man. J Clin Invest 1954; 33: 891–900.
21. Hanzel GS, Harrity PJ, Schreiber TL, O'Neill WW. Retrograde percutaneous aortic valve implantation for critical aortic stenosis. Catheter Cardiovasc Interv 2005; 64: 322–6.
22. Cribier A, Eltchaninoff H, Tron C et al. Early experience with percutaneous transcatheter implantation of heart valve prosthesis for the treatment of end-stage inoperable patients with calcific aortic stenosis. J Am Coll Cardiol 2004; 43: 698–703.
23. Cribier A. Update on percutaneous aortic valve replacement. Oral session at EuroPCR. Paris, France, May 2004.
24. Cribier A, Eltchaninoff H, Tron C et al. Treatment of calcific aortic stenosis with the percutaneous heart valve: mid-term follow-up from the initial feasibility studies, the French experience. J Am Coll Cardiol 2006; 47: 1214–23.
25. Berman M, Stamler A, Sahar G, et al. Validation of the 2000 Bernstein-Parsonnet score versus the EuroSCORE as a prognostic tool in cardiac surgery. Ann Thorac Surg 2006; 81: 537–40.
26. Grube E, Laborde JC, Zickman B et al. First report on a human percutaneous transluminal implantation of a self-expanding valve prosthesis for interventional treatment of aortic valve stenosis. Catheter Cardiovasc Interv 2005; 66: 465–9.

19

Acute coronary dissection, occlusion, and perforation during percutaneous coronary intervention: surgical, percutaneous, or medical management

Goran Stankovic and Antonio Colombo

Acute coronary dissections • Acute closure • Coronary perforation • Vessel rupture • Wire perforations • Pericardial drainage

ACUTE CORONARY DISSECTIONS

Historically the occurrence of a dissection following coronary angioplasty had a double connotation. In a classic study by Gruentzig the best long-term results occurred in lesions which had a residual gradient less than 15 mmHg and had a visible dissection.[1] On the other side the presence of a dissection was a risk factor for acute and subacute vessel closure and this was one of the main reasons for referral to emergency surgery.[2–6] The National Heart, Lung and Blood Institute (NHLBI) classification system for intimal tears, developed by the Coronary Angioplasty Registry, is proposed for the classification of dissection types (dissections are graded based upon their angiographic appearances as types A to F).[3]

The advent of routine stent implantation has completely changed this view, and nowadays we can summarize the issue in one statement: *dissection prior to stenting (following predilatation when performed) has no practical value, while dissection post-stenting should not be present and should be corrected.*

There are a number of studies that demonstrate that a residual persistent dissection constitutes a risk factor for stent closure.[3] The operator should make any possible effort to correct this condition by implanting another stent. In some circumstances, and prior to the introduction of drug-eluting stents, there was the need to limit stent length to the minimum needed. The concept of 'spot stenting' allowed the presence of persistent dissections, provided an evaluation with intravascular ultrasound (IVUS) demonstrated the presence a sufficiently large residual lumen.[7,8] We have previously shown that IVUS evaluation may identify a non-obstructive dissection which can be left untreated when final IVUS area stenosis is less than 60% at the site of a dissection.[8]

At present, the introduction of drug-eluting stents has lowered the impact of stent length on the risk of restenosis, and the implantation of an additional stent to fully cover any residual dissection appears the most practical approach.[9]

Every operator now knows all the tricks to negotiate a stent in a distal location, such as usage of short stents, buddy wire, or buddy balloons techniques, usage of low-friction ring design stents etc. There are extreme conditions when a stent cannot be advanced distally, and in these situations additional pharmacotherapy is the only additional approach.[10]

The presence of a dissection always needs to be evaluated, not only in the context of residual lumen but also of examining the distal flow pattern (Thrombolysis in Myocardial Infarction (TIMI) flow). In very rare, currently unheard of conditions in our experience, the presence of a non-correctible dissection involving a major epicardial vessel may require surgical revascularization.

ACUTE CLOSURE

Acute vessel closure is the most feared complication of coronary artery dissection, and in the pre-stent era occurred in up to 11% of all elective percutaneous transluminal coronary angioplasty (PTCA), while with the advent of coronary stents, the incidence of acute closure in elective percutaneous coronary intervention (PCI) is now less than 1%.[3,11] The problem of acute stent closure has emerged even following implantation of drug-eluting stents.[11] There is no clear explanation for this type of event, but a few elements need to be examined and looked at:

- the presence of a residual dissection
- reduced distal run-off due to embolization, spasm, or false lumen stenting
- inadequate anticoagulation or antiplatelet therapy.

The fact that acute stent closure is a rare event means many operators are not sufficiently concerned about this complication, and its occurrence is frequently never fully investigated. The most important element is always to correct and prevent any possible risk factor. Anticoagulation monitoring by the activated clotting time (ACT) and distal flow evaluation are key elements to be studied prior to stenting. There is no reason to proceed to additional stenting if the distal run-off appears poor. The illusion that implanting a proximal stent to correct any possible non-critical stenosis will improve the distal run-off is an unrewarding approach (Figure 19.1). Before proceeding with any further intervention, the operator needs to understand the reason for the reduced run-off. Selective injection through a multifunction probing catheter can help to establish if the problem is in the distal or proximal bed. The use of pharmacological agents such as nitroprusside, adenosine, verapamil or a combination of these can be of importance.[13] In conditions that are poor to resolve, the insertion of a balloon pump can be the most practical approach. As previously stated, stent closure needs to be prevented.

If closure does occur, it is then important to re-open the stent and to understand why the complication manifested. Thrombus formation remains the main reason for stent closure. All known measures to deal with acute thrombosis should therefore be put into action. In addition to heparin anticoagulation, selective injection of abciximab into the occluded vessel has been proposed. Thrombus aspiration, with or without distal protection, the use of Possis thrombus removal etc, depend on local expertise, availability, and extension of the thrombus and its location.

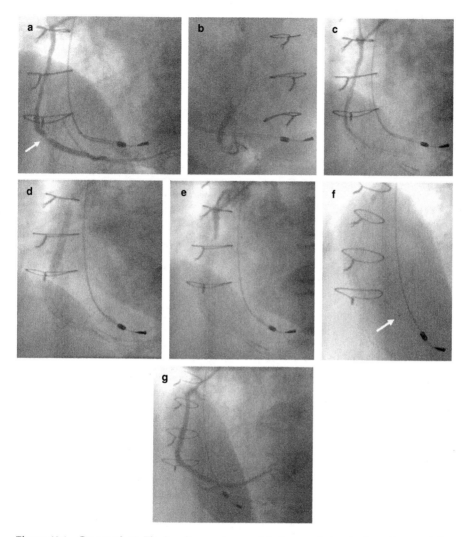

Figure 19.1 Case study 1. The baseline angiogram (a), shows a lesion in the mid-part of the saphenous vein graft to the right coronary artery with TIMI 3 flow. Following direct stent implantation there is a reduction of the flow to TIMI 2 ((b) and (c)). The operator believed that the reduction in distal flow was the result of the presence of proximal disease and proceeded with implantation of another stent more proximally (d). The following injection showed a further reduction of flow, now without opacification of the distal bed (e). Finally the multifunction-probing catheter was advanced in the graft (arrow indicates the tip of the probing catheter) and 200 μg of nitroprusside selectively injected (f), which has resulted in prompt restoration of TIMI 3 flow (g).

CORONARY PERFORATION

Coronary perforation remains one of the most serious complications in the catheterization laboratory, with multiple studies demonstrating very poor outcomes, particularly in relation to myocardial infarction (MI) and death.[14–19] Angiographic evidence of perforation has been reported in 0.1% to 3.0% of lesions treated with various

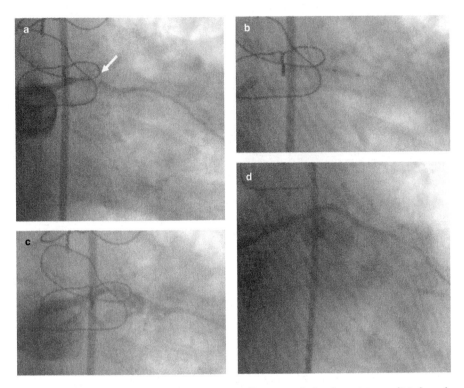

Figure 19.2   Case study 2. A baseline angiogram illustrates a lesion in an intermediate branch in a patient with prior bypass surgery (a, arrow). The operator assumed that the vessel was fibrotic and elected to use a cutting balloon (3×10 mm) (b) which created a coronary rupture (c). Following unsuccessful prolonged balloon inflation, a PTFE-covered stent was deployed with complete sealing of the leakage (d).

intervention techniques,[14,15,18–23] and even today accounts for 20% of referrals for emergency bypass surgery.[24] Patients who are especially at risk are elderly, female, those with calcified and tortuous arteries,[15,18,19,22] and those in whom atheroablative devices are used.[18–21,25,26] In our own series, we noted an 8% incidence of death, 18% incidence of MI, and a 13% need for emergency coronary bypass surgery.[19]

Adverse clinical events following coronary perforations are related to their angiographic severity.[14–17,19] Ellis et al first reported that class III perforations (extravasation through a frank ≥1 mm perforation) were associated with a very high incidence of major adverse events (death, 19%; emergency CABG, 63%; Q-wave MI, 15%; cardiac tamponade, 63%).[15]

Regarding the treatment options, there are several proposed algorithms for percutaneous management of coronary perforations.[18,19,22] Prevention, early diagnosis, adjusted risk evaluation, and immediate implementation of therapeutics resources are the keys to coronary perforation control. Prevention is especially important in situations that potentially increase the risk of perforation (as the high-risk patient or lesion subsets, or use of debulking techniques or hydrophilic, taper, or stiff guidewires). Early diagnosis is based on the correct evaluation of symptoms and careful monitoring of clinical signs, such as a puncture-like chest pain during guidewire advancement, or with resistance to wire and device progression.

Perforations can occur due to vessel rupture or to distal guidewire vessel perforation.

VESSEL RUPTURE

Traditionally, perforation has been associated with usage of new devices such as atherectomy (rotational and directional), laser angioplasty, and cutting balloon angioplasty (Figure 19.2).[19,21–23,27] The slow disappearance of these devices seems to lead to a decrease in the incidence of this complication.[19] Despite the above consideration, we cannot dismiss that coronary perforation can occur at the time of lesion predilatation, or when expanding a stent. Treatment of more complex lesions located at sharp bends, and dilatation of hard calcific lesions remain important risk factors. The first golden rule remains to avoid using compliant or semicompliant balloons in calcific or fibrotic lesions, or to try to overcome a lesion which cannot be dilated at high pressure by using an oversized balloon. The use of IVUS to appropriately evaluate the vessel size, and strict adherence to the information obtained is of paramount importance. There is no reason why a cardiac catheterization lab should not have modern non-compliant balloons available to be utilized in these circumstances.

When, despite all possible precautions, coronary perforation occurs, the first step is not to lose control of the situation, in particular not to lose the access of the artery. In any risky condition it remains imperative to deflate the balloon and wait to remove it until a contrast injection has shown the absence of perforation. The immediate inflation of the balloon at low pressure remains the first simple step to avoid immediate consequences. When possible, a prolonged balloon inflation should be attempted. If the patient is unable to tolerate ischemia during balloon inflation, a perfusion balloon should be used. Perfusion balloons allow distal vessel perfusion, thereby reducing ischemia during prolonged inflations. The implantation of a polytetrafluoroethylene (PTFE)-covered stent remains the last resort.[17] The use of autologous vein-covered stents has been reported, but remains impractical due to the prolonged time required for vein harvest and suturing of the vein graft to a stent before deployment.[3,28,29]

We are less enthusiastic about the need for and safety of heparin neutralization, especially following implantation of drug-eluting stents. If the operator considers performing a prolonged balloon inflation or using a perfusion balloon, the safety of using protamine to neutralize the heparin given to the patient becomes questionable. Recently we have seen three cases of stent thrombosis occurring following neutralization of heparin in the context of treatment of a perforation. The use of glycoprotein IIb/IIIa inhibitors or direct thrombin inhibitors poses additional problems regarding the treatment of coronary perforations. Platelet transfusion should be employed for reversal of an abciximab antiplatelet effect. In the presence of normal renal function, infusions of small-molecule glycoprotein IIb/IIIa inhibitors such as eptifibatide and tirofiban may be stopped with prompt reversal given their short half-lives (wait a few hours, maybe dialyze).

In cases where sealing of the perforation by conservative measures cannot be achieved, urgent bypass surgery must be performed.

WIRE PERFORATIONS

These types of perforations can occur while treating a chronically occluded artery, or while performing standard angioplasty with stent implantation.

Perforations occurring during treatment of chronic occlusions have usually been benign, and have been termed wire exits rather than perforations. The operator knows about the risk and avoids advancing a balloon over the wire in an incorrect position. In our own series we also observed an increase in the rate of guidewire perforations in recent years (1998 onwards), which may coincide with the introduction of hydrophilic coronary wires and special stiff wires designed to recanalize chronic total occlusions.[19] The risk of this complication is in direct relation to the magnitude of the perforation.

Distal wire perforations are more subtle because frequently the operator is not aware of their occurrence. They tend to manifest more frequently with the use of hydrophilic wires that have been advanced too distally. The most common approach is to immediately exchange any hydrophilic wire for a regular wire in order to avoid such risk. These findings stress the importance of careful fluoroscopic observation of the progress of a guidewire through the arterial tree, as well as the need for frequent change in magnification in order to monitor guidewire position in the distal coronary artery when hydrophilic, taper, or stiff wires are used.

If distal perforation occurs, the operator can perform distal balloon inflation, coil embolization, or microparticle injections.[30–32] Cases have been reported about using autologous thrombus injected distally as an effective approach. In rare circumstances, implantation of a PTFE stent to divert the flow into a branch can exclude blood flow to the perforated segment. Surgical ligation remains a therapeutic option if other methods fail.

PERICARDIAL DRAINAGE

Treatment of impending tamponade may be an essential part of the approach to treating a coronary perforation. Every operator needs to be familiar with pericardial drainage and have all the necessary tools including a long needle to access obese patients or patients with a large anterior–posterior (AP) diameter. Operators also need to be familiar with techniques involving autotransfusion of aspirated blood into a central vein. It is also important to understand that completed removal of the blood from the pericardium may not always be the best approach, because the presence of a large pressure gradient between the perforation and the pericardium may delay spontaneous closure of the leak. Adequate fluid and pressure support of the patient may minimize the need to aggressively remove all the blood from the pericardium, therefore helping the closure of the perforation.

REFERENCES

1. Leimgruber PP, Roubin GS, Hollman J, et al. Restenosis after successful coronary angioplasty in patients with single-vessel disease. Circulation 1986; 73: 710–17.
2. Holmes DR Jr, Holubkov R, Vlietstra RE et al. Comparison of complications during percutaneous transluminal coronary angioplasty from 1977 to 1981 and from 1985 to 1986: the National Heart, Lung, and Blood Institute Percutaneous Transluminal Coronary Angioplasty Registry. J Am Coll Cardiol 1988; 12: 1149–55.
3. Rogers JH, Lasala JM. Coronary artery dissection and perforation complicating percutaneous coronary intervention. J Invasive Cardiol 2004; 16: 493–9.
4. Detre KM, Holmes DR Jr, Holubkov R et al. Incidence and consequences of periprocedural occlusion. The 1985–1986 National Heart, Lung, and Blood Institute Percutaneous Transluminal Coronary Angioplasty Registry. Circulation 1990; 82: 739–50.

5. Bell MR, Reeder GS, Garratt KN et al. Predictors of major ischemic complications after coronary dissection following angioplasty. Am J Cardiol 1993; 71: 1402–7.

6. Sharma SK, Israel DH, Kamean JL, Bodian CA, Ambrose JA. Clinical, angiographic, and procedural determinants of major and minor coronary dissection during angioplasty. Am Heart J 1993; 126: 39–47.

7. Colombo A, De Gregorio J, Moussa I et al. Intravascular ultrasound-guided percutaneous transluminal coronary angioplasty with provisional spot stenting for treatment of long coronary lesions. J Am Coll Cardiol 2001; 38: 1427–33.

8. Nishida T, Colombo A, Briguori C et al. Outcome of nonobstructive residual dissections detected by intravascular ultrasound following percutaneous coronary intervention. Am J Cardiol 2002; 89: 1257–62.

9. Biondi-Zoccai GG, Agostoni P, Sangiorgi GM et al. Incidence, predictors, and outcomes of coronary dissections left untreated after drug-eluting stent implantation. Eur Heart J 2006; 27: 540–6.

10. Islam MA, Blankenship JC, Balog C et al. Effect of abciximab on angiographic complications during percutaneous coronary stenting in the Evaluation of Platelet IIb/IIIa Inhibition in Stenting Trial (EPISTENT). Am J Cardiol 2002; 90: 916–21.

11. Lincoff AM, Popma JJ, Ellis SG, Hacker JA, Topol EJ. Abrupt vessel closure complicating coronary angioplasty: clinical, angiographic and therapeutic profile. J Am Coll Cardiol 1992; 19: 926–35.

12. Chieffo A, Bonizzoni E, Orlic D et al. Intraprocedural stent thrombosis during implantation of sirolimus-eluting stents. Circulation 2004; 109: 2732–6.

13. Kelly RV, Cohen MG, Stouffer GA. Incidence and management of 'no-reflow' following percutaneous coronary interventions. Am J Med Sci 2005; 329: 78–85.

14. Ajluni SC, Glazier S, Blankenship L, O'Neill WW, Safian RD. Perforations after percutaneous coronary interventions: clinical, angiographic, and therapeutic observations. Cathet Cardiovasc Diagn 1994; 32: 206–12.

15. Ellis SG, Ajluni S, Arnold AZ et al. Increased coronary perforation in the new device era. Incidence, classification, management, and outcome. Circulation 1994; 90: 2725–30.

16. Alfonso F, Goicolea J, Hernandez R et al. Arterial perforation during optimization of coronary stents using high-pressure balloon inflations. Am J Cardiol 1996; 78: 1169–72.

17. Briguori C, Nishida T, Anzuini A et al. Emergency polytetrafluoroethylene-covered stent implantation to treat coronary ruptures. Circulation 2000; 102: 3028–31.

18. Dippel EJ, Kereiakes DJ, Tramuta DA et al. Coronary perforation during percutaneous coronary intervention in the era of abciximab platelet glycoprotein IIb/IIIa blockade: an algorithm for percutaneous management. Catheter Cardiovasc Interv 2001; 52: 279–86.

19. Stankovic G, Orlic D, Corvaja N et al. Incidence, predictors, in-hospital, and late outcomes of coronary artery perforations. Am J Cardiol 2004; 93: 213–16.

20. Bittl JA, Ryan TJ Jr, Keaney JF Jr et al. Coronary artery perforation during excimer laser coronary angioplasty. The percutaneous Excimer Laser Coronary Angioplasty Registry. J Am Coll Cardiol 1993; 21: 1158–65.

21. Holmes DR Jr, Reeder GS, Ghazzal ZM et al. Coronary perforation after excimer laser coronary angioplasty: the Excimer Laser Coronary Angioplasty Registry experience. J Am Coll Cardiol 1994; 23: 330–5.

22. Gruberg L, Pinnow E, Flood R et al. Incidence, management, and outcome of coronary artery perforation during percutaneous coronary intervention. Am J Cardiol 2000; 86: 680–2.

23. Gunning MG, Williams IL, Jewitt DE et al. Coronary artery perforation during percutaneous intervention: incidence and outcome. Heart 2002; 88: 495–8.

24. Seshadri N, Whitlow PL, Acharya N et al. Emergency coronary artery bypass surgery in the contemporary percutaneous coronary intervention era. Circulation 2002; 106: 2346–50.

25. Carrozza JP Jr, Baim DS. Complications of directional coronary atherectomy: incidence, causes, and management. Am J Cardiol 1993; 72: 47E–54E.

26. Cohen BM, Weber VJ, Relsman M, Casale A, Dorros G. Coronary perforation complicating rotational ablation: the U.S. multicenter experience. Cathet Cardiovasc Diagn 1996; Suppl(3): 55–9.

27. Ramana RK, Arab D, Joyal D et al. Coronary artery perforation during percutaneous coronary intervention: incidence and outcomes in the new interventional era. J Invasive Cardiol 2005; 17: 603–5.

28. Stefanadis C, Toutouzas K, Tsiamis E, et al. Stents covered by autologous venous grafts: feasibility and immediate and long-term results. Am Heart J 2000; 139: 437–45.

29. Stefanadis C, Toutouzas K, Vlachopoulos C, et al. Autologous vein graft-coated stent for treatment of coronary artery disease. Cathet Cardiovasc Diagn 1996; 38: 159–70.

30. Dixon SR, Webster MW, Ormiston JA, Wattie WJ, Hammett CJ. Gelfoam embolization of a distal coronary artery guidewire perforation. Catheter Cardiovasc Interv 2000; 49: 214–17.

31. Gaxiola E, Browne KF. Coronary artery perforation repair using microcoil embolization. Cathet Cardiovasc Diagn 1998; 43: 474–6.

32. Yoo BS, Yoon J, Lee SH et al. Guidewire-induced coronary artery perforation treated with transcatheter injection of polyvinyl alcohol form. Catheter Cardiovasc Interv 2001; 52: 231–4.

20

Septal ablation for hypertrophic cardiomyopathy: to whom, when, and how?

Muzaffer Degertekin, Tugrul Okay,
Fatih Bayrak, and Bülent Mutlu

Patient selection for percutaneous transluminal septal myocardial ablation (indications and contraindications) • **Technique for percutaneous transluminal septal myocardial ablation** • **Complications and follow-up after percutaneous transluminal septal myocardial ablation** • **Results of percutaneous transluminal septal myocardial ablation** • **Summary**

Hypertrophic cardiomyopathy (HCM) is a genetic cardiac disease with heterogeneous clinical course and expression. The clinical course is variable, and patients may remain stable over long periods without any symptoms; however the course of some patients may be punctuated by adverse clinical events, such as sudden death, stroke, chest pain, and heart failure.[1,2]

A fundamental goal of treatment in HCM is the alleviation of symptoms related to heart failure. Medical therapy with beta-blockers, verapamil, and disopyramide has been the initial therapeutic approach for relieving symptoms. Unfortunately, in about 10% of patients with left ventricle outflow obstruction, severe symptoms are unresponsive to medical therapy.[3] For these patients, surgical therapy has been the cornerstone of treatment for decades, with a reported mortality of <2% in highly experienced centers.[4-6]

The idea of a percutaneous septal ablation was first considered in the 1980s. Percutaneous transluminal septal myocardial ablation (PTSMA) aims to reduce left ventricle outflow tract gradient by reducing the interventricular septum thickness through alcohol-induced occlusion of a septal branch, resulting with a circumscribed infarction.[7] The first successful PTSMA was reported by Sigwart,[8] and this technique has gained great popularity in the past few years, especially in European countries.

PATIENT SELECTION FOR PERCUTANEOUS TRANSLUMINAL SEPTAL MYOCARDIAL ABLATION (INDICATIONS AND CONTRAINDICATIONS)

According to recently published American College of Cardiology (ACC)/European Society of Cardiology (ESC) consensus document, all candidates for PTSMA should have severe symptoms (New York Heart Association (NYHA) class III or IV) refractory to all medications utilized in hypertrophic cardiomyopathy (HCM), as well as a

Table 20.1   Indications for percutaneous transluminal septal myocardial ablation

Clinical indications
- NYHA class III–IV patients with drug-refractory symptoms or intolerant to drugs
- NYHA class II patients with high-risk features such as recurrent exercise-induced syncopes
- Failure of prior myectomy
- High surgical risk because of comorbidities

Hemodynamic indications
- Symptomatic patients with left ventricle outflow gradient higher than 50 mmHg at rest or during provocation (Valsalva, post-extrasystole, post-exercise).

Morphological indications
- Septal thickness >18 mm
- Subaortic systolic anterior motion-associated gradient
- Mid-cavitary gradient
- Absence of co-existent organic valvular disease necessitating surgery
- Absence of co-existent severe coronary artery disease necessitating surgery
- Absence of abnormal subvalvular aparatus necessitating surgery
- Suitable coronary anatomy

Patient preference
- With patient discussion that describes surgery as the gold standard

subaortic gradient of 50 mmHg or more measured with Doppler echocardiography either under basal conditions and/or physiological provocative maneuvers during exercise.[9] Doppler measurements should also be done within 2 h after oral 250 mg disopyramide administration, because if the gradient falls it is accepted as a sign of succesful PTSMA. A comprehensive evaluation should be carried out before intervention. Co-existence of valvular or subvalvular abnormalities or severe coronary artery disease requiring surgical correction should be excluded. Anomalous papillary muscle insertion can cause subvalvular or mid-cavitary obstruction that may not respond to PTSMA. Systolic anterior motion causes severe mitral regurgitation in some patients with high left ventricle outflow gradients. The jet of the mitral regurgitation due to systolic anterior motion is late systolic, and is directed posterolaterally. Jets in other directions should prompt the diagnosis of primary mitral valve disease. Transeusophageal echocardiography (TEE) also has an important role in decision making, particularly in patients with poor images, and with complex leaflet anatomy. Any suspicion of a subaortic membrane is also a very important indication for TEE.

There are not sufficient data avaible to perform this procedure on patients who do not meet these criteria; however, as the procedure is relatively easy to perform, the criteria for intervention have been relaxed. Patients with symptoms less than NYHA class III should only be treated if they have high gradients and high risk factors, such as recurrent exercise-induced syncope. The patient selection criteria for PTSMA are outlined in Table 20.1. HCM without obstruction and/or without symptoms is a clear contraindication for PTSMA. If myocardial contrast echocardiography (MCE) fails to identify a target septal artery, and if balloon positioning bears a risk of alcohol reflux, alcohol should not be injected.

In cases with single coronary artery disease suitable for stenting, a combined procedure (percutaneous transluminal coronary angioplasty (PTCA) and PTMSA) can be performed.[10]

TECHNIQUE FOR PERCUTANEOUS TRANSLUMINAL SEPTAL MYOCARDIAL ABLATION

Hemodynamics should be investigated before the intervention. A gradient of more than 50 mmHg either at rest or during provocation should be confirmed at the time of cardiac catheterization, before proceeding with septal ablation. It should be kept in mind that gradients obtained during catheterization may be lower than echocardiographic measurements, because of supine position and sedation of the patient. An end-hole catheter at the left ventricle apical position, and a separate ascending aortic catheter are optimally used for gradient assessment. A separate venous access site should be available for positioning a temporary transvenous pacemaker to be used if ablation is performed. It is better to choose the jugular vein as the venous access site for early mobilization of the patient. Selective coronary angiography is performed, and the first septal perforator artery is identified. The size and distribution of the septal perforator arteries vary widely. Although the first septal perforator arises from the proximal left anterior descending artery in most cases, occasionally it arises as a separate branch from the left main coronary, left circumflex, ramus intermedius arteries, or the right coronary artery.

Singh et al studied 10 fresh autopsy hearts from patients who did not have either hypertrophic obstructive cardiomyopathy or coronary artery disease.[11] They found substantial anatomical variation in the first septal perforated artery; in two patients it supplied the free wall of the right ventricle, and in four patients it incompletely supplied the basal septum. These data have important implications for alcohol septal ablations, indicating that successful septal ablation may not be possible if only the first septal perforator is injected, and that alcohol infusion has the potential to create large infarctions, not only of the interventricular septum but also of the right ventricle.

In some patients, the septal perforator artery bifurcates more proximally than usual, in which case both branches should be checked with contrast agent. If both of the septal branches supply the basal septum, then the balloon catheter may be placed in the most proximal branch. Otherwise, both branches should be cannulated separately. Access to the first septal perforator may be difficult, depending on the size and the angulation. Various guidewire bends may be required. The best and most effective way is to make a double curve. The width of the second curve depends on the caliber of the left anterior descending artery. Wire control catheters may be used for severely angulated septal branches. If the angle is severe, it may be difficult to advance a balloon over the wire; in this case, the wire may consistently prolapse from the septal into the distal left anterior descending coronary artery. Placement of a stiffer guidewire, as far distal as possible, into the septal artery facilitates positioning of the balloon. We most prefer BMW and Extra-Support 0.014 wires (Guidant USA). During the whole procedure, a good guiding catheter support is crucial for the safety and success of the intervention.

There are important technical details that should be taken into consideration in balloon selection. A short over-the-wire angioplasty balloon (8–10 mm in length and 1.5–2.5 mm in diameter) is generally used. A balloon catheter with a thin and flexible

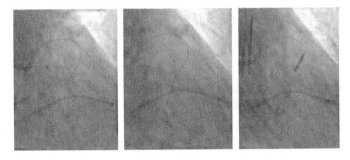

Figure 20.1   Access of guidewire to septal perforator; introduction and inflation of the balloon is demonstrated.

shaft can bend at the left anterior descending–septal artery bifurcation after removal of the guidewire, which may lead to alcohol reflux. In order to overcome this problem, we use balloon catheters with more and stiffer shafts – Occam Concerto Balloons (Occam International BV, The Netherlands). The balloon must be placed so that during inflation, the left anterior descending coronary artery is not compromised, and is sized so that the septal artery is completely occluded. The size of the septal arteries can be underestimated due to compression of the severe hypertrophied septum. In most cases a 2.0 mm balloon catheter is a suitable size. Figure 20.1 demonstrates access of the guidewire and balloon into the septal perforator.

An essential component of the procedure is evaluation of the myocardial distribution of the septal perforator artery. This is assessed either with angiographic contrast medium or with echocardiographic contrast medium or, optimally, with both. The appropriately sized balloon, with a balloon:artery ratio of approximately 1.3:1, is inflated. During inflation, the left ventricular outflow tract (LVOT) gradient is assessed continually; it may decrease substantially, which is an excellent sign confirming that the correct target septal branch has been chosen.[12] In selected patients, the gradient may only decrease by 75% with prolonged balloon inflation. During this time, or subsequently with alcohol injection, atrioventricular block may occur, which requires a normally functioning temporary pacemaker. After balloon inflation, the guidewire is removed, and a selective septal angiogram is performed: 1–2 ml of angiographic contrast medium is injected slowly under fluoroscopy through the balloon lumen, to prevent ventricular fibrillation. If the contrast medium washes out rapidly, the clinician should be alert in respect of collateral flow presence and right coronary artery amgiography should be performed while the inflated balloon is in the septal artery to demonstrate the retrograde filling of septal artery by collateral flow (Figure 20.2). The total volume of alcohol may need to be decreased when contrast medium washout is limited. Echocardiographic contrast medium is then delivered through the same inflated balloon catheter, during which time echocardiographic monitoring is performed. The location of contrast medium in the septum is assessed from an apical long-axis view (Figure 20.3). The contrast medium should enhance the proximal hypertrophied septum at the point of maximal systolic anterior motion of the anterior mitral valve leaflet, with associated septal contact. If contrast medium enhances the septal myocardium distal to this point, alcohol should not be administered. Sometimes the contrast medium enhances the right ventricular free wall through a moderator band or enhances one of the left ventricular papillary muscles. In these situations, alcohol ablation should

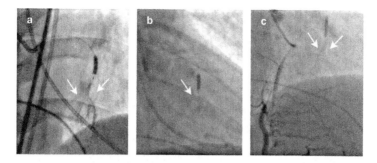

Figure 20.2 (a) The contrast medium does not wash out from the septal artery if no collateral flow is present. (b) The contrast medium washes out rapidly from the septal artery; (c) Right coronary artery angiography demonstrating the retrograde filling of septal artery by collateral flow while the inflated balloon is in the septal artery.

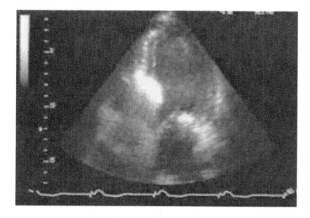

Figure 20.3 Myocardial contrast echocardiography demonstrating enhanced contrast of the base of the hypertrophied septum at the point where maximal systolic anterior motion occurs.

not be attempted. Instead, the balloon should be deflated and repositioned in another proximal branch of the septal perforator, or in another septal perforator, and the process repeated. If no location is identified that results in enhanced contrast of the base of the hypertrophied septum at the point where maximal systolic anterior motion occurs, the procedure should be terminated. If the right ventricular site of the basal septum, at the point of the septal contact, opacifies, alcohol can be delivered. In these cases the symptomatic improvement and septal thinning do not differ during long-term follow-up.

After the appropriate position has been identified, inflation of the balloon should be maintained. It is essential to document that the left anterior descending coronary artery is not compromised by the proximal portion of the inflated balloon, and that the temporary pacemaker has excellent capture thresholds. Typically, additional anesthesia is given for pain control, and 96% absolute alcohol is then delivered through the balloon catheter. The specific protocols for the volume of alcohol as well as for the speed of delivery vary among institutions. This variability is based on practice patterns, not on scientific, well-controlled data. We typically inject 1–2.5 ml

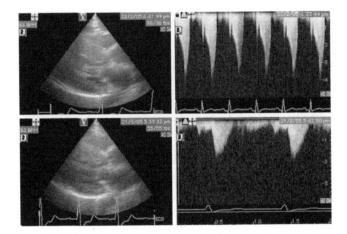

Figure 20.4 Comparision of pre- (upper panel) and post- (lower panel) PTSMA two-dimensional echocardiographic and Doppler echocardiographic images of a patient.

of alcohol over approximately 5 min, depending on the size of the septal perforator artery and the volume of septum to be ablated. Recent studies have reported a lower incidence of complete heart block when the alcohol is injected slowly instead of as a bolus;[12-14] however, there is no agreement on what constitutes a slow injection, and it may be left to the operator's discretion depending on the septal anatomical features and the rate of contrast medium washout; for example, according to Chang et al, slow injection of alcohol encompassed 30–60 s,[14] and according to Bhagwandeen et al, it was 1–5 min.[12] During this time, the gradient is measured continuously. If the resting gradient is more than 30 mmHg, the goal is to decrease it to less than 10 mmHg. If the resting gradient is less than 30 mmHg at baseline, but there is a significant provokable gradient, the goal is to decrease that provokable gradient by more than 50%. After instillation of the alcohol, the balloon is usually left inflated for an additional 3–5 min. The catheter is flushed with saline before the balloon is deflated, to avoid alcohol leakage into the left anterior descending artery, and it is withdrawn after inserting the guidewire. Final angiography is performed to identify that the septal artery has been occluded, and that the left anterior descending coronary artery has not been disrupted. In Figure 20.4 pre- and post-procedural two-dimensional and Doppler echocardiograhic images are demonstrated.

COMPLICATIONS AND FOLLOW-UP AFTER PERCUTANEOUS TRANSLUMINAL SEPTAL MYOCARDIAL ABLATION

In a recent study, patients with higher baseline gradients, fewer septal perforators injected with alcohol, lower peak creatine kinase (CK) levels (<1300 U/l), smaller septal areas opacified by MCE, and higher residual gradients in the catheterization lab remained symptomatic after the procedure.[15]

Following PTSMA, conduction disturbances are the most common complications observed. Predominantly right bundle branch block may be observed in up to 80% of the cases. Complete atrioventricular (AV) block is the most concerning conduction disturbance, which was observed in up to 50% of the first series. Slow

Table 20.2 Baseline characteristics and complications observed in 66 patients successfully treated with percutaneous transluminal septal myocardial ablation in our series

Parameters	Mean ± standard deviation (range)
Age (years)	47.8 ± 14 (21–74)
Septum diameter pre-procedure (cm)	2.6 ± 0.6 (4.6–1.8)
Septum diameter and follow-up	1.8 ± 0.5 (3.1–1.3)
Gradient pre-procedure (mmHg)	45 ± 16 (85–20)
Gradient at follow-up	12 ± 8 (4–40)
Post-procedure peak CK-MB (U/l)	296 ± 143 (96–676)

CK-MB, creatine kinase MB.

injection of smaller amounts of alcohol, and common use of MCE have decreased the incidence of this complication to less than 5%,[16] to a nearly post-surgical rate, and the need for permanent pacemaker after the procedure is about 2–10%. In an 8-year period the pacemaker implantation rate in our series was 12.1% in the first 33 cases (5–6 ml alcohol used), and 3% in the last 33 (2–3 ml alcohol). Female sex, bolus injection of alcohol, injection of more than one septal artery, and the presence of underlying left bundle branch block, and first-degree heart block were found to be independent predictors of complete heart block after ablation.[14] Other reported complications include ventricular arrhythmias, infarctions due to alcohol leakage or damage, acute mitral regurgitation due to ruptured papillary muscle, and remote infarction especially in the region of the right coronary artery. Remote infarction is mostly unpredictable, and using contrast agent does not always help to prevent this complication. In our series we have seen 4 cases (6%) in 66 patients. Baseline characteristics of the patients in our series are shown in Table 20.2. The mortality rate after PTSMA is between 1% and 2%, similar to that of surgery.[17–19]

The hospitalization duration after PTSMA varies from 48 h to 14 days, depending on the practice. Patients should be monitored for 48–72 h in the coronary care unit, with a temporary pacemaker. If no high-degree AV block is observed, the pacemaker may be removed at 48 h.

RESULTS OF PERCUTANEOUS TRANSLUMINAL SEPTAL MYOCARDIAL ABLATION

After PTSMA, acute reduction of gradient is observed in up to 90% of the patients.[8,20–25] Often, a biphasic response of the gradient is observed in which an acute reduction (due to stunning of the myocardium) is followed by a rise of about 50% of the pre-procedure level in the next day, but within the next months it may fall to greatly reduced levels. A progressive gradient reduction occurs up to 6–12 months after the procedure, as result of scar remodeling.[24] The thinning of the basal septum largely depends on the magnitude of the creatine kinase MB (CK-MB) rise. The mean decrease of the septum thickness is mostly around 5–7 mm. Figure 20.5 shows two-dimensional echocardiographic images of a patient with astonishing septal thinning at 6-year follow-up.

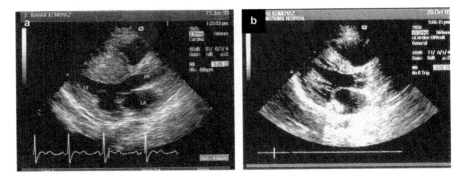

Figure 20.5 Two-dimensional echocardiographic images of a patient with astonishing septal thinning at 6-year follow-up. (a) Pre procedure; (b) 6 years after procedure.

SUMMARY

PTSMA is becoming a common procedure in the treatment of severely symptomatic patients with hypertrophic obstructive cardiomyopathy, but the surgical myectomy still remains to be the gold standard of therapy. If patient selection is correct, PTSMA offers an excellent improvement in gradient and symptoms.

REFERENCES

1. Maron BJ, McKenna WJ, Danielson GK, et al. American College of Cardiology/European Society of Cardiology clinical expert consensus document on hypertrophic cardiomyopathy. A report of the American College of Cardiology Foundation Task Force on Clinical Expert Consensus Documents and the European Society of Cardiology Committee for Practice Guidelines. J Am Coll Cardiol 2003; 42: 1687–713.
2. Maron BJ. Hypertrophic cardiomyopathy: a systematic review. JAMA 2002; 287: 1308–20.
3. Maron BJ. Appraisal of dual-chamber pacing therapy in hypertrophic cardiomyopathy: too soon for a rush to judgment? J Am Coll Cardiol 1996; 27: 431–2.
4. Robbins RC, Stinson EB. Long-term results of left ventricular myotomy and myectomy for obstructive hypertrophic cardiomyopathy. J Thorac Cardiovasc Surg 1996; 111: 586–94.
5. Heric B, Lytle BW, Miller DP, et al. Surgical management of hypertrophic obstructive cardiomyopathy. Early and late results. J Thorac Cardiovasc Surg 1995; 110: 195–206; discussion 206–8.
6. Schoendube FA, Klues HG, Reith S, et al. Long-term clinical and echocardiographic follow-up after surgical correction of hypertrophic obstructive cardiomyopathy with extended myectomy and reconstruction of the subvalvular mitral apparatus. Circulation 1995; 92 (9 Suppl): II122–7.
7. Seggewiss H. Current status of alcohol septal ablation for patients with hypertrophic cardiomyopathy. Curr Cardiol Rep 2001; 3: 160–6.
8. Sigwart U. Non-surgical myocardial reduction for hypertrophic obstructive cardiomyopathy. Lancet 1995; 346: 211–14.
9. Maron BJ. Role of alcohol septal ablation in treatment of obstructive hypertrophic cardiomyopathy. Lancet 2000; 355: 425–6.
10. Seggewiss H, Faber L, Meyners W, et al. Simultaneous percutaneous treatment in hypertrophic obstructive cardiomyopathy and coronary artery disease: a case report. Cathet Cardiovasc Diagn 1998; 44: 65–9.

11. Singh M, Edwards WD, Holmes DR, Jr, et al. Anatomy of the first septal perforating artery: a study with implications for ablation therapy for hypertrophic cardiomyopathy. Mayo Clin Proc 2001; 76: 799–802.
12. Bhagwandeen R, Woo A, Ross J, et al. Septal ethanol ablation for hypertrophic obstructive cardiomyopathy: early and intermediate results of a Canadian referral centre. Can J Cardiol 2003; 19: 912–17.
13. Lakkis NM, Nagueh SF, Kleiman NS, et al. Echocardiography-guided ethanol septal reduction for hypertrophic obstructive cardiomyopathy. Circulation 1998; 98: 1750–5.
14. Chang SM, Nagueh SF, Spencer WH, 3rd, Lakkis NM. Complete heart block: determinants and clinical impact in patients with hypertrophic obstructive cardiomyopathy undergoing nonsurgical septal reduction therapy. J Am Coll Cardiol 2003; 42: 296–300.
15. Chang SM, Lakkis NM, Franklin J, Spencer WH, 3rd, Nagueh SF. Predictors of outcome after alcohol septal ablation therapy in patients with hypertrophic obstructive cardiomyopathy. Circulation 2004; 109: 824–7.
16. Schulte HD, Gramsch-Zabel H, Schwartzkopff B. [Hypertrophic obstructive cardiomyopathy: surgical treatment]. Schweiz Med Wochenschr 1995; 125: 1940–9.
17. Shamim W, Yousufuddin M, Wang D, et al. Nonsurgical reduction of the interventricular septum in patients with hypertrophic cardiomyopathy. N Engl J Med 2002; 347: 1326–33.
18. Faber L, Seggewiss H, Gleichmann U. Percutaneous transluminal septal myocardial ablation in hypertrophic obstructive cardiomyopathy: results with respect to intraprocedural myocardial contrast echocardiography. Circulation 1998; 98: 2415–21.
19. Qin JX, Shiota T, Lever HM, et al. Outcome of patients with hypertrophic obstructive cardiomyopathy after percutaneous transluminal septal myocardial ablation and septal myectomy surgery. J Am Coll Cardiol 2001; 38: 1994–2000.
20. Ruzyllo W, Chojnowska L, Demkow M, et al. Left ventricular outflow tract gradient decrease with non-surgical myocardial reduction improves exercise capacity in patients with hypertrophic obstructive cardiomyopathy. Eur Heart J 2000; 21: 770–7.
21. Knight C, Kurbaan AS, Seggewiss H, et al. Nonsurgical septal reduction for hypertrophic obstructive cardiomyopathy: outcome in the first series of patients. Circulation 1997; 95: 2075–81.
22. Lakkis N, Kleiman N, Killip D, Spencer WH, 3rd. Hypertrophic obstructive cardiomyopathy: alternative therapeutic options. Clin Cardiol 1997; 20: 417–18.
23. Bhargava B, Agarwal R, Kaul U, Manchanda SC, Wasir HS. Transcatheter alcohol ablation of the septum in a patient of hypertrophic obstructive cardiomyopathy. Cathet Cardiovasc Diagn 1997; 41: 56–8.
24. Gietzen FH, Leuner CJ, Raute-Kreinsen U, et al. Acute and long-term results after transcoronary ablation of septal hypertrophy (TASH). Catheter interventional treatment for hypertrophic obstructive cardiomyopathy. Eur Heart J 1999; 20: 1342–54.
25. Faber L, Meissner A, Ziemssen P, Seggewiss H. Percutaneous transluminal septal myocardial ablation for hypertrophic obstructive cardiomyopathy: long term follow up of the first series of 25 patients. Heart 2000; 83: 326–31.

21

End-stage left ventricular failure: potential catheter-based therapeutic strategies

Emerson C Perin, Guilherme V Silva, and Pilar Jimenez-Quevedo

'No-option' patients • New strategies for treatment

Cardiovascular disease is increasing in epidemic proportions in developed countries and is the leading cause of mortality in the United States. The most common type of cardiovascular disease is coronary artery disease: approximately 13 million Americans have a history of a myocardial infarction (MI), angina pectoris, or both.[1] Coronary artery disease is one of the main causes of congestive heart failure (CHF). About 22% of men and 46% of women with MIs will be disabled by CHF within 6 years after the infarction.[1] Currently, 4.6 million Americans have CHF, and 550 000 new cases are added annually.[2] This is the only type of cardiovascular disease whose prevalence, incidence, and mortality has generally increased over the past 25 years. With the aging of the Western population and the decline in mortality related to other types of cardiovascular disease, CHF can be expected to take an even greater toll on public health.

This chapter concentrates on patients with end-stage CHF who are no longer candidates for standard therapies, and it discusses the alternative strategies that have been developed during the last few decades.

'NO-OPTION' PATIENTS

Percutaneous coronary intervention (PCI) and coronary artery bypass grafting are effective at relieving symptoms and improving outcomes in patients with coronary artery disease. Despite advances in medical treatment and revascularization, some patients with symptomatic coronary artery disease are no longer candidates for percutaneous or surgical revascularization. These 'no-option' patients may account for up to 12% of those referred for diagnostic catheterization.[3] Their number is growing, mainly because life expectancy is increasing, even in patients with advanced disease. Many of these patients have already undergone multiple PCIs or previous surgical revascularization and, thus, are not candidates for additional procedures. Other conditions that result in no-option status include diffuse coronary artery disease (Figure 21.1), small distal vessels, recurrent in-stent restenosis, chronic total occlusion, and comorbidities that preclude any conventional revascularization technique.

However, no-option patients are a heterogeneous group. Viable myocardium identifies two different clinical and prognostic patterns in this population. The first group

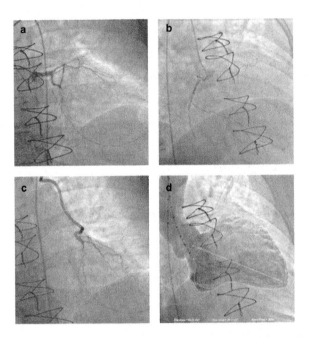

Figure 21.1   Coronary angiography showing the coronary anatomy of a patient without the option for myocardial revascularization with surgery or angioplasty. (a) Left coronary tree, with occluded left anterior descending (LAD) and circumflex arteries; (b) occlusion of the mid-segment of the right coronary artery; (c) the left internal mammary artery graft to the LAD is patent, but the distal part of the native LAD is diffusely diseased and occluded; (d) left ventriculogram analysis showing an ejection fraction of 39%.

includes patients with a substantial amount of viable myocardium, in whom angina is the predominant symptom. In these patients, improved myocardial perfusion may relieve symptoms, improve the left ventricular ejection fraction (LVEF), reverse ventricular remodeling, and increase survival. Conversely, the second group includes patients with limited or no myocardial viability, in whom heart failure symptoms predominate. This group has a poorer response to increased myocardial perfusion.

We believe that the heterogeneity of the underlying state of the myocardium has largely to do with the presence or absence of collateral circulation. Often, patients who develop extensive collateral circulation may depend on one or two patent coronary arteries or saphenous vein grafts to supply their entire myocardium. They typically have refractory angina (reflecting a significant amount of viable myocardium) but are not at significantly lower risk than patients who have multiple prior myocardial infarcts, more extensive scarring (less viable myocardium) due to the lack of collateral circulation, and, typically, more heart failure symptoms.

Establishing the no-option status requires a multidisciplinary approach, which should include cardiologists and cardiac surgeons. It is important to ensure that all conventional medical therapies are applied at the maximally tolerated dose. These therapies include anti-anginal agents (beta-blockers, calcium-channel blockers, nitrates), antiplatelet agents, angiotensin-converting enzyme inhibitors, statins, and diuretics. In addition, the patient's lifestyle must be modified, and secondary causes of angina such as anemia and uncontrolled hypertension must be excluded. Despite optimal conventional therapy, many patients continue to have not only severe symptoms that limit their quality of life but also a poor long-term clinical outcome with an increased incidence of MI and mortality.

NEW STRATEGIES FOR TEATMENT

Transmyocardial laser revascularization

Transmyocardial laser revascularization (TMLR) uses laser ablation to create transmural channels in the ischemic myocardium in order to restore myocardial perfusion. The physiological premise behind the application of TMLR is based on the work of investigators who were seeking to emulate the reptilian circulation in the mammalian heart by creating conduits for blood to flow from the ventricular cavity into the myocardium.

The mechanism of action of TMLR is still uncertain. The laser may destroy sympathetic nerve endings, thus resulting in a form of sympathectomy; it may improve myocardial perfusion secondary to angiogenesis; or it may simply have a placebo effect. At present, two types of lasers are being evaluated in the treatment of refractory angina: the carbon dioxide and the holmium:yttrium aluminium garnet (Ho:YAG) laser. Animal experiments have shown that both lasers produce histological effects after 6 weeks, but that thermoacoustic damage is greater with the Ho:YAG device.[4]

Several randomized trials evaluating surgical TMLR in no-option versus medically treated patients have shown symptomatic improvement after TMLR. In the first study, Schofield and associates randomly assigned 188 patients to either the TMLR or the medical group.[5] At 1 year, the TMLR patients had better angina scores and less need for anti-anginal medications but no improvement in exercise capacity. Frazier and colleagues randomized 192 patients to receive either TMLR or medical therapy.[6] At 12 months, the TMLR group had a significant improvement in angina class, quality-of-life scores, and cardiac perfusion, as assessed by single-photon emission computed tomography (SPECT). Similarly, Burkhoff and coworkers reported better total exercise tolerance and quality of life at 1 year but no intergroup differences in myocardial perfusion or ejection fraction.[7] Allen and coauthors demonstrated that patients randomized to undergo TMLR versus medical treatment had a significantly increased Kaplan–Meier survival rate.[8] Interestingly, however, neither group had an improvement in myocardial perfusion. Finally, a meta-analysis of seven randomized trials, involving TMLR in 1053 patients, showed that TMLR significantly improved the angina class but not the survival rate.[9] In all these trials, post-TMLR complications were almost always cardiac and included MI, left ventricular failure, atrial fibrillation, and ventricular arrhythmias. The peri-operative mortality has ranged from 3% to 5% in most reports, but rates as high as 12% have been described.

Recently, percutaneous TMLR has been advocated to reduce the peri-operative mortality of surgical TMLR. The results after percutaneous TMLR are similar to those seen in open-chest studies.[10]

In conclusion, TMLR causes clinical improvement but does not increase survival. Moreover, it is impossible to judge how large a role the placebo effect plays, as symptomatic benefits do not always correlate with objective findings (improved LVEF or myocardial perfusion). Therefore, measurable physiological benefits will have to be demonstrated, beyond any placebo effect, before TMLR can become an established option for treating coronary artery disease.

Enhanced external counterpulsation

Enhanced external counterpulsation (EECP) uses three sets of cuffs to compress the vascular beds of the leg and thigh in a sequential manner timed to the patient's electrocardiogram. The cuffs are wrapped around the patient's legs and, using compressed air, sequential pressure (300 mmHg) is applied from the lower legs to the lower and upper thighs during early diastole to propel blood back to the heart. This technique increases the mean arterial blood pressure and the retrograde aortic blood flow during diastole, causing diastolic augmentation and coronary perfusion. In a multicenter randomized, controlled trial (Multicenter Study of Enhanced External Counterpulsation [MUST-EECP]), 139 patients with angina and documented ischemia on treadmill testing were randomized to receive 35 h of active counterpulsation (300 mmHg of cuff pressure) or inactive counterpulsation (75 mmHg of cuff pressure) for 4–7 weeks.[11] The active group had a significant decrease in angina episodes and nitroglycerin usage. Moreover, the time to ≥1 mm ST segment depression also increased in the active group compared with the inactive group. Other registries have shown the same results: most of the patients (including diabetic persons) treated with EECP have experienced a significant reduction in angina and improvement in quality of life that has persisted for more than 2 years.[12–15] Despite reports of clinical improvement, more clinical data are required before EECP can be recommended as standard therapy.[16]

Neurostimulation

Neurostimulation methods attempt to palliate angina by interrupting or modulating the afferent neural signals through which pain is perceived. There are two modalities of neurostimulation: transcutaneous electrical nerve stimulation (TENS) and spinal cord stimulation (SCS).

Based on the 'gate-control theory', TENS provides transcutaneous stimulation at large, high-frequency, non-nociceptive myelinated type A fibers. It also inhibits the neural impulse through smaller unmyelinated type C fibers, reducing the activation of central pain receptors. In addition, TENS reduces sympathetic discharge, leading to a decrease in the cardiac workload and myocardial oxygen demand. Increased exercise capacity and reduced ischemia have been noted on the exercise electrocardiogram (ECG), along with decreased angina and reduced nitrate use.[17]

In SCS, the epidural space is punctured at the level of the fourth or sixth thoracic vertebra, and an electrode is introduced to the level of the T_1 to T_2 dorsal epidural space. An electrode stimulator is then placed subcutaneously in the upper left side of the abdomen. Stimulation of this electrode suppresses the capacity of intrinsic cardiac sympathetic neurons to generate activity during myocardial ischemia, thereby decreasing pain and redistributing myocardial blood flow from non-ischemic to ischemic areas.[18,19] Initial studies documented a reduction in anginal symptoms, an increase in exercise capacity, and a reduction in the degree of ST-segment depression at a given workload.[20] Later, Hautvast and coworkers showed decreased ischemic ECG changes during ambulatory 48-h monitoring in patients with refractory angina.[21] Greco and associates reported a significant decrease in the New York Heart Association (NYHA) functional class without any effect on mortality.[22] Spinal cord stimulation does not induce adverse effects in patients with transient ischemia, who retain their capacity to sense angina during an increased workload.[23,24] This method prevents hospital admissions without leading to silent infarctions and also reduces the mean duration of hospitalization.[25]

The only randomized trial of SCS, the Electrical Stimulation versus Coronary Bypass Surgery (ESBY) trial, showed that SCS is equivalent to coronary artery bypass grafting in terms of symptom relief.[26] However, the bypass group had a better exercise capacity and less ST segment depression at maximum and comparable workloads. The bypass group also had a higher 6-month mortality and more cerebrovascular events. Therefore, the researchers concluded that SCS is an alternative to coronary artery bypass grafting in patients at high operative risk.

In summary, symptoms and ischemia seem to improve with either TENS or SCS, but the SCS data are more convincing. On the other hand, neither of these methods has any effect on survival, MI, left ventricular function, or the need for repeat revascularization. Concerns about neurostimulation include the invasive nature of SCS and cutaneous side-effects of TENS, as well as a strong placebo effect.[27] In fact, the 2002 American College of Cardiology (ACC)/American Heart Association (AHA) guidelines on the treatment of chronic stable angina state that more data are needed about intermediate and long-term outcomes before neurostimulation can be accepted as a standard treatment for refractory angina.[16]

Percutaneous *in situ* coronary venous arterialization

Percutaneous *in situ* coronary venous arterialization (PICVA) supplies blood to the ischemic myocardium retrogradely through the venous system or redirects arterial blood flow from the occluded artery into an adjacent coronary vein, thereby arterializing the vein and retroperfusing the ischemic myocardium. Percutaneous *in situ* coronary artery bypass (PICAB) is a variant of PICVA, in which arterial blood flow is redirected from a diseased artery to an adjacent coronary vein and is then rerouted back to the original artery, to a position beyond the lesion.[27,28] Although still at an experimental stage, these technologies currently offer a feasible alternative for no-option patients with refractory angina and may have great potential for the future.

Gene therapy

To treat refractory angina, gene transfer technology with growth factors has been proposed to induce angiogenesis and arteriogenesis. The following substances have been shown to stimulate these processes: vascular endothelial growth factor (VEGF), fibroblast growth factor (FGF), platelet-derived growth factor, platelet-activating factor, angioproteins, cytokines such as interleukins, master switch genes, hypoxia-inducible factor-1 alpha, and nitric oxide. The safest, most effective delivery strategy for inducing angiogenesis in ischemic myocardium is uncertain and needs further study.

By increasing the rate of endothelial cell proliferation, VEGF improves myocardial perfusion and the angina functional class. This growth factor has been used intramuscularly as plasmid-encoding VEGF and with adenoviral vectors. All patients have reported symptomatic improvement with no evidence of systemic or cardiac toxicity.[29–31]

Fibroblast growth factor also increases the rate of endothelial cell proliferation. Basic FGF, delivered in sustained-release microcapsules, improved patient perception of angina.[32] Recombinant FGF, studied via the intracoronary and intravenous routes, improved SPECT perfusion abnormalities.[33] The first randomized, double-blinded, placebo-controlled trial of gene therapy was performed with intracoronary delivery of recombinant adenovirus 5 FGF-4.[34] The treatment group had a greater improvement in exercise duration than did the placebo group, but the latter group had a marked improvement from baseline, demonstrating an important placebo effect.

Because of the lack of randomized trials, the true efficacy of gene therapy cannot be definitively evaluated. Researchers still do not know whether the improvements in myocardial perfusion can be attributed to angiogenesis. Potential complications include aberrant vascular proliferation, increased vascular permeability leading to edema, triggering of unrecognized neoplasms, proatherogenic effects, and induction of immune or inflammatory responses.

Cardiac stem cell therapy

Clinical trials of cardiac stem cell therapy

The most clinically utilized approach in stem cell therapy for patients with endstage ischemic heart failure is the transendocardial delivery of autologous bone marrow mononuclear cells. The following discussion will detail that experience.

Tse et al have reported that transendocardial injection of autologous bone marrow mononuclear cells (BMMNCs) in eight patients with severe ischemic heart disease led to preserved left ventricular function.[35] At 3-month follow-up, heart failure symptoms and myocardial perfusion had improved, especially in the ischemic region as shown by cardiac magnetic resonance imaging.

Fuchs and associates studied the clinical feasibility of transendocardial delivery of filtered unfractionated autologous bone marrow-derived (not mononuclear) cells in 10 patients with severe, symptomatic, chronic myocardial ischemia not amenable to conventional revascularization.[36] Twelve targeted injections (0.2 ml each) were administered into ischemic, non-infarcted myocardium identified previously by SPECT perfusion imaging. No serious adverse effects (i.e. arrhythmia, infection, myocardial inflammation, or increased scar formation) were noted. Moreover, even though the treadmill exercise duration did not change significantly (391 ± 155 vs. 485 ± 198 s; $P = 0.11$), there was improvement in Canadian Cardiovascular Society angina scores (3.1 ± 0.3 vs. 2.0 ± 0.94; $P = 0.001$) and in stress scores in segments within the injected regions (2.1 ± 0.8 vs. 1.6 ± 0.8; $P < 0.001$).

Our group performed the first clinical trial of transendocardial injection of autologous BMMNCs to treat heart failure patients.[37] This study, performed in collaboration with physicians and scientists at the Hospital Pro-Cardiaco in Rio de Janeiro, Brazil, used electromechanical mapping (EMM)-guided transendocardial delivery of stem cells. The results of 2- and 4-month non-invasive and invasive follow-up evaluations and of 6- and 12-month follow-up evaluations have already been published.[37,38]

A total of 21 patients were enrolled. The first 14 patients comprised the treatment group, and the last 7 patients the control group. Baseline evaluations included complete clinical and laboratory tests, exercise stress (ramp treadmill) studies, two-dimensional Doppler echocardiography, SPECT perfusion scanning, and 24-h Holter monitoring. Autologous BMMNCs were harvested, isolated, washed, and resuspended in saline for injection via NOGA catheter (15 injections of 0.2 ml, totalling 30×10^6 cells per patient) in viable myocardium (UniV voltage ≥ 6.9 mV). All patients underwent non-invasive follow-up tests at 2 months, and the treatment group also underwent invasive studies at 4 months, using standard protocols and the same procedures as at baseline. The demographic and exercise test variables did not differ significantly between the treatment and control groups. There were no procedural complications. At 2 months,

Table 21.1 Comparison of clinical values for the treatment and control groups at baseline, 2 months, 6 months, and 12 months

	Baseline		2 months		6 months		12 months		P^a
	Treatment	Control	Treatment	Control	Treatment	Control	Treatment	Control	
SPECT									
Total reversible defect (%)	14.8 ± 14.5	20 ± 25.4	4.45 ± 11.5	37 ± 38.4	8.8 ± 9	32.7 ± 37	11.3 ± 12.8	34.3 ± 30.8	0.01
Total fixed defect (50%) (%)	42.6 ± 10.3	38 ± 12	39.8 ± 6.9	39.1 ± 11.2	38 ± 6.7	36.4 ± 12	38.2 ± 8.5	35.2 ± 9.3	0.3
Ramp treadmill									
$\dot{V}o_2$ max (ml/kg/min)	17.3 ± 8	17.5 ± 6.7	23.2 ± 8	18.3 ± 9.6	24.15 ± 7	17.3 ± 6	25.1 ± 8.7	18.2 ± 6.7	0.03
METS	5.0 ± 2.3	5.0 ± 1.91	6.6 ± 2.3	5.2 ± 2.7	7.19 ± 2.4	4.92 ± 1.7	7.2 ± 2.5	5.1 ± 1.9	0.02
LVEF	30 ± 6	37 ± 14	37 ± 6	27 ± 6	30 ± 10	28 ± 4	35.1 ± 6.9	34 ± 3	0.9
Functional class									
NYHA	2.2 ± 0.9	2.7 ± 0.8	1.5 ± 0.5	2.4 ± 1.0	1.3 ± 0.6	2.4 ± 0.5	1.4 ± 0.7	2.7 ± 0.5	0.01
CCSAS	2.6 ± 0.8	2.9 ± 1.0	1.8 ± 0.6	2.5 ± 0.8	1.4 ± 0.5	2 ± 0.1	1.2 ± 0.4	2.7 ± 0.5	0.002
PVC (n)	2507 ± 6243	672 ± 1085	901 ± 1236	2034 ± 4528	3902 ± 8267	1041 ± 1971	–	–	0.4
dQRS (ms)	136 ± 15	145 ± 61	145.9 ± 25	130 ± 27	144.8 ± 25	140 ± 61	–	–	0.62
LAS 40 (ms)	50 ± 24	70 ± 76	54 ± 33	48 ± 20	25 ± 25	66 ± 79	–	–	0.47
RMS 40 (μV)	22.2 ± 22	23.3 ± 23	23.3 ± 19	24.6 ± 28	25 ± 25	30 ± 27	–	–	0.7

CCSAS, Canadian Cardiovascular Society Angina Score; dQRS, filtered QRS duration; LAS 40, duration of terminal low-amplitude signal less than 40 mV; METS, metabolic equivalents; NYHA, New York Heart Association; PVC, premature ventricular contraction; RMS 40, root mean square voltage in the terminal 40 ms of the QRS complex; SPECT, single-photon emission computed tomography; $\dot{V}o_2$ max, maximum oxygen consumption.

$^a P$ for comparisons between treatment and control groups by analysis of variance.

Table 21.2   Correlation of bone marrow mononuclear cell subpopulations and reduction in total reversible perfusion defects

Cell population and phenotype	r	P
Hematopoietic progenitor cells (CD45^{lo}CD34$^+$)	0.6	0.04
Early hematopoietic progenitor cells (CD45^{lo}CD34$^+$HLA-DR$^-$)	0.6	0.04
CD4$^+$ T cells (CD45$^+$CD3$^+$CD4$^+$)	0.5	0.1
CD8$^+$ T cells (CD45$^+$CD3$^+$CD8$^+$)	0.5	0.07
B cells (CD45$^+$CD19$^+$)	0.7	0.02
Monocytes (CD45$^+$CD14$^+$)	0.8	0.03
NK cells (CD45$^+$CD56$^+$)	0.1	0.9
B-cell progenitors (CD34$^+$CD19$^+$)	0.5	0.3
CFU-F	0.7	0.06

r, Pearson correlation coefficient; CFU-F, fibroblast colony-forming unit; NK, natural killer.

there was a significant reduction in the total reversible defect in the treatment group and in the treatment versus the control group ($P = 0.02$) on quantitative SPECT analysis. At 4 months, the left ventricular ejection fraction (LVEF) improved from a baseline of 20% to 29% ($P = 0.003$), and the end-systolic volume decreased ($P = 0.03$) in the treated patients. Electromechanical mapping revealed significant mechanical improvement in the injected segments ($P < 0.0005$). In our opinion, these findings established the safety of transendocardial injection of autologous BMMNCs and warranted further investigation of this therapy's efficacy endpoints. This trial was important because, for the first time, myocardial perfusion and cardiac function were observed to improve in a group of severely impaired patients treated solely with stem cells. The significant improvement seen at 2 and 4 months was maintained at 6 and 12 months, even as exercise capacity improved slightly (Table 21.1). Monocyte, B-cell, hematopoietic progenitor cell, and early hematopoietic progenitor cell subpopulations correlated with improvement in reversible perfusion defects at 6 months (Table 21.2).

Clinical trials of skeletal myoblasts have focused on the treatment of patients with ischemic cardiomyopathy and systolic dysfunction. Overall, these trials have resulted in improved segmental contractility and a better global LVEF. The preferred delivery route has been surgical intramyocardial injection, and one feasibility trial of transendocardial injection has been reported in the literature so far.

Safety of cardiac stem cell therapy

With regard to left ventricular function, cardiac stem cell therapy is well tolerated overall. No pro-arrhythmic effects have been observed with autologous BMMNC therapy, although other deleterious effects are possible. Early concerns about abnormal transdifferentiation and tumorigenesis have subsided, but the potential for accelerated atherogenesis remains, given the limited clinical experience and small number of patients treated. Because atherosclerosis is an inflammatory disease triggered and sustained by cytokines, adhesion molecules, and cellular components such as monocytes and macrophages, intracoronary delivery is potentially risky.

Myoblast therapy raises the possibility of arrhythmogenic effects. Consequently, many clinical studies require the placement of cardiac defibrillators in patients receiving myoblasts.

REFERENCES

1. American Heart Association. Heart Disease and Stroke Statistics – 2005 update. Dallas, TX: American Heart Association, 2005: 2–16.
2. Cooper R, Cutler J, Desvigne-Nickens P et al. Trends and disparities in coronary heart disease, stroke, and other cardiovascular diseases in the United States: findings of the national conference on cardiovascular disease prevention. Circulation 2000; 102: 3137–47.
3. Mukherjee D, Bhatt DL, Roe MT, Patel V, Ellis SG. Direct myocardial revascularization and angiogenesis – how many patients might be eligible? Am J Cardiol 1999; 84: 598–600.
4. Fisher PE, Khomoto T, DeRosa CM et al. Histologic analysis of transmyocardial channels: comparison of CO_2 and holminum:YAG lasers. Ann Thorac Surg 1997; 64: 466–72.
5. Schofield PM, Sharples LD, Caine N et al. Transmyocardial laser revascularisation in patients with refractory angina: a randomised controlled trial. Lancet 1999; 353: 519–24.
6. Frazier OH, March RJ, Horvath KA. Transmyocardial revascularization with a carbon dioxide laser in patients with end-stage coronary artery disease. N Engl J Med 1999; 341: 1021–8.
7. Burkhoff D, Schmidt S, Schulman SP et al. Transmyocardial laser revascularisation compared with continued medical therapy for treatment of refractory angina pectoris: a prospective randomised trial. ATLANTIC Investigators. Angina Treatments-Lasers and Normal Therapies in Comparison. Lancet 1999; 354: 885–90.
8. Allen KB, Dowling RD, Angel WW et al. Transmyocardial revascularization: 5-year follow-up of a prospective, randomized multicenter trial. Ann Thorac Surg 2004; 77: 1228–34.
9. Liao L, Sarria-Santamera A, Matchar DB et al. Meta-analysis of survival and relief of angina pectoris after transmyocardial revascularization. Am J Cardiol 2005; 95: 1243–5.
10. Oesterle S, Sanborn T, Ali N et al. Percutaneous transmyocardial laser revascularisation for severe angina: the PACIFIC randomised trial. Lancet 2000; 356: 1705–10.
11. Arora RR, Chou TM, Jain D et al. The multicenter study of enhanced external counterpulsation (MUST-EECP): effect of EECP on exercise-induced myocardial ischemia and anginal episodes. J Am Coll Cardiol 1999; 33: 1833–40.
12. Lawson WE, Hui JC, Lang G. Treatment benefits in the enhanced external counterpulsation consortium. Cardiology 2000; 94: 31–5.
13. Linnemeier G, Rutter MD, Barsness G, Kennard ED, Nesto RW. Enhanced external counterpulsation for the relief of angina in patients with diabetes: safety, efficacy and 1-year clinical outcomes. Am Heart J 2003; 146: 453–8.
14. Lawson WE, Hui JC, Cohn PF. Long-term prognosis of patients with angina treated with enhanced external counterpulsation: five year follow-up study. Clin Cardiol 2000; 23: 254–8.
15. Michaels AD, Linnemeier G, Soran O, Kelsey SF, Kennard ED. Two-year outcomes after enhanced external counterpulsation for stable angina pectoris (from the International EECP Patient Registry (IEPR)). Am J Cardiol 2004; 93: 461–4.
16. Gibbons RJ, Abrams J, Chatterjee K et al. American College of Cardiology; American Heart Association Task Force on Practice Guidelines. Committee on the Management of Patients With Chronic Stable Angina. ACC/AHA 2002 guideline update for the management of patients with chronic stable angina – summary article: a report of the American College of Cardiology/American Heart Association Task Force on Practice Guidelines (Committee on the Management of Patients With Chronic Stable Angina). Circulation 2003; 107: 149–58.
17. Hautvast RW, Brouwer J, DeJongste MJ, Lie KI. Effect of spinal cord stimulation on heart rate variability and myocardial ischemia in patients with chronic intractable angina pectoris - a prospective ambulatory electrocardiographic study. Clin Cardiol 1998; 21: 22–8.
18. Foreman RD, Linderoth B, Ardell JL et al. Modulation of intrinsic cardiac neurons by spinal cord stimulation: implications for its therapeutic use in angina pectoris. Cardiovasc Res 2000; 47: 367–75.
19. Murray S, Collins PD, James MA. Neurostimulation treatment for angina pectoris. Heart 2000; 83: 217–20.
20. Mannheimer C, Augustinsson LE, Carlsson CA, Manhem K, Wilhelmsson C. Epidural spinal electrical stimulation in severe angina pectoris. Br Heart J 1988; 59: 56–61.

21. Hautvast RW, DeJongste MJ, Staal MJ, van Gilst WH, Lie KI. Spinal cord stimulation in chronic intractable angina pectoris: a randomized, controlled efficacy study. Am Heart J 1998; 136: 1114–20.
22. Greco S, Auriti A, Fiume D et al. Spinal cord stimulation for the treatment of refractory angina pectoris: a two-year follow-up. Pacing Clin Electrophysiol 1999; 22: 26–32.
23. Sanderson JE, Brooksby P, Waterhouse D, Palmer RB, Neubauer K. Epidural spinal electrical stimulation for severe angina: a study of its effects on symptoms, exercise tolerance and degree of ischaemia. Eur Heart J 1992; 13: 628–33.
24. Mannheimer C, Eliasson T, Andersson B et al. Effects of spinal cord stimulation in angina pectoris induced by pacing and possible mechanisms of action. BMJ 1993; 307: 477–80.
25. Murray S, Carson KG, Ewings PD, Collins PD, James MA. Spinal cord stimulation significantly decreases the need for acute hospital admission for chest pain in patients with refractory angina pectoris. Heart 1999; 82: 89–92.
26. Mannheimer C, Eliasson T, Augustinsson LE et al. Electrical stimulation versus coronary artery bypass surgery in severe angina pectoris: the ESBY study. Circulation 1998; 97: 1157–63.
27. Kim MC, Kini A, Sharma SK. Refractory angina pectoris: mechanism and therapeutic options. J Am Coll Cardiol 2002; 39: 923–4.
28. Gowda RM, Khan IA, Punukollu G, Vasavada BC, Nair CK. Treatment of refractory angina pectoris. Int J Cardiol 2005; 101: 1–7.
29. Baumgartner I, Pieczek A, Manor O et al. Constitutive expression of phVEGF165 after intramuscular gene transfer promotes collateral vessel development in patients with critical limb ischemia. Circulation 1998; 97: 1114–23.
30. Losordo DW, Vale PR, Symes JF et al. Gene therapy for myocardial angiogenesis: initial clinical results with direct myocardial injection of phVEGF165 as sole therapy for myocardial ischemia. Circulation 1998; 98: 2800–4.
31. Rosengart TK, Lee LY, Patel SR et al. Angiogenesis gene therapy: phase I assessment of direct intramyocardial administration of an adenovirus vector expressing VEGF121 cDNA to individuals with clinically significant severe coronary artery disease. Circulation 1998; 100: 468–74.
32. Laham RJ, Sellke FW, Edelman ER et al. Local perivascular delivery of basic fibroblast growth factor in patients undergoing coronary bypass surgery: results of a phase I randomized, double-blind, placebo-controlled trial. Circulation 1999; 100: 1865–71.
33. Udelson JE, Dilsizian V, Laham RJ et al. Therapeutic angiogenesis with recombinant fibroblast growth factor-2 improves stress and rest myocardial perfusion abnormalities in patients with severe symptomatic chronic coronary artery disease. Circulation 2000; 102: 1605–10.
34. Grines CL, Watkins MW, Helmer G et al. Angiogenic Gene Therapy (AGENT) trial in patients with stable angina pectoris. Circulation 2002; 105: 1291–7.
35. Tse HF, Kwong YL, Chan JK, Lo G, Ho CL, Lau CP. Angiogenesis in ischaemic myocardium by intramyocardial autologous bone marrow mononuclear cell implantation. Lancet 2003; 361: 47–9.
36. Fuchs S, Satler LF, Kornowski R et al. Catheter-based autologous bone marrow myocardial injection in no-option patients with advanced coronary artery disease: a feasibility study. J Am Coll Cardiol 2003; 41: 1721–4.
37. Perin EC, Dohmann HF, Borojevic R et al. Transendocardial, autologous bone marrow cell transplantation for severe, chronic ischemic heart failure. Circulation 2003; 107: 2294–302.
38. Perin EC, Dohmann HF, Borojevic R et al. Improved exercise capacity and ischemia 6 and 12 months after transendocardial injection of autologous bone marrow mononuclear cells for ischemic cardiomyopathy. Circulation 2004; 110: II213–18.

22

Massive pulmonary embolism: the potential of catheter-based strategies

Phillip T Zeni Jr

Diagnosis • Systemic thrombolysis • Catheter-directed thrombolyis • Percutaneous mechanical thrombectomy • Technique • Inferior vena cava filters • Conclusion

Deep venous thrombosis (DVT) and pulmonary embolism (PE) continue to be a significant cause of morbidity and mortality despite improvements in diagnostic imaging and anticoagulation regimens. Pulmonary embolism is the most severe complication from DVT, and is diagnosed in over 600 000 patients a year with as many as 150 000 deaths per year.[1] This makes pulmonary embolism the third leading cause of death behind heart disease and cancer. Pulmonary embolism has a high mortality rate with an approximately 10% immediate mortality, and a 30% mortality rate for those who survive the initial event. Patients' symptoms range from completely asymptomatic to cardiogenic shock and sudden death.[2] Seventy-five percent (75%) of the patients who die from this disease do so during their initial admission.[3]

The categorization of PE has traditionally been restricted to massive and non-massive PE. Massive PE is defined as the occlusion of two or more lobar segments.[4] In 2000, the European Society of Cardiology Task Force on Pulmonary Embolism published guidelines on the diagnosis and stratification of acute pulmonary embolism.[5] They suggested three different categories including massive, non-massive, and sub-massive. This task force defined massive pulmonary embolism as patients having pulmonary embolism and hypotension resulting in a systolic blood pressure of less than 90 mmHg not caused by another factor. All other patients with emboli were categorized as non-massive. The subcategory of sub-massive was used to describe patients with pulmonary embolism and right ventricular dysfunction by echocardiography.[5]

Low-risk patients with small emboli with normal left ventricular function and hemodynamic stability are usually treated with intravenous unfractionated heparin or subcutaneous low-molecular-weight heparin (LMWH) injection with subsequent administration of oral warfarin.

Patients at moderate risk with sub-massive emboli demonstrating right ventricular dysfunction, but who are hemodynamically stable, also undergo treatment with intravenous unfractionated heparin or LMWH followed by oral warfarin; however, some authors have recommended the use of intravenous thrombolytic therapy to improve pulmonary perfusion and decrease right heart strain. The administration of intravenous thrombolytics has shown to produce more rapid clot lysis and improve pulmonary perfusion more than anticoagulation alone.[6]

In patients at high risk with massive pulmonary embolisms and hemodynamic instability, more aggressive treatment options are considered. Systemic thrombolytic therapy has often been used to improve pulmonary perfusion. Concomitant intravenous

Table 22.1 Treatment options for pulmonary embolism

Category	Treatment options
Low risk (small emboli, normal right ventricular function, hemodynamically stable)	• Intravenous unfractionated heparin or subcutaneous low-molecular-weight heparin • Followed by oral warfarin
Moderate risk (sub-massive emboli, right heart strain,[a] hemodynamically stable)	• Intravenous unfractionated heparin or subcutaneous low-molecular-weight heparin • Followed by oral warfarin • Intravenous thrombolysis
High risk (massive PE, hemodynamically unstable)	• Intravenous unfractionated heparin or subcutaneous low-molecular-weight heparin after thrombolysis • Followed by oral warfarin • Intravenous thrombolysis, or • Catheter-directed thrombolysis, or • Surgical embolectomy, or • Percutaneous mechanical thrombectomy

[a]By echocardiography.

unfractionated heparin has been used as well. Patients with massive life-threatening pulmonary embolisms may benefit from surgical pulmonary embolectomy, dependent upon symptomatology.[7] However, there are a number of minimally invasive devices that can rapidly restore pulmonary perfusion through percutaneous technique. Also, catheter-directed intrapulmonary thrombolysis may result in more rapid dissolution of pulmonary emboli than intravenous thrombolytics (Table 22.1).

DIAGNOSIS

Due to the high mortality rate, patients suspected of PE should be screened as rapidly as possible by either ventilation/perfusion scintigraphy or spiral computed tomography. The role of spiral computed tomography has been greatly enhanced in the diagnosis of PE over the last decade, due to the fact that approximately 20% of patients with a non-diagnostic radionuclide lung scan and a normal lower extremity duplex sonogram will have PE.[8] Spiral computed tomography is between 53% and 99% sensitive. Pitfalls can occur and are often due to inadequate contrast, rapid breathing, and cardiac motion (although less likely with multislice detector scanners), and lung consolidation.

Patients with large pulmonary emboli needing additional therapy should undergo confirmation and evaluation with pulmonary arteriography (the gold standard). The mortality rate from pulmonary arteriography is less than 0.5%, with a morbidity of less than 5%. These numbers are increased in patients with massive PE. Once arteriography establishes PE is present, the number of occluded segments should be determined. Patients with occlusion of two or more lobar segments are classified as massive PE.[4] All other patients are classified as non-massive. Also, as suggested by the European Society of Cardiology Task Force on Pulmonary Embolism, an echocardiogram should be obtained to evaluate for right heart strain. Those patients with non-massive PE and right heart strain should be classified as sub-massive. While echocardiography is useful in confirming the diagnosis of PE and in the evaluation of right heart strain, its low sensitivity has precluded it being used as a screening modality for PE.[9] Since it is estimated that 95% of all pulmonary emboli are from the lower extremities, all patients with PE should have bilateral lower-extremity duplex sonography to evaluate for residual thrombus.

SYSTEMIC THROMBOLYSIS

Thrombolytic therapy is approved by the US Food and Drug Administration (FDA) for the treatment of acute PE. The only currently available agents approved for thrombolysis in patients with pulmonary embolism are recombinant tissue plasminogen activator (rt-PA) (alteplase) and streptokinase. Traditionally, urokinase has been used, but it was made temporarily unavailable from the manufacturers resulting in increasing popularity of other thrombolytics. Although widely used for arterial and venous thrombolysis, r-PA (reteplase) is not yet approved by the US FDA for intrapulmonary thrombolysis. Tenecteplase (TNK) has also not yet been approved in the treatment of pulmonary embolism or deep venous thrombosis. The current recommended dose for acute PE is 50 mg of r-PA.[10]

CATHETER-DIRECTED THROMBOLYSIS

Direct intrapulmonary delivery of thrombolytics has often been thought of as more advantageous, resulting in more rapid breakdown of pulmonary emboli, although no data support these claims. Verstraete et al published the results of a multicenter trial, and demonstrated no significant benefit by giving rt-PA intrapulmonary versus intravenously.[11] However, direct delivery of the thrombolytic agent to the thrombus may result in more of the drug targeting the actual pulmonary embolus instead of being redirected to areas of normal perfusion. Some *in vitro* studies have shown that the administration of thrombolytics into the perfusion stream results in thrombolytics only reaching the periphery of the thrombus, instead of direct catheter administration resulting in increased contact with the thrombus.[7]

PERCUTANEOUS MECHANICAL THROMBECTOMY

Percutaneous mechanical thrombectomy (PMT) offers many advantages in the treatment of massive pulmonary embolism. PMT is especially useful in patients with massive PE who have contraindications to thrombolytic therapy. Previous studies have demonstrated that up to 50% of patients with PE have significant contraindications to thrombolytic therapy.[12] In acute massive PE, the goals of mechanical thrombectomy include increasing pulmonary artery perfusion, reducing pulmonary arterial pressures, improving oxygenation, and reducing right heart strain. Also, the embolic burden does not necessarily have to be removed from the patient to make a significant difference in outcome. If the large obstructing central thrombus can be fragmented into multiple smaller emboli, these will embolize into the smaller peripheral branches, resulting in increased lung perfusion. The surface area of the distal pulmonary arterial bed is so great that a large amount of central thrombus can be fragmented, and pulmonary perfusion essentially restored to normal without removal of thrombus. A number of devices have been used for mechanical thrombectomy. These include the Oasis and Greenfield suction catheter (Medi-tec/Boston Scientific, USA), the pig-tail rotational catheter (Cook-Europe, the Netherlands), the Amplatz thrombectomy device (Bard-Microvena, USA), the AngioJet Expedior (Possis Medical, USA), the Hydrolyser (Cordis-Europe, Netherlands), and the Aspirex (Straub Medical, Switzerland).

The ability to immediately restore pulmonary perfusion with essentially no risk of intracranial hemorrhage is obviously advantageous; however, there are risks from using mechanical thrombectomy devices, including pulmonary arterial rupture, arrhythmias, hemoptysis (although common in massive PE), and the associated risks of contrast injection. Another complication of these devices is hemolysis with subsequent hemoglobinuria. In patients who have undergone mechanical thrombectomy, and have adjuvant thrombolytic infusion, it may be difficult to distinguish hemoglobinuria from hematuria.

Although no large studies have been performed, multiple small retrospective studies have been performed showing the safe and effective use of these devices in this highly unstable patient population.[13-16] The ideal thrombectomy catheter would be easy to use, easy to deliver and direct, completely remove large amounts of thrombus, be low profile and low cost.[7] No catheter meets all of these criteria at the current time.

In the author's clinical experience, the two most useful devices are the Angio-Jet (Possis Medical, Minneapolis, MN) and the Amplatz thrombectomy device (Bard-Microvena, USA). Both catheters can be delivered successfully percutaneously from the groin. The AngioJet catheter has the benefit of being able to be positioned over the wire, while the Amplatz thrombectomy device needs to be placed through a guiding sheath. The AngioJet catheter works on the Bernoulli principle, with clot being aspirated into a waste bag. One lumen of the AngioJet catheter carries high-pressure/high-velocity saline, which loops back at the distal end, redirecting flow through a gap into the second lumen. The flow of saline across this gap creates a low-pressure area that aspirates thrombus and macerates it.[7] Aspirated material flows into a collection bag that is not connected to suction. The Amplatz thrombectomy device relies on an impeller, resulting in fragmentation and break-down of the thrombus. One significant advantage of the Amplatz device is the large open end which allows relatively large amounts of thrombus to be fragmented.

In the author's experience, both devices do well in fragmenting the large central emboli, although neither will remove 100% of the patient's thrombus burden. There is often residual thrombus which embolizes to the periphery (Figure 22.1). In addition, balloon catheters are able to fragment these large central emboli as well, and if no other mechanical thrombectomy catheter is available, a simple balloon angioplasty catheter can be used to improve pulmonary perfusion. Some authors have also described the use of metallic stents to increase pulmonary perfusion.[7]

TECHNIQUE

The author's technique for treatment of massive PE is to perform pulmonary arteriography from the groin placing a 6Fr sheath in the right common femoral vein using sonographic guidance. A 5Fr pig-tail catheter is used to select each main pulmonary artery, and pulmonary arterial pressures are measured. Subsequently, non-ionic

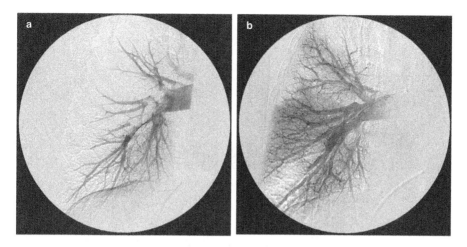

Figure 22.1   (a) Pulmonary arteriogram before treatment demonstrates thrombus in the right pulmonary artery; (b) right pulmonary artery immediately after AngioJet treatment shows clearing of central thrombus. Note residual distal thrombus.

contrast (iodixanol, 320 mg/ml, Nycomed, Princeton, NJ, USA) is injected. The usual injection rate is 15 ml/s for 2 s, but this may be decreased in patients with significant pulmonary hypertension. If mechanical thrombectomy is to be performed, the pig-tail catheter is removed and an 8Fr 65 cm or 80 cm sheath (Super Arrow Flex; Arrow International, Reading, PA, USA) is placed over a 0.035 guidewire. The thrombectomy device is advanced into the thrombus and activated. Contrast is injected through the sheath during the procedure, to monitor progress. If thrombolytic infusion is to be performed a multiside hole infusion catheter is placed through the area of thrombus with delivery of the thrombolytic agent overnight and close monitoring of the patient including fibrogen levels every 6 h. If fibrinogen levels fall 30–40% from baseline, the thrombolytic is held until a repeat arteriogram can be obtained. If bilateral emboli are present, then two catheters are placed, one in each pulmonary artery, for overnight infusion (Figure 22.2).

INFERIOR VENA CAVA FILTERS

Inferior vena cava (IVC) filters play an important role in the management of deep venous thrombosis and pulmonary embolism. The traditional indications for permanent IVC filter implantation have been: contraindication to anticoagulation with known deep venous thrombosis, recurrent thromboembolism despite anticoagulation, large free-floating iliocaval thrombosis, and patients with limited pulmonary reserve. All patients with massive pulmonary embolism should have an IVC filter placed. In this high-risk population, the pulmonary reserve is so limited that the benefits clearly outweigh the risks. In patients with non-massive pulmonary embolism, a duplex of the lower extremities should be obtained, and those patients with deep venous thrombosis and a contraindication to anticoagulation should also receive a filter. The decision to place a filter in a patient with sub-massive PE depends not only on the duplex findings, and the patient's ability to tolerate

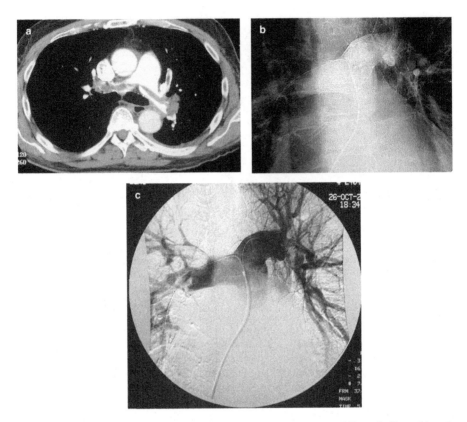

Figure 22.2 (a) Spiral computed tomography showing a large saddle embolism; (b) pulmonary arteriogram with guiding sheath in the main pulmonary artery and bilateral infusion catheters; (c) pulmonary arteriogram showing large bilateral pulmonary emboli with infusion catheters in place.

anticoagulation, but also the amount of right heart strain by echocardiography. A new option for patients is the temporary filter. In the past, physicians were reluctant to place IVC filters in patients, due to the possibility of filter failure and fracture after long-term implantation. However, with new temporary filters, these complications may be avoided. The current recommended indications for temporary IVC filter implantation are patients who cannot receive anticoagulation, patients older than 45 years who have poor cardiopulmonary reserve, patients who have had one or more of the following injuries: closed head injury, spinal cord injury, complex pelvic fractures, and multiple long bone fractures. Three filters are available for temporary implantation, the Recovery filter by Bard, the Gunther–Tulip filter by Cook, Inc, and the OptEase filter by Cordis. These filters have shown encouraging initial results regarding embolic protection, with a low rate of filter migration and IVC thrombosis. The Recovery filter has been removed over 400 days after implantation. With the advent of temporary filters, the indication for filter implantation has been greatly increased.

CONCLUSION

In conclusion, massive PE is an extremely common problem, and is difficult to diagnosis and treat. Most patients with suspected PE are currently diagnosed with spiral CT. This is often enough to characterize the patient as having massive or non-massive PE. Adjuvant deep venous studies of the lower extremities should be obtained as well. Patients who have massive PE and have residual thrombus within the lower extremities should undergo IVC filter placement. Those patients with sub-massive PE should at least have intravenous thrombolytics administered, if not catheter-directed thrombolytics. Those patients who are unstable and have massive PE diagnosed by spiral CT may benefit from either surgical embolectomy, or catheter-directed mechanical thrombectomy. In the author's experience, fragmenta-tion of the large central emboli is usually enough therapy to improve the patient's pulmonary perfusion, decreasing mortality in this high-risk population. Some authors have advocated the increased use of surgical pulmonary embolectomy for massive PE. The high mortality rate often quoted for surgical pulmonary embolec-tomy may be much lower with modern surgical techniques.[17] Twenty-four hour, seven day a week coverage for surgical pulmonary embolectomy is usually only available in large tertiary care centers, and may not be available in smaller hospitals.

Although there are multiple catheters on the market for mechanical thrombec-tomy, each with their own advantages and disadvantages, none of the catheters are approved for use in the pulmonary arteries. The specific device and technique used will depend on the expertise of the operator. In patients when heparin alone is insuf-ficient, thrombolysis is contraindicated, and if the patient has not become dependent on systemic pressors, percutaneous catheter intervention should be considered.

Acknowledgement

To my loving wife with whom everything is possible.

REFERENCES

1. Ferris EJ. Deep venous thrombosis and pulmonary embolism: correlative evaluation and therapeutic implications. Am J Roentgenol 1992; 159: 1149–55.
2. Kasper W, Konstantinides S, Geibel A et al. Mangement strategies and determinants of outcome in acute major pulmonary embolism: results of a multicenter registry. J Am Coll Cardiol 1997; 30: 1165–71.
3. Goldhaber SZ. Pulmonary embolism. N Engl J Med 1998; 339: 93–104.
4. Walsh P, Greenspan R, Morris S et al. The Urokinase Pulmonary Embolism Trial: a national cooperative study. Circulation 1973; 47 (Suppl): II101–II108.
5. Torbicki A, van Beek EJR, Charbonnier B et al, for the Task Force on Pulmonary Embolism, European Society of Cardiology. Task force report: guidelines on diagnosis and manage-ment of acute pulmonary embolism. Eur Heart J 2000; 21: 1301–36.
6. Konstantinides S, Geibel A, Heusel G et al. Heparin plus alteplase compared with heparin alone in patients with submassive pulmonary embolism. N Engl J Med 2002; 347: 1143–50.
7. Uflacker R. Interventional Therapy for Pulmonary Embolism. J Vasc Interv Radiol 2001; 12: 147–64.
8. Turkstra F, Kuijer PM, van Beek EJ et al. Diagnostic utility of ultrasonography of leg veins in patients suspected of having pulmonary embolism. Ann Intern Med 1997; 126: 775–81.

9. Perrier A, Tamm C, Unger PF, Lerch R, Sztajzel J. Diagnostic accuracy of Doppler-echocardiography in unselected patients with suspected pulmonary embolism. Int J Cardiol 1998; 65: 101–9.
10. British Thoracic Society Standards of Care Committee Pulmonary Embolism Guideline Development Group. British Thoracic Society guidelines for the management of suspected acute pulmonary embolism. Thorax 2003; 58: 470–83.
11. Verstraete M, Miller GAH, Bounameaux H et al. Intravenous and intrapulmonary recombinant tissue-type plasminogen activator in the treatment of acute massive pulmonary embolism. Circulation 1988; 77: 353–60.
12. Terrin M, Goldhaber SZ, Thompson B. Selection of patients with acute PE for thrombolytic therapy: Thrombolysis in PE (TIPE) patients survey. The TIPE Investigators. Chest 1989; 95 (Suppl 5): 279S–281S.
13. Zeni PT Jr, Blank BG, Peeler DW. Use of rheolytic thrombectomy in treatment of acute massive pulmonary embolism. J Vasc Interv Radiol 2003; 14: 1511–15.
14. Uflacker R, Strange C, Vujic I. Massive pulmonary embolism: preliminary results of treatment with the Amplatz thrombectomy device. J Vasc Interv Radiol 1996; 7: 519–28.
15. Fava M, Loyola S, Huete I. Massive pulmonary embolism: treatment with the hydrolyser thrombectomy catheter. J Vasc Interv Radiol 2000; 11: 1159–64.
16. Schmitz-Rode T, Günther RW, Pfeffer JG et al.. Acute massive pulmonary embolism: use of a rotatable pigtail catheter for diagnosis and fragmentation therapy. Radiology 1995; 197: 157–62.
17. Doerge H, Schoendube FA, Voss M, Seipelt R, Messmer BJ. Surgical therapy of fulminant pulmonary embolism: early and late results. Thorac Cardiovasc Surg 1999; 47: 9–13.

23

Large thrombus burden, slow flow, no-reflow, and distal embolization

Jose A Silva and Christopher J White

Large thrombus burden • Pharmacological approaches • Mechanical approaches • Slow-flow, no-reflow • Distal embolization • Summary

Thrombus-containing lesions often represent the pathological substrate of a group of clinical entities known as acute coronary syndromes (ACS). Acute coronary syndromes may present with clinical manifestations which range from unstable angina pectoris, non-ST segment elevation myocardial infarction (NSTEMI), or the classic 'transmural' or ST segment elevation myocardial infarction (STEMI). They all share a common pathophysiology, namely, a 'vulnerable' atherosclerotic coronary plaque suddenly ruptures, exposing thrombogenic material to circulating platelets and coagulation factors, which ultimately lead to the formation of thrombus.[1-4] Depending upon the thrombus size, the intrinsic fibrinolytic system, platelet activation, and collateral flow, among others, the clinical presentation will differ in each instance.

The treatment of thrombotic lesions, those with a large thrombus burden in particular, is challenging because revascularization is associated with procedural complications such as abrupt occlusion, MI, the need for emergent bypass surgery, and death.[5,6] In addition, percutaneous coronary intervention (PCI) of thrombus-containing lesions makes distal embolization and development of slow- or no-reflow more likely.[7,8] Furthermore, the presence of thrombus appears to play an important role in late restenosis.[9,10] Consequently, removal of coronary thrombi prior to intervention is desirable.

In the present chapter we will review the most important treatment modalities for coronary lesions with a large thrombus burden, as well as some of its more common complications such as no-reflow and distal embolization.

LARGE THROMBUS BURDEN

The treatment of thrombus-containing lesions includes both pharmacological and mechanical approaches. Pharmacological options include antiplatelet agents (i.e. aspirin, the ADP inhibitors ticlopidine and clopidogrel, and glycoprotein platelet (GP) IIb/IIIa receptor inhibitors), direct thrombin inhibitors (i.e. hirudin and argatroban), indirect thrombin inhibitors (unfractionated heparin (UFH) or low-molecular-weight heparins (LMWH)), and plasminogen activators (i.e. thrombolytic agents). It is beyond the scope of the present review to address the pharmacology of all of these agents, but due to the importance of thrombolytic agents as well as the overwhelming evidence of benefit of the GP IIb/IIIa inhibitors in the setting of acute coronary syndromes with or without PCI, we will highlight their importance. Mechanical approaches to treating or removing thrombus include mechanical disruption (i.e. balloon angioplasty, stenting), direct removal with atherectomy, maceration, and suction with a transluminal extraction catheter device (TEC) (Interventional Technologies, Inc, San Diego, California), aspiration with the AngioJet system (Possis Medical, Minneapolis, Minnesota, USA), or the X-sizer thrombectomy system (X-Sizer catheter system; eV3, White Bear Lake, Minnesota, USA), and vibrational disintegration with the Acolysis Device (Acolysis System, Angiosonics, Morrisville, North Carolina, USA). Distal protection devices for the treatment of thrombotic lesions will be discussed in the sections on no-reflow and distal embolization.

PHARMACOLOGICAL APPROACHES

Thrombolytic agents

Until the advent of the thrombectomy devices, intracoronary thrombolysis remained the cornerstone of the treatment for thrombus-containing lesions. Intracoronary urokinase has been used with mixed results.[11,12] In one report of 48 patients (90%, native coronary arteries), who had thrombus accumulation during percutaneous transluminal coronary angioplasty (PTCA) in patients ACS, an intracoronary urokinase infusion (141 000 units during an average period of 34 min) resulted in thrombus resolution in 90% of the patients.[11] When the same thrombolytic agent was used to treat saphenous vein grafts (SVG) with angiographic evidence of thrombus prior to stenting, there was an increase in procedural complications and stent thrombosis.[13]

Although urokinase may have a place in treating thrombus-containing lesions, its prophylactic use, to prevent thrombus formation in ACS, has proven to be deleterious. The Thrombolysis and Angioplasty in Unstable Angina (TAUSA) investigators randomized more than 400 patients with unstable or post-infarction angina to receive urokinase or placebo.[14] The group that received urokinase had an increased incidence of abrupt occlusion (10.2% vs. 4.3%; $P < 0.04$), which resulted in an increased incidence of the composite of ischemia, MI, or emergent bypass surgery (12.9% vs. 6.3%; $P < 0.02$).

Chronic intracoroanry urokinase infusions have successfully been used to recanalize chronic occlusions in native coronary arteries and SVG.[15,16] In 60 patients with chronically occluded native coronary arteries, urokinase was infused over 8 h after failed attempts to recanalize them with standard angioplasty techniques. After the urokinase infusion, 53% of the vessels were successfully recanalized.[15] Similarly, the Royal Brompton and UCL Study of Thallium and Technetium (ROBUST) investigators attained successful recanalization in 69% of chronically occluded SVG after a mean infusion dose of 3.7 million units of urokinase over an average infusion duration of 25.4 h.[16]

Urokinase can also be delivered directly onto the surface of the thrombus with a Dispatch catheter, or urokinase-coated hydrogel balloons. The Dispatch catheter was tested by Glazier et al, showing angiographic resolution of thrombus in both native coronary arteries and SVG.[17] Similarly, the urokinase-coated hydrogel balloon inhibited platelet deposition, and caused thrombolysis in an animal model, without evidence of angiographic distal embolization in patients with intracoronary thrombus.[18,19] The main disadvantages of the thrombolytic approach are the time required to achieve thrombus resolution and the cost of the agents.

The glycoprotein IIb/IIIa inhibitors

This group of agents are highly effective platelet inhibitors, since they interact and block the binding of the active form of the IIb/IIIa platelet receptor with fibrinogen and von Willebrand factor among other platelet-binding molecules that inhibit platelet aggregation, regardless of the stimuli. There are three GP IIb/IIIa inhibitors clinically available, which vary in structure, molecular size, specificity, and pharmacodynamics.[20]

In contrast to intracoronary thrombolysis that yielded mixed results with thrombus-containing lesions, the GP IIb/IIIa inhibitors have uniformly been effective in decreasing the procedural complication rate and the incidence of major adverse cardiovascular events (MACE). Over 30 000 patients have been treated with these agents in nine clinical trials, demonstrating a 19% reduction in death or MI at the 30-day follow-up.[21] These agents have also been demonstrated to be beneficial in patients with STEMI when used as adjunctive therapy to PCI, or in combination with low-dose thrombolytic agents (Table 23.1).[22]

The mechanism by which these GP IIb/IIIa platelet receptor inhibitors 'passivate' the complex, thrombus-laden, coronary plaque remains unclear. There is evidence showing angiographic resolution of thrombus in patients with ACS, or of preventing intracoronary thrombus developing as a complication of coronary angioplasty, when these agents are given systemically or locally.[23-25] More recently, abciximab (Reopro) has been found to be highly effective for reducing angiographic thrombus burden when delivered on the thrombus surface with the Dispatch catheter.[26]

Despite evidence of thrombus resolution with the use of GP IIb/IIIa inhibitors, the clinical benefit of these agents in the presence of large thrombus burden remains uncertain.[23-26] A study with pooled data from eight prospective randomized trials, not only confirmed that PCI of angiographic thrombotic lesions remains a predictor for increased in-hospital and 6-month death and MI, but that the use of GP IIb/IIIa inhibitors had no benefit for the same outcomes when PCI was performed in lesions with evidence of angiographic thrombus.[27] An angiographic subanalysis of the Platelet Receptor Inhibition in Ischemic Syndrome Management in Patients (PRISM-PLUS) trial, demonstrated that the combination of tirofiban plus heparin significantly reduced the intracoronary thrombus burden, however, the persistence of angiographic thrombus, was predictive of 30-day MACE despite treatment with tirofiban.[28] Further, a subanalysis from the ReoPro in Acute Myocardial Infarction and Primary PTCA Organization and Randomized Trial (RAPPORT) trial showed that the presence of angiographic thrombus was a predictor for abnormal Thrombolysis in Myocardial Infarction (TIMI) flow, despite the use of abciximab.[29] A negligible benefit has also been reported with the adjunctive use of the GP IIb/IIIa inhibitor, tirofiban, with PCI in the setting of STEMI with a large thrombus burden.[30]

MECHANICAL APPROACHES

Balloon angioplasty and stenting

The treatment of thrombus-containing lesions with balloon angioplasty alone is considered a high-risk procedure, as it is associated with increased procedural complications such as abrupt occlusion, distal embolization, no-reflow and need for emergent revascularization procedures. Using coronary angioscopy, White et al found that the presence of thrombus increased the in-hospital composite endpoint of death, MI, or

Table 23.1   Clinical trials of intravenous glycoprotein IIb/IIIa inhibitors in acute ST elevation myocardial infarction

Total (number of patients)	Protocol	Clinical presentation	Study details	Primary endpoint	Clinical outcome (%)
RAPPORT (483)	Abciximab bolus + infusion	ST elevation MI	Primary PTCA within 12 h of drug therapy	Death or MI at 6 months	5.8, ↓48
	Placebo				11.2
IMPACT-AMI (230)	Eptifibatide + rt-PA + heparin	ST elevation MI	Combination therapy	90-min TIMI 3 flow	52.0, ↓25
	Placebo + rt-PA + heparin				39.0
ADMIRAL (300)	Abciximab bolus + infusion	ST elevation MI	Therapy prior to PTCA and stent	Death, MI, or urgent revascularization at 30 days	10.7 ↓46
	Placebo				20
TIMI 14 (888)	Full-dose t-PA	ST elevation MI	Dose-finding and confirmation trial	90-min TIMI 3 flow	62.0, ↑19
	Abciximab + t-PA				77
	Abciximab + streptokinase				80
SPEED (305)	Full-dose r-PA	ST elevation MI		60- to 90-min TIMI 3 flow	48.0, ↑23
	Abciximab + r-PA		Various doses of r-PA; full dose of abciximab		63

(continued)

Table 23.1 Continued

Total (number of patients)	Protocol	Clinical presentation	Study details	Primary endpoint	Clinical outcome (%)
INTRO-AMI (305)	High-dose infusion eptifibatide+t-PA 50 mg t-PA full dose	ST elevation MI	Eptifibatide double bolus 180/90 μg/kg and 2.0 μg/kg/min t-PA	60-min TIMI 3 flow	56, ↑40 40
CADILLAC (2082)	PTCA or stenting+abciximab; PTCA or stenting alone	ST elevation MI	PTCA+abciximab Stenting+abciximab PTCA alone Stenting alone	Death, MI, stroke or repeat revascularization at 6 months	16.5 10.2 20 11.5

Key to trials:
RAPPORT   ReoPro in Acute Myocardial Infarction and Primary PTCA Organization and Randomized Trial
IMPACT-AMI   Integrilin to Minimize Platelet Aggregation and Coronary Thrombosis-Acute Myocardial Infarction
ADMIRAL   Abciximab before direct Angioplasty and Stenting in Myocardial Infarction Regarding Acute and Long-term Follow-up
TIMI 14   Thrombolysis in Myocardial Infarction 14
SPEED   Strategies for Patency Enhancement in the Emergency Department
INTRO-AMI   Integrilin and Reduced Dose of Thrombolytics in Acute Myocardial Infarction
TNT   Tirofiban and Thrombolysis
CADILLAC   Controlled Abciximab and Device Investigation to Lower Late Angioplasty Complications

MI, myocardial infarction; PTCA, percutaneous transluminal coronary angioplasty; r-PA, reteplase; TNK-tPA, tenecteplase-tissue plasminogen activator; t-PA, tissue plasminogen activator.

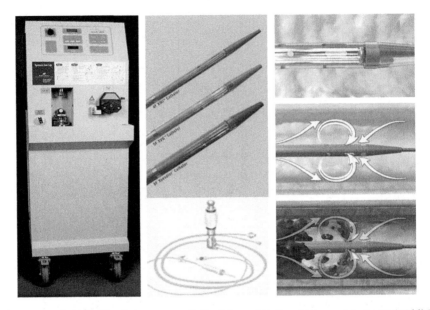

Figure 23.1   AngioJet Rheolytic system, with the drive unit (left), catheters and pump set (middle).

emergent bypass surgery, when compared with target lesions without angioscopic thrombus (14% vs. 2%; $P = 0.03$).[5] These finding have been confirmed by other investigators.[6] In addition, coronary thrombi, appear to increase the late restenosis rate.[7,8]

The landmark study by Colombo et al,[31] and several other studies have shown that in STEMI patients, primary stenting using a high-pressure balloon inflation in combination with an adequate antiplatelet regimen is associated with a high technical success and a decrease in hospital complications and late restenosis rates.[32–35] Nevertheless, most studies of STEMI with stent placement have not included a significant number of patients with large thrombus burden, and therefore the results are difficult to extrapolate to this patient population.

Atherectomy

Despite initial enthusiasm for the use of directional coronary atherectomy (DCA) in thrombus-containing lesions,[36] larger studies have found an increased complication rate.[37–39] Although removal of thrombus can be accomplished with the transluminal extraction catheter (TEC), the incidence of distal embolization is significant.[40–44] In one prospective study of TEC in STEMI, an incidence of distal embolization and abrupt closure of up 12% was reported.[45]

Thombus aspiration

AngioJet rheolytic thrombectomy

Rheolytic thrombectomy with the AngioJet (Possis, Minneapolis, MN, USA) has been shown to be a safe and effective tool for the treatment of thrombus-containing saphenous vein graft lesions. The system works by applying the Venturi–Bernoulli principle: high-speed saline jets create a low-pressure region at the tip (about

Table 23.2 VeGAS 2: principal effectiveness and safety results; all randomized patients treated (349 patients, 352 lesions)

Efficacy measures	AngioJet (*n* = 180)	Urokinase (*n* = 169)	Significant
Lesion success (%)	87.6	80.1	No
Procedure success (%)	86.3	72.7	Yes
Device success (%)	87.4	75.8	Yes
Post-procedure MLD (mm)	2.59±0.82	2.45±1.08	No
Post-procedure % DS	22±21	28±29	No
TLR-free at 30 days (%)	96.6	95.8	No
TVR-free at 30 days (%)	94.9	95.2	No
TVF-free at 30 days (%)	84.9	76.9	No
MACE-free at 30 days (%)	84.9	76.9	Yes
Primary endpoint: event free at 30 days (%)	70.9	70.8	No
Safety measures and other clinical events			
In-hospital MACE (%)	13.9	32.5	Yes
Out-of-hospital MACE to 30 days (%)	3.9	1.8	No
Abrupt closure (%)	3.3	4.7	No
Subacute closure (%)	2.8	4.1	No
Bleeding complications (%)	5.0	11.8	Yes
Vascular complications (%)	4.4	17.8	Yes
CVA to 30 days (%)	1.7	1.2	No
Length of stay (days mean±SD)	2.5±2.3	3.5±2.6	Yes

CVA, cerebrovascular accident; DS, diameter stenosis; MACE, major adverse cardiovascular effect; MLD, minimal lumen diameter ; SD, standard deviation, TLR, target lesion revascularization; TVF, target vessel failure; TVR, target vessel revascularization.

−760 mmHg), which act to pull the thrombus into the catheter exhaust lumen and propel it from the vessel (Figure 23.1).

In the Vein Graft AngioJet Study (VeGAS 2) trial, 346 patients with an angiographically visible thrombus-containing lesion were randomized to either a urokinase infusion or mechanical thrombectomy with the AngioJet system.[46] Procedural success, in-hospital major cardiovascular events, bleeding and vascular complications were significantly better in the AngioJet group (Table 23.2 and Figure 23.2).

Rheolytic thrombectomy has also been tested in 70 STEMI patients (16% with cardiogenic shock) with a large angiographic thrombus burden.[47] TIMI 3 coronary flow was obtained in 88% of this group of patients. The 30-day freedom from MACE was 93%. A randomized trial of 100 STEMI patients comparing rheolytic thrombectomy prior to stenting versus stenting alone, showed earlier ST segment resolution (90% vs. 72%; $P = 0.22$), a lower corrected TIMI frame count (18 ± 8 vs. 23 ± 11; $P = 0.032$), and a smaller infarct size in the rheolytic thrombectomy group (Figure 23.3).[48] The AngioJet has also been shown to be effective for the treatment of coronary stent thrombosis, another condition that carries significant mortality and morbidity. In one published report of 18 patients treated with the AngioJet for acute coronary stent thrombosis, no patient died or required emergent bypass surgery. Acute MI evolved in 10 patients, but only one patient developed Q-wave MI.[49]

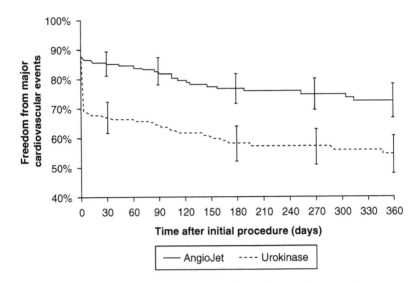

Figure 23.2   VeGAS 2 randomized trial: freedom from MACE at 360 days of follow-up.

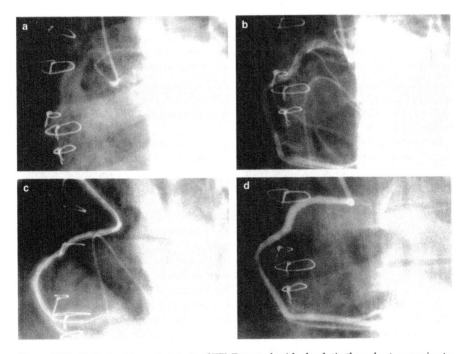

Figure 23.3   Patient with acute interior STEMI treated with rheolytic thrombectomy prior to stenting.

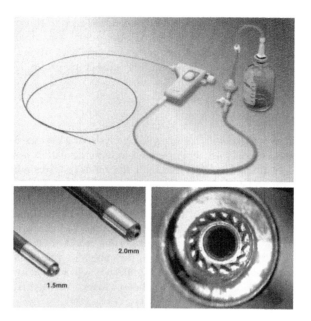

Figure 23.4 X-Sizer thrombectomy system, catheter, and cutter (bottom right).

Despite these favorable results, the AngioJet Rheolytic Thrombectomy In Patients Undergoing Primary Angioplasty for Acute Myocardial Infarction (AIMI) Study, a multicenter prospective randomized trial of patients with STEMI treated with rheolytic thrombectomy ($n = 240$) or conventional PCI ($n = 240$), failed to show any advantage with the use of rheolytic thrombectomy. Final TIMI 3 coronary flow was higher in the group treated with conventional PCI (97% vs. 92%, $P = 0.02$). In addition, the 30-day major cardiovascular event rate was higher in the rheolytic thrombectomy group (6.7% vs. 1.7%; $P < 0.01$). It was postulated that distal embolization was responsible for the adverse events.[50]

X-Sizer thrombectomy

The X-sizer thrombectomy system (X-Sizer catheter system; eV3, White Bear Lake, Minnesota, USA) consists of a two-lumen over-the-wire catheter, with a helical shape cutter (available 1.5 and 2.0, and 2.3 mm) at its distal tip. The cutter rotates at 2100 rpm, and is activated by a hand-held battery motor unit. One catheter lumen contains the guidewire, and the other lumen is connected to a 250 ml vacuum bottle, which draws thrombus toward the cutter, where it is macerated and aspirated for collection in the bottle (Figure 23.4).

In a multicenter prospective randomized study, 797 patients (839 vessels) with stenotic saphenous vein grafts (73%) or thrombus-containing native coronary arteries (17%), were randomized to thrombectomy plus PCI compared to PCI alone. The 30-day (16.8% vs. 17.1%; $P = 0.92$) and 1-year (31.3% vs. 28.2%; $P = 0.35$) MACE was not different. However, the incidence of large MI (creatine phosphokinase-MB isoenzyme $> 8 \times$ upper limit of normal) was reduced in the thrombectomy group (5.5% vs. 9.6%; $P = 0.002$).[51] In the setting of STEMI, the X-Sizer was tested in a prospective randomized trial of 201 patients. The patients were assigned to thrombectomy prior to stenting or stenting alone. ST segment resolution >50% was more frequent (68% vs. 53%; $P = 0.037$), and distal embolization was lower (2% vs. 10%; $P = 0.033$) in the X-Sizer group compared to the PCI without thrombectomy group. MACE occurred in 13% of each group at 6 months of follow-up.[52]

Ultrasound thrombolysis

Thrombolysis can be induced with the Acolysis (Acolysis, Angiosonics, Morrisville, NC, USA) device. The device operates by ultrasound-induced cavitation, bubble generation and implosion at the tip of the probe, leading to thrombus lysis/disintegration.[53,54] In a small study of 20 thrombotic lesions in SVG, device success was obtained in 70% with a residual stenosis of $65 \pm 28\%$.[55] The median age of the thrombus was 6 days. All patients required adjunctive treatment with PTCA or stenting. Procedural success was attained in only 65% of the patients. Distal embolization was observed in one patient, and two patients developed no-reflow. Finally, in a prospective randomized trial of Acolysis or abciximab, followed by PCI in angiographic thrombotic lesions of saphenous vein grafts, the group assigned to Acolysis had a significantly lower procedural success (63% vs. 82%; $P = 0.008$), and a significantly higher incidence of MACE (25% vs. 12%, $P = 0.036$).[56]

SLOW-FLOW, NO-REFLOW

The no-reflow (or slow-flow) phenomenon refers to a condition of decreased or absent myocardial perfusion following transient coronary occlusion, despite the absence of mechanical obstruction in the coronary artery supplying that territory.[57] It was initially described in the coronary circulation by Krug et al, 50 years ago after temporary coronary occlusion, in a dog model.[58]

The no-reflow phenomenon occurs in 0.7–5% of the patients undergoing elective PCI.[59,60] It may occur in as many as 30–40% of patients undergoing PCI for STEMI or for the treatment of degenerated saphenous vein grafts.[60–62] It is more common in patients with diabetes, following treatment with rotational atherectomy, and in patients without pre-infarction angina.[63]

The interventionalist must be vigilant, and must be ready to begin therapy without delay when this condition arises, because patients who develop no-reflow during PCI have a significantly higher incidence of in-hospital and long-term complications such as MI, heart failure, negative ventricular remodeling, ventricular tachycardia, and death.[61–65] In one study, patients who developed no-reflow during PCI had a five-fold increase of MI and a four-fold increase of death.[63]

Diagnosis of no-reflow

It is important to recognize that although the no-reflow phenomenon implies ischemia at the myocardial tissue level, the diagnosis of this phenomenon has historically been based on decreased or absent antegrade flow as judged by coronary arteriography.[59] It is now well-known that angiographic flow velocity in an epicardial coronary artery may remain normal, despite impaired or absent myocardial tissue perfusion.[66] This concept is of particular importance during reperfusion therapy for STEMI, where 20–30% of patients with successful reperfusion after acute MI and restoration of TIMI 3 coronary flow will have myocardial no-reflow demonstrated by myocardial contrast echocardiography.[61,66,67] Furthermore, it has been demonstrated that all patients with TIMI 2 coronary flow have abnormal myocardial perfusion.[68] These findings have been confirmed using other diagnostic modalities to assess myocardial tissue perfusion, such as myocardial scintigraphy, intracoronary Doppler, ST segment resolution in the 12-lead electrocardiogram (ECG), and myocardial blush during the myocardial phase of coronary angiography.[68–71] Consequently, the interventionalist must keep in mind the relatively low sensitivity of coronary angiography for diagnosing the no-reflow phenomenon, and patients with TIMI 3 coronary flow but persistent ST elevation or abnormal myocardial blush during the myocardial phase of coronary angiography must be considered as having the no-reflow phenomenon.

Pathophysiology of no-reflow

In the dog model, an ischemic time of between 40 and 90 min is necessary for the development of the no-reflow phenomenon.[57,58] This is not the case in humans in whom this complication may develop after only brief (< 60 s) interruptions of epicardial coronary flow. For this reason, some investigators believe that there are different mechanisms accounting for no-reflow in animal models and in humans.[72] Other investigators have proposed a classification of this phenomenon as experimental no-reflow, MI reperfusion no-reflow, and angiographic no-reflow.[73]

The pathophysiology of no-reflow is complex, multifactorial, and incompletely understood. In humans, it appears to be a combination of distal embolization, and microvascular spasm. Distal embolization appears to be an important component for the development of no-reflow following PCI.[59,60] Aspiration of coronary arteries in patients with thrombotic lesions and no-reflow showed embolic debris in the majority of cases, containing both thrombi and atheromatous gruel.[74] In addition, microvascular constriction induced by serotonin, angiotensin II, and α-adrenergic agonists appear to play a role in the development of no-reflow.[75] Other mechanisms implicated include oxidative stress, reperfusion injury, endothelial dysfunction, neutrophil infiltration, platelet aggregation, thromboxane production, plasminogen activator inhibitor-1, tissue factor and inflammatory factors (sCD40L, soluble E-selectin).[73,76,77]

Treatment of no-reflow

Because one of the predominant abnormalities during no-reflow appears to be microvascular vasoconstriction, several studies have reported that the use of intracoronary vasodilators that relieve spasm in the microvascular circulation, such as calcium-channel blockers (verapamil, 100–900 µg) or adenosine (18–24 µg bolus repeated as needed (10 to 30 doses) until flow is re-established) are often effective.[59,62,78] However, verapamil may be ineffective in 10–30% of the cases,[59,62] and adverse effects such as hypotension, prolonged heart block, and a negative inotropic effect may also occur. Adenosine, which has a very short half-life (usually a few seconds), appears to be more potent than verapamil for relieving microvascular spasm, and, at the doses mentioned above, is well tolerated without significant side-effects.[78] More recently, it has been reported that intracoronary nitroprusside in doses of 50–1000 µg is beneficial for the treatment of the no-reflow in both native coronaries and saphenous vein grafts.[79]

There are also anecdotal reports regarding the use of antiplatelet agents (abciximab) to treat no-reflow after failed treatment with intracoronary verapamil in native coronary arteries.[80] In addition, a recent report has found that the GP IIb/IIIa inhibitors tirofiban and eptifibatide improve the bioavailability of vascular nitric oxide in patients with coronary artery disease, by blocking platelet–endothelial interactions, which may potentially add vasodilator properties to these agents.[81] Nevertheless, a small group of patients do not respond to any of these pharmacological measures. Almost all of them develop MI, and some progress to cardiogenic shock requiring inotropic support and/or balloon counterpulsation. The prognosis of these patients, once cardiogenic shock has developed, is poor, and many of them expire.

Prevention of no-reflow

The GP IIb/IIIa inhibitors have been shown to reduce the incidence of no-reflow in patients with acute coronary syndromes and STEMI undergoing PCI.[82,83] In addition, a recent meta-analysis of six large prospective randomized trials of 937 STEMI treated with PCI found that early use of these agents (prior to arrival to the catheterization suite), resulted in a higher TIMI 3 coronary flow (20.3% vs. 12.2%; $P < 0.01$), without a reduction in mortality (3.4% vs. 4.7%; P = not significant), compared to the group of patients who received GP IIb/IIIa inhibitors in the catheterization suite.[84] Other antiplatelet agents such as clopidogrel, when added to aspirin and fibrinolytic therapy, has been shown in a recent prospective randomized trial to improve myocardial TIMI 3 perfusion grade compared to placebo.[85]

The use of distal protection devices has decreased the incidence of no-reflow during PCI in several studies, and confirmed the role of distal embolization in the development of this complication. The PercuSurge (Export, PercuSurge, Sunnyvale, CA, USA) device consists of latex balloon on wire (Guardwire), which allows distal occlusion and aspiration of thrombotic and non-thrombotic debris. This device was tested in the Saphenous vein graft Angioplasty Free of Emboli Randomized (SAFER) trial in patients undergoing stent placement in saphenous vein grafts with (n = 273) and without (n = 278) Guardwire. The group treated with PercuSurge had a 42% reduction of MACE at 1 month (Figure 23.5), with most of the reduction being in post-procedure MI (8.6% vs. 16.4%) and no-reflow (3% vs. 8%; P = 0.025).[86] Interestingly, a recent study has suggested that the PercuSurge might be more effective than the filter-based distal protection devices, because the PercuSurge aspiration catheter is capable of retrieving not only atherosclerotic debris and thrombus, but also many vasoactive and inflammatory mediators that potentially induce the no-reflow phenomenon.[77]

However, the use of distal emboli protection devices in the setting of STEMI has not been shown to provide additional benefits to primary PCI alone. An initial report of 53 patients with acute STEMI, treated with PCI and a filter-based distal protection device, showed improved TIMI 3 myocardial blush and ST segment resolution.[87] Two subsequent prospective randomized trials testing balloon occlusion- and filter-based emboli protection prior to stenting failed to show improvement in ST segment resolution or TIMI 2/3 myocardial blush in the group treated with distal protection prior to stent placement, compared to group treated with stent placement alone (see below).[88,89]

DISTAL EMBOLIZATION

The concept of microvascular embolization of platelet-rich thrombus was initially described in experimental studies of endothelial injury.[90] The importance of distal embolization, as a result of mechanical manipulation of atherosclerotic coronary arteries during PCI, was under-recognized and underestimated.[91] The work of Abdelmeguid et al 10 years ago demonstrated, that 'mild' elevations of creatine

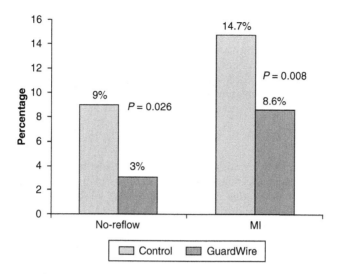

Figure 23.5   No-reflow and myocardial incidence in the SAFER trial.

phosphokinase (CPK)-MB during PCI were associated with mortality and the development of cardiovascular events.[92]

The implementation of new cardiovascular imaging modalities, as well as the introduction of more sensitive markers of myocardial necrosis such as troponin, have helped to confirm the original observations regarding the negative impact of distal embolization, and its correlation with abnormal myocardial tissue perfusion.[93-96]

Pharmacological therapy

Although the GP IIb/IIIa inhibitors appear to contribute to the dissolution of angiographic thrombus, their clinical benefits in the treatment of large thrombus burden remains to be proven. Conversely, there is a great deal of evidence showing that these agents play an important role in the treatment of distal embolization. Neumann et al showed improved myocardial perfusion in 200 patients treated with primary stenting, randomized to abciximab or placebo.[97] The coronary flow velocity in the infarct zone as well as the segmental wall motion and left ventricular function were significantly better in patients that received abciximab. The Evaluation of Platelet IIb/IIIa Inhibitor for Stenting (EPISENT) investigators showed a 55% reduction in large (>5-fold CPK-MB) procedural MI, and a 57% reduction in the 1-year mortality (2.4% for stent–placebo, and 1.0% for stent abciximab).[98] In addition, in patients who have already developed distal embolization after an ACS as judged by CPK-MB elevation, the benefit conferred by these agents is greater in patients with a higher creatine phosphokinase-MB.[99] Although the mechanism of protection remains speculative, it is possible that these agents may improve microvascular flow by facilitating platelet disaggregation and unplugging capillaries. It is possible that a similar mechanism of protection may operate when using other antiplatelet agents such as clopidogrel or thrombin inhibitors for the treatment of ACS.[100-104]

Several studies have demonstrated that patients with ACS have a decrease in major cardiovascular events with early and intensive lipid lowering therapy,[105,106] and that the use of lipid-lowering agents prior to PCI decreases distal embolization. In the Atorvastatin for Reduction of Myocardial Damage during Angioplasty (ARMYDA) study, 153 patients with chronic stable angina were randomized to atorvastatin versus placebo.[107] MI by creatine kinase-MB determination was markedly reduced after PCI in the atorvastatin group (5% vs. 18%; $P = 0.025$).

Mechanical therapy

Antiplatelet and antithrombotic agents may have a role in the treatment of distal embolization by promoting dissolution of the thrombus that plugs the myocardial microcirculation; however, they would have no effect on the atherosclerotic debris. This has been demonstrated during PCI of SVG, where the majority of the particulate debris was found to be atherosclerotic material.[108] Furthermore, the GP IIb/IIIa inhibitors have not been shown to decrease major cardiovascular events after PCI of SVG.[109,110]

Emboli protection devices were created to capture particulate matter during PCI. They fall into two general categories: (1) distal balloon-occlusion, by which a balloon occludes the arterial flow distal to the target lesion, PCI is performed, and a catheter aspirates the debris; and (2) distal filter devices, by which a filter traps the debris during PCI and is then withdrawn from the vessel with the embolic material. The major disadvantage of the balloon-occlusion system is that arterial occlusion may cause intolerable ischemia, as well as decreased angiographic visualization while performing PCI. It has the theoretical advantage of a more complete removal of embolic material. The filter-based systems allow myocardial perfusion during PCI, but may allow passage of debris smaller than the filter pores (80–150 μm).

Several studies have demonstrated the safety and effectiveness of these devices in retrieving embolic material,[108,111] and later documented reduction in major cardiovascular events in prospective randomized trials.[108,111] In the SAFER trial (partially discussed in the section on no-reflow), 406 patients of the group assigned to Percusurge had a 42% relative reduction in major cardiovascular events (Figure 23.6).[86] The Filterwire EX Randomized Evaluation (FIRE) trial demonstrated comparable protection from distal embolization of the balloon-occlusion system (Percusurge) and the filter-based device (FilterWire EX) in the treatment of 682 SVG, with a 30-day incidence of MACE (11.6% and 9.9% respectively, $P = 0.53$).[112] There are ongoing studies testing the effectiveness of different distal protection devices, in different clinical conditions.[113]

Whereas distal protection devices appear highly effective in reducing cardiac events during PCI of SVG, their effectiveness in improving clinical outcomes in the treatment of STEMI remains unproven. In a prospective study, 501 patients with STEMI were randomized to primary stenting and conventional treatment, with or without distal protection. Although visible debris was retrieved in 73% of the patients assigned to distal protection (balloon-occlusion and aspiration system), complete ST segment resolution (63% vs. 62%) and infarct size (12% vs. 9.5%), as well as the 6-month MACE (10% vs. 11%) were similar in both groups.[88] In another study of acute MI with (69%) or without (31%) ST segment elevation, 200 patients were randomized to primary stenting, with or without a filter-based distal protection system. Although debris was captured by the filters in 60% of the cases, the maximal adenosine-induced Doppler-flow velocity (34 ± 17 vs. 36 ± 20 cm/s), infarct size (12 ± 9% vs. 10 ± 9%), and 30-day mortality (2% vs. 3%) were similar in both groups.[89]

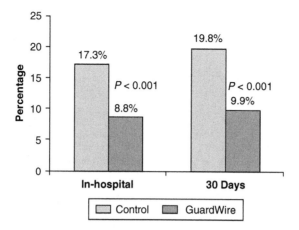

Figure 23.6 Major cardiovascular events in the SAFER trial.

The results of these two prospective randomized trials contrast with an earlier small, non-randomized study of 53 patients, which showed improvement in ST segment resolution as well as TIMI frame count in the patients treated with distal protection.[87] It is possible that in the setting of STEMI, prevention of distal embolization of thrombotic debris adds little or negligible benefit to a microcirculation that is already damaged or affected by reperfusion injury. Further research is necessary to clarify this issue.

The use of covered stents to exclude degenerated or thrombotic material from the vessel lumen was conceived as a strategy that might potentially lead to decreased distal embolization, with initial encouraging reports.[114–116] However, prospective randomized trials have shown that covered stents do not decrease distal embolization when compared to bare-metal stents, and at present are not useful for this purpose.[117–119]

SUMMARY

Percutaneous treatment of thrombus-containing lesions is associated with an increased incidence of no-reflow, distal embolization, and MACE. The use of intracoronary fibrinolysis for these lesions has shown mixed results. Potent antiplatelet agents such as the GP IIb/IIIa inhibitors decrease MACE in the setting of ACS; however, in the treatment of lesions with a large thrombus burden or SVG, these agents have not conferred additional benefit compared to PCI alone. The use of mechanical thrombectomy devices to remove thrombus prior to PCI is associated with clinical benefit.

The no-reflow phenomenon occurs as a result of microvascular vasoconstriction and distal embolization, and is more frequent during PCI of thrombotic lesions such as STEMI, and during percutaneous revascularization of SVG. Intracoronary administration of calcium-channel antagonists, adenosine, and nitroprusside are often useful to treat this complication. The use of distal protection devices appears to decrease the incidence of no-reflow.

Distal embolization is a common occurrence after PCI of SVG, and has been shown to carry negative short- and long-term prognosis. The use of aggressive lipid-lowering (statin) therapy prior to PCI may decrease the incidence of distal embolization, and ideally, all patients who tolerate these medications should receive them prior to the procedure. Emboli protection devices decrease distal embolization during PCI of SVG. Although these devices do capture debris during primary PCI for STEMI in native coronary arteries, they have not yet been shown to improve clinical outcomes, when compared with PCI without distal protection.

REFERENCES

1. Davies MJ, Thomas AC. Plaque fissuring – the cause of acute myocardial infarction, sudden ischaemic death, and crescendo angina. Br Heart J 1985; 53: 363–73.
2. Davies MJ, Bland JM, Hangartner JR, Angelini A, Thomas AC. Factors influencing the presence or absence of acute coronary artery thrombi in sudden ischemic death. Eur Heart J 1989; 10: 203–8.
3. Fuster VS. Conner Memorial Lecture. Mechanisms leading to myocardial infarction: Insights from studies of vascular biology. Circulation 1994; 90: 2126–46.
4. Oliver MF, Davies MJ. The atheromatous lipid core. Eur Heart J 1998; 19: 16–18.
5. White CJ, Ramee SR, Collins TJ et al. Coronary thrombi increase PTCA risk. Angioscopy as a clinical tool. Circulation 1996; 93: 253–8.
6. Waxman S, Sassower MA, Mittleman MA et al. Angioscopic predictors of early adverse outcome after coronary angioplasty in patients with unstable angina and non-Q-wave myocardial infarction. Circulation 1996; 93: 2106–13.
7. Okamatsu K, Takano M, Sakai S et al. Elevated troponin T levels and lesion characteristics in non-ST-elevation acute coronary syndromes. Circulation 2004; 109: 465–70.
8. Tanaka A, Kawarabayashi T, Nishibori Y et al. No-reflow phenomenon and lesion morphology in patients with acute myocardial infarction. Circulation 2002; 105: 2148–52.
9. Violaris AG, Melkert R, Herrman JP, Serruys PW. Role of angiographically identifiable thrombus on long-term luminal renarrowing after coronary angioplasty: a quantitative angiographic analysis. Circulation 1996; 93: 889–7.
10. Bauters C, Lablanche JM, McFadden EP, Hamon M, Bertrand ME. Relation of coronary angioscopic findings at coronary angioplasty to angiographic restenosis. Circulation 1995; 92: 2473–9.
11. Schieman G, Cohen BM, Kozina J et al. Intracoronary urokinase for intracoronary thrombus accumulation complicating percutaneous transluminal coronary angioplasty in acute ischemic syndromes. Circulation 1990; 82: 2052–60.
12. Vaitkus PT, Laskey WK. Efficacy of adjunctive thrombolytic therapy in percutaneous transluminal coronary angioplasty. J Am Coll Cardiol 1994; 24: 1415–23.
13. Denardo SJ, Morris NB, Rocha-Singh KJ et al. Safety and efficacy of extended urokinase infusion plus stent deployment for treatment of obstructed, older saphenous vein grafts. Am J Cardiol 1995; 76 :776–80.
14. Ambrose JA, Almeida OD, Sharma SK et al. Adjunctive thrombolytic therapy during angioplasty for ischemic rest angina. Results of the TAUSA Trial. TAUSA Investigators. Thrombolysis and Angioplasty in Unstable Angina trial. Circulation 1994; 90: 69–77.
15. Zidar FJ, Kaplan BM, O'Neill WW et al. Prospective, randomized trial of prolonged intracoronary urokinase infusion for chronic total occlusions in native coronary arteries. J Am Coll Cardiol 1996; 27: 1406–12.
16. Hartmann JR, McKeever LS, O'Neill WW et al. Recanalization of Chronically Occluded Aortocoronary Saphenous Vein Bypass Grafts With Long-Term, Low Dose Direct Infusion of Urokinase (ROBUST): a serial trial. J Am Coll Cardiol 1996; 27: 60–6.
17. Glazier JJ, Kiernan FJ, Bauer HH et al. Treatment of thrombotic saphenous vein bypass grafts using local urokinase infusion therapy with the Dispatch catheter. Cathet Cardiovasc Diagn 1997; 41: 261–7.
18. Mitchel JF, Fram DB, Palme DF II et al. Enhanced intracoronary thrombolysis with urokinase using a novel, local drug delivery system. In vitro, in vivo, and clinical studies. Circulation 1995; 91: 785–93.

19. Mitchel JF, Azrin MA, Fram DB et al. Inhibition of platelet deposition and lysis of intracoronary thrombus during balloon angioplasty using urokinase-coated hydrogel balloons. Circulation 1994; 90: 1979–88.
20. Scarborough RM, Kleiman NS, Phillips DR. Platelet glycoprotein IIb/IIIa antagonists. What are the relevant issues concerning their pharmacology and clinical use? Circulation 1999; 100: 437–44.
21. Topol EJ. Toward a new frontier in myocardial reperfusion therapy: emerging platelet preeminence. Circulation 1998; 97: 211–18.
22. Eisenberg MJ, Jamal S. Glycoprotein IIb/IIIa inhibition in the setting of acute ST-elevation myocardial infarction. J Am Coll Cardiol 2003; 42: 1–6.
23. Simoons ML, de Boer MJ, van den Brand MJ et al. Randomized trial of a GPIIb/IIIa platelet receptor blocker in refractory unstable angina. European Cooperative Study Group. Circulation 1994; 89: 596–603.
24. Muhlestein JB, Karagounis LA, Treehan S, Anderson JL. 'Rescue' utilization of abciximab for the dissolution of coronary thrombus developing as a complication of coronary angio-plasty. J Am Coll Cardiol 1997; 30: 1729–34.
25. Bailey SR, O'Leary E, Chilton R. Angioscopic evaluation of site-specific administration of ReoPro. Cathet Cardiovasc Diagn 1997; 42: 181–4.
26. Barsness GW, Buller C, Ohman EM et al. Reduced thrombus burden with abciximab delivered locally before percutaneous intervention in saphenous vein grafts. Am Heart J 2000; 139: 824–9.
27. Singh M, Reeder GS, Ohman EM et al. Does the presence of thrombus seen on coronary angiogram affect the outcome after percutaneous coronary angioplasty? An angiographic trials pool data experience. J Am Coll Cardiol 2001; 38: 624–30.
28. Zhao XQ, Theroux P, Snapinn SM, Sax FL, for the PRISM-PLUS Investigators. Intracoronary thrombus and platelet glycoprotein IIb/IIIa receptor blockade with tirofiban in unstable angina or non-Q-wave myocardial infarction. Angiographic results from the PRISM-PLUS Trial (Platelet Receptor Inhibition for Ischemic Syndrome Management in Patients Limited by Unstable Signs and Symptoms). Circulation 1999; 100: 1609–15.
29. Cura FA, L'Allier PL, Kapadia SR et al. Predictors of TIMI ≥2 coronary flow after primary angioplasty in patients with acute myocardial infarction (Abstract). J Am Coll Cardiol 2000; 35: 20A.
30. Yip HK, Wu CJ, Chang HW et al. Impact of tirofiban on angiographic morphologic features of high-burden thrombus formation during direct percutaneous coronary inter-vention and short-term outcomes. Chest 2003; 124: 962–8.
31. Colombo A, Hall P, Nakamura S et al. Intracoronary stenting without anticoagulation accomplished with intravascular ultrasound guidance. Circulation 1995; 91: 1676–88.
32. Schömig A, Neumann F-J, Kastrati A et al. A randomized comparison of antiplatelet and anticoagulant therapy after the placement of coronary-artery stents. N Engl J Med 1996; 334: 1084–9.
33. Stone GW, Brodie BR, Griffin JJ et al. Prospective, multicenter study of the safety and feasibility of primary stenting in acute myocardial infarction: in-hospital and 30-day results of the PAMI stent pilot trial. Primary Angioplasty in Myocardial Infarction Stent Pilot Trial Investigators. J Am Coll Cardiol 1998; 31: 23–30.
34. Stone GW, Grines CL, Cox DA et al, for the CADILLAC Investigators. Comparison of angioplasty with stenting, with or without abciximab, in acute myocardial infarction. N Engl J Med 2002; 346: 957–66.
35. Montalescot G, Barragan P, Wittenberg O et al, for the ADMIRAL Investigators. Platelet glycoprotein IIb/IIIa inhibition with coronary stenting for acute myocardial infarction. N Engl J Med 2001; 344: 1895–903.
36. Holmes DR, Ellis SG, Garrats KN. Directional coronary atherectomy for thrombus containing lesions (abstract). Circulation 1991; 84 (Suppl II): II-26.
37. Kurisu S, Sato H, Tateishi H et al. Directional coronary atherectomy for the treatment of acute myocardial infarction. Am Heart J 1997; 134: 345–50.

38. Saito S, Arai H, Kim K, Aoki N, Sakurabayashi T, Miyake S. Primary directional coronary atherectomy for acute myocardial infarction. Cathet Cardiovasc Diagn 1994; 32: 44–8.
39. Emmi R, Movsowitz H, Manginas A et al. Directional coronary atherectomy in lesions with coexisting thrombus (abstract). Circulation 1993; 88 (Suppl I): I-596.
40. Kaplan BM, Safian RD, Goldstein JA, Grines CL, O'Neill WW. Efficacy of angioscopy in determining the effectiveness of intracoronary urokinase and TEC atherectomy thrombus removal from an occluded saphenous vein graft prior to stent implantation. Cathet Cardiovasc Diagn 1995; 36: 335–7.
41. Popma JJ, Leon MB, Mintz GS et al. Results of coronary angioplasty using the transluminal extraction catheter. Am J Cardiol 1992; 70: 1526–32.
42. Safian RD, Grines CL, May MA et al. Clinical and angiographic results of transluminal extraction coronary atherectomy in saphenous vein bypass grafts. Circulation 1994; 89: 302–12.
43. Safian RD, May MA, Lichtenberg A et al. Detailed clinical and angiographic analysis of transluminal extraction coronary atherectomy for complex lesions in native coronary arteries. J Am Coll Cardiol 1995; 25: 848–54.
44. Braden GA, Xenopoulos NP, Young T et al. Transluminal extraction catheter atherectomy followed by immediate stenting in treatment of saphenous vein grafts. J Am Coll Cardiol 1997; 30: 657–63.
45. Kaplan BM, Larkin T, Safian RD et al. Prospective study of extraction atherectomy in patients with acute myocardial infarction. Am J Cardiol 1996; 78: 383–8.
46. Kuntz RE, Baim DS, Cohen DJ et al. A trial comparing rheolytic thrombectomy with intracoronary urokinase for coronary and vein graft thrombus (the Vein Graft AngioJet Study (VeGAS 2)). Am J Cardiol 2002; 89: 326–30.
47. Silva JA, Ramee SR, Cohen DJ et al. Rheolytic thrombectomy during percutaneous revascularization for acute myocardial infarction: experience with the AngioJet catheter. Am Heart J 2001; 141: 353–9.
48. Antonucci D, Valenti R, Migliorini A et al. Comparison of rheolytic thrombectomy before direct infarct artery stenting versus direct stenting alone in patients undergoing percutaneous coronary intervention or acute myocardial infarction. Am J Cardiol 2004; 93: 1033–5.
49. Silva JA, White CJ, Ramee SR et al. Rheolytic thrombectomy for the treatment of stent thrombosis: results from a multicenter experience. Cathet Cardiovasc Intervent 2003; 58: 11–17.
50. Ali A, Cox D, Dib N et al. for the AIMI Investigators. Rheolytic thrombectomy with percutaneous coronary intervention for infarct size reduction in acute myocadial infarction. 30-day results from a multicenter randomized study. J Am Coll Cardiol 2006; 48: 244–52.
51. Stone GW, Cox DA, Babb J et al, for the X-TRACT Investigators. Prospective, randomized evaluation of thrombectomy prior to percutaneous intervention in diseased saphenous vein grafts and thrombus-containing coronary arteries. J Am Coll Cardiol 2003; 42: 2007–13.
52. Lefebre T, Garcia E, Reimers B et al, on behalf of the X AMINE ST Investigators. X-sizer for thrombectomy in acute myocardial infarction improves ST-segment resolution. Results of the X-Sizer in AMI for Negligible Embolization and Optimal ST Resolution (X AMINE ST) Trial. J Am Coll Cardiol 2005; 46: 246–52.
53. Miller DL, Thomas RM, Williams AR. Mechanisms for hemolysis by ultrasonic cavitation in the rotating exposure system. Ultrasound Med Biol 1991; 17: 171–8.
54. Miller DL, Williams AR. Bubble cycling as the explanation of the promotion of ultrasonic cavitation in a rotating tube exposure system. Ultrasound Med Biol 1989; 15: 641–8.
55. Rosenschein U, Gaul G, Erbel R et al. Percutaneous transluminal therapy of occluded saphenous vein grafts: can the challenge be met with ultrasound thrombolysis? Circulation 1999; 99: 26–9.
56. Singh M, Rosenschein U, Ho KK et al. Treatment of saphenous vein bypass grafts with ultrasound thrombolysis: a randomized study (ATLAS). Circulation 2003; 107: 2331–6.

57. Klonner RA, Ganote CE, Jennings RB. The 'no-reflow' phenomenon after temporary coronary occlusion in the dog. J Clin Invest 1974; 54: 1496–508.
58. Krug A, de Rochemont WM, Korb G. Blood supply of the myocardium after temporary coronary occlusion. Circ Res 1966; 19: 57–62.
59. Piana RN, Paik GY, Moscucci M et al. Incidence and treatment of no-reflow after percutaneous coronary intervention. Circulation 1994; 89: 2514–18.
60. Abbo KM, Dooris M, Glazier S et al. Features and outome of no-reflow after percutaneous coronary intervention. Am J Cardiol 1995; 75: 778–82.
61. Ito H, Maruyama A, Iwakura K et al. Clinical implications of the 'no reflow' phenomenon. A predictor of complications and left ventricular remodeling in reperfused anterior wall myocardial infarction. Circulation 1996; 93: 223–8.
62. Kaplan BM, Benzuly KH, Kinn JW et al. Treatment of no-reflow in degenerated saphenous vein graft interventions: comparison of intracoronary verapamil and nitroglycerin. Cathet Cardiovasc Diag 1996; 39: 113–18.
63. Kaul S, Ito H. Microvasculature in acute myocardial ischemia: part II. Evolving concepts in pathophysiology. Circulation 2004; 109: 310–15.
64. Morishima I, Sone T, Okumura et al. Angiographic no-reflow phenomenon as a predictor of long-term outcome in patients treated with percutaneous transluminal coronary angioplasty for first acute myocardial infarction. J Am Coll Cardiol 2000; 36: 1202–9.
65. Resnic FS, Wainstein M, Lee MKY et al. No-reflow is an independent predictor of death and myocartdial infarction. Am Heart J 2003; 145: 42–6.
66. Ito H, Iwakura K. Assessing the relation between coronary reflow and myocardial reflow. Am J Cardiol 1998; 81(12A): 8G–12G.
67. Ito H, Okamura A, Iwakura K et al. Myocardial perfusion patterns related to thrombolysis in myocardial infarction grades after coronary angioplasty in patients with acute anterior wall myocardial infarction. Circulation 1996; 93: 1993–9.
68. Iwakura K, Ito H, Takiuchi S et al. Alternation in the coronary flow velocity pattern in patients with no reflow and reperfused acute myocardial infarction. Circulation 1996; 94: 1269–75.
69. Schofer J, Montz R, Mathey D. Scintigraphy evidence of the 'no reflow' phenomenon in human beings after coronary thrombolysis. J Am Coll Cardiol 1985; 5: 593–8.
70. Santoro GM, Valenti R, Buonamici P et al. Relation between ST-segment changes and myocardial perfusion evaluated by myocardial contrast echocardiography in patients with acute myocardial infarction. Am J Cardiol 1998; 82: 932–7.
71. Gibson CM, Cannon CP, Murphy SA et al. Relationship of the TIMI myocardial perfusion grades, flow grades, frame count and percutaneous coronary intervention to long-term outcomes after thrombolytic administration in acute myocardial infarction. Circulation 2002; 105: 1909–13.
72. Kelly RV, Cohen MG, Runge MS et al. The no-reflow phenomenon in coronary arteries. J Thromb Haemost 2004; 2: 1903–7.
73. Eeckhout E, Kern MJ. The no-reflow phenomenon: a review of mechanisms and therapies. Eur Heart J 2001; 22: 729–39.
74. Kotani J, Nanto S, Mintz GS et al. Plaque gruel of atheromatous coronary lesion may contribute to no-reflow phenomenon in patients with acute coronary syndrome. Circulation 2002; 106: 1672–9.
75. Wilson RF, Laxson DD, Lesser JR, White CW. Intense microvascular constriction after angioplasty of acute thrombotic coronary arterial lesions. Lancet 1989; I: 807–11.
76. Rezkalla SH, Kloner RA. No-reflow phenomenon. Circulation 2002; 105: 656–62.
77. Salloum J, Tharpe C, Vaughan D et al. Release and elimination of soluble vasoactive factors during percutaneous coronary intervention of saphenous vein grafts: analysis using the PercuSurge GuardWire distal protection device. J Invasive Cardiol 2005; 17: 575–9.
78. Fischell TA, Carter AJ, Foster MT et al. Reversal of 'no-reflow' during vein graft stenting using high velocity boluses of intracoronary adenosine. Cathet Cardiovasc Diagn 1998; 45: 360–5.

79. Hillegas WB, Dean NA, Liao L et al. Treatment of no-reflow and impaired flow with the nitric oxide donor nitroprusside following percutaneous coronary interventions: initial human clinical experience. J Am Coll Cardiol 2001; 37: 1335–43.

80. Rawitscher D, Levin TN, Cohen I, Feldman T. Rapid reversal of no-reflow using abciximab after coronary device intervention. Cathet Cardiovasc Diagn 1997; 42: 187–90

81. Heitzer T, Ollman I, Koke K et al. Platelet glycoprotein IIb/IIIa receptor blockade improves vascular nitric oxide bioavailability in patients with coronary artery disease. Ciculation 2003; 108: 536–41.

82. De Lemos JA, Antman EM, Gibson CM et al. Abciximab improves both epicardial flow and myocardial perfusion in ST-elevation myocardial infarction. Observations from the TIMI 14 trial. Circulation 2000; 101: 239–43.

83. Whorle J, Grebe OC, Nusser T et al. Reduction of major cardiac events with intracoronary compared with intravenous bolus application of abciximab in patients with acute myocardial infarction or unstable angina undergoing coronary angioplasty. Circulation 2003; 107: 1840–3.

84. Montalescot G, Borentain M, Payot L et al. Early versus late administration of glycoprotein IIb/IIIa inhibitors in primary percutaneous coronary intervention of acute ST-segment elevation myocardial infarction. JAMA 2004; 292: 362–6.

85. Sabatine MS, Cannon CP, Gibson CM et al. For the CLARITY-TIMI 28 Investigators. Addition of clopidogrel to aspirin and fibrinolytic therapy for myocardial infarction with ST-segment elevation. N Engl J Med 2005; 352: 1179–89.

86. Baim DS, Dennis W, George B et al. On behalf of the Saphenous vein graft Angioplasty Free of Emboli Randomized (SAFER) Trial investigators. Randomized trial of a distal embolic protection device during percutaneous intervention of saphenous vein aorto-coronary bypass grafts. Circulation 2002; 105: 1285–90.

87. Limbruno U, Micheli A, De Carlo M et al. Mechanical prevention of distal embolization during primary angioplasty: safety, feasibility, and impact on myocardial reperfusion. Circulation 2003; 108: 171–6.

88. Stone GW, Webb J, Cox DA et al. Ennhanced Myocardial Efficacy and Recovery by Aspiration of Liberated Debris (EMERALD) Investigators. Distal microcirculatory protection during epicutaneous coronary intervention in acute ST-segment elevation myocardial infarction: a randomized controlled trial. JAMA 2005; 293: 1116–18.

89. Gick M, Jander N, Bestehom HP et al. Randomized evaluation of the effect of filter-based distal protection on myocardial perfusion and infarct size after primary percutaneous catheter intervention in myocardial infarction with and without ST-segment elevation. Circulation 2005; 112: 1462–9.

90. Edith JF, Allison P, Noble S et al. Thrombin is an important mediator of platelet aggregation in stenosed canine coronary arteries with endothelial injury. J Clin Invest 1989; 84: 18–27.

91. Topol EJ, Yadav JS. Recognition of the importance of embolization in atherosclerotic vascular disease. Circulation 2000; 101: 570–80.

92. Abdelmeguid AE, Topol EJ, Whitlow PL et al. Significance of mild transient release of creatine kinase-MB fraction after percutaneous coronary interventions. Circulation 1996; 94: 1528–36.

93. Ravkilde J, Nissen H, Mickley H et al. Cardiac troponin T and CK-MB mass release after visually successful percutaneous transluminal coronary angioplasty in stable angina pectoris. Am Heart J 1994; 127: 13–20.

94. Stubbs P, Collison P, Moseley D et al. Prognostic significance of admission troponin T concentrations in patients with myocardial infarction. Circulation 1996; 94: 1291–7.

95. Hong MK, Mehran R, Dangas G et al. Creatine kinase-MB elevation following successful saphenous vein graft intervention is associated with late mortality. Circulation 1999; 100: 2400–5.

96. Wong GC, Morrow DA, Murphy S et al. For the TACTICS-TIMI 18 Study Group. Elevations in troponin T are associated with abnormal tissue level perfusion. A TACTICS-TIMI 18 Substudy. Circulation 2002; 106: 202–7.

97. Neumann FJ, Blasini R, Schmitt C et al. Effects of glycoprotein IIb/IIIa receptor blockade on recovery of coronary flow and left ventricular function after the placement of coronary-artery stents in acute myocardial infarction. Circulation 1998; 98: 2695–701.
98. EPISTENT Investigators. Randomized controlled trial to assess safety of coronary stenting with the use of abciximab. Lancet 1998; 352: 85–90.
99. Hamm CW, Heeschen C, Goldmann B et al. Benefit of abciximab in patients with refractory unstable angina in relation to serum troponin T levels. N Engl J Med 1999; 340: 1623–6.
100. Yusuf S, Zhao F, Mehta SR et al, for the Clopidogrel in Unstable Angina to Prevent Recurrent Events Trial Investigators. Effects of clopidogrel in addition to aspirin in patients with acute coronary syndromes without ST-segment elevation. N Engl J Med 2001; 345: 494–502.
101. Mehta SR, Yusuf S, Peters RJ et al. Effects of pretreatment with clopidogrel and aspirin followed by long-term therapy in patients undergoing percutaneous coronary intervention. Lancet 2001; 358: 527–33.
102. Antman EM, McCabe CH, Gurfinkel EP et al. Enoxaparin prevents death and cardiac ischemic events in unstable angina/non-Q-wave myocardial infarction. Results of the Thrombolysis in Myocardial Infarction (TIMI) 11B Trial. Circulation 1999; 100: 1593–601.
103. Cohen M, Demers C, Gurfinkel EP et al. A comparison of low-molecular-weight heparin with unfractionated heparin for unstable coronary artery disease. Efficacy and Safety of Subcutaneous Enoxaparin in Non-Q-Wave Coronary Events Study Group. N Engl J Med 1997; 337: 447–52.
104. The Direct Thrombin Inhibitor Trialists' Collaborative Group. Direct thrombin inhibitors in acute coronary syndromes: principal results of a meta-analysis based on individual patients' data. Lancet 2002; 359: 294–302.
105. Okazaki S, Yokoyama T, Miyauchi K et al. Early statin treatment in patients with acute coronary syndrome. Demonstration of the beneficial effect on atherosclerotic lesions by serial volumetric intravascular ultrasound analysis duing half a year after coronary event: The ESTABLISH Study. Circulation 2004; 110: 1061–8.
106. Cannon CP, Braunwald E, McCabe CH et al, for the Pravastatin or Atorvastatin Evaluation and Infection Therapy – Thrombolysis in Myocardial Infarction 22 Investigators. Intensive versus moderate lipid lowering with statins after acute coronary syndromes. N Engl J Med 2004; 350: 1495–504.
107. Pasceri V, Patti G, Nusca A et al, on behalf of the ARMYDA Investigators. Randomized trial of atorvatastin for reduction of myocardial damage during coronary intervention. Results from the ARMYDA (Atorvatastin for Reduction of Myocardial Damage during Angioplasty) Study. Circulation 2004; 110: 674–8.
108. Webb JG, Carere RG, Virmani R et al. Retrieval and analysis of particulate debris after saphenous vein intervention. J Am Coll Cardiol 1999; 34: 468–75.
109. Mak K-H, Challapalli R, Eisenberg MJ et al, for the EPIC Investigators. Effect of platelet glycoprotein IIb/IIIa receptor inhibition on distal embolization during percutaneous revascularization of aortocoronary saphenous vein grafts. Am J Cardiol 1997; 80: 985–8.
110. Ellis SG, Lincoff AM, Miller D, Tcheng JE et al. Reduction of complications of angioplasty with abciximab occurs largely independently of baseline lesion morphology. J Am Coll Cardiol 1998; 32: 1619–23.
111. Carlino M, De Gregorio J, Di Mario C et al. Prevention of distal embolization during saphenous vein graft lesion angioplasty. Experience with a new temporary occlusion and aspiration system. Circulation 1999; 99: 3221–3.
112. Stone GW, Rogers C, Hermiller J et al, for the FilterWire EX Randomized Evaluation (FIRE) Investigators. Randomized comparison of distal protection with a filter-based catheter and a balloon occlusion and aspiration system during percutaneous intervention of diseased saphenous vein aorto-coronary bypass grafts. Circulation 2003; 108: 548–53.
113. Gorog DA, Foale RA, Malik I. Distal myocardial protection during percutaneous coronary intervention. When and where? J Am Coll Cardiol 2005; 46: 1434–45.

114. Gurbel PA, Criado FJ, Curnutte EA, Patten P, Secada-Lovio J. Percutaneous revascularization of an extensively diseased saphenous vein bypass graft with a saphenous vein-covered Palmaz stent. Cathet Cardiovasc Diagn 1997; 40: 75–8.
115. Stefanadis C, Toutouzas K, Tsiamis E et al. Total reconstruction of a diseased saphenous vein graft by means of conventional and autologous tissue-coated stents. Cathet Cardiovasc Diagn 1998; 43: 318–21.
116. Stefanadis C, Tsiamis E, Vlachopoulos C et al. Autologous vein graft-coated stents for the treatment of thrombus-containing coronary artery lesions. Cathet Cardiovasc Diagn 1997; 40: 217–22.
117. Stankovic G, Colombo A, Presbitero P et al. Randomized evaluation of polytetrafluoroethylene-covered stents in saphenous vein grafts: The Randomized Evaluation of polytetrafluoroethylene COVERed stent in saphenous vein grafts (RECOVERS) Trial. Circulation 2003; 108: 37–42.
118. Schanchinger V, Hamm CW, Munzel T et al. A randomized trial of polytetrafluoroethylene-membrane-covered stents compared with conventional stents in aorto-coronary saphenous vein grafts. J Am Coll Cardiol 2003; 42: 1360–9.
119. Blackman DJ, Choudhury RP, Banning AP et al. Failure of the symbiot PTFE-covered stent to reduce distal embolization during percutaneous coronary intervention in saphenous vein grafts. J Invasive Cardiol 2005; 17: 609–12.

24

The role of interventional cardiology in functional coronary stenosis

Eulógio E Martinez, Nestor F. Mercado, Pedro A Lemos, and Antonio Esteves Filho

Myocardial bridges • Coronary spasm

Coronary angiography is almost always performed as a last step in the diagnostic chain of suspected heart atherosclerotic disease. In this context, finding a luminal stenosis is frequently considered as a pathognomonic sign of coronary atherosclerosis. However, other potential causes of coronary stenosis have been reported increasingly, in association or not with atherosclerosis. It is important to note that the correct recognition of the nature of the luminal obstruction has a profound impact on the diagnostic and therapeutic management of the patient. In this chapter, therefore, we revise two important forms of *functional* coronary obstruction: myocardial bridging, and coronary spasm.

MYOCARDIAL BRIDGES

Myocardial bridges are bands of cardiac muscle that overlay an intramural segment of a coronary artery.

They are predominantly found in the left anterior descending (LAD), but not infrequently in diagonal branches, in the posterior descending right coronary artery, or in marginal branches of the circumflex artery.

Although in pathological series the incidence of intramyocardial segments ranges from 15% to 85%, the identification of myocardial bridges in diagnostic catheterization is relatively infrequent, ranging from 0.5% to 2.5% in different angiographic series.[1-8] This indicates that the vast majority of muscle bands overlying coronary artery segments do not provoke the milking effect typical of angiographic myocardial bridges.

There are difficulties in diagnosing myocardial bridging as a cause of myocardial ischaemia, considering that there seems to be little correlation between the severity of systolic narrowing and clinical symptoms, and that most myocardial bridges are found in asymptomatic individuals. Furthermore, it seems theoretically unlikely that a purely systolic narrowing will be of pathophysiological relevance when coronary blood flow is predominantly diastolic. On the other hand, there are patients with a myocardial bridge as the only detectable abnormality in whom clinical problems like acute coronary syndromes and severe arrhythmias have been reported.[9]

In studies published more than 20 years ago, some diastolic abnormalities were detected in patients with myocardial bridges. These abnormalities included an extension of the obstruction into diastole, and a time-lag of up to one-third of diastole before flow returned to normal following systolic compression.[10,11]

In the last decade, new techniques such as quantitative coronary angiography (QCA), intravascular ultrasound (IVUS), and intracoronary pressure and flow measurements have improved our understanding of the pathophysiology of symptomatic muscle bridges.[12–16]

QCA measurements in patients with myocardial bridges and systolic narrowing revealed diastolic diameter reductions maintained until mid- to late diastole.[13,14,17] Results from IVUS studies revealed that the systolic compression is usually eccentric and confirmed the delayed relaxation and reduction of vessel lumen diameter in diastole.[18,19] Aditionally, in symptomatic patients, IVUS studies have shown a high incidence of atherosclerotic plaques in the coronary artery segment immediately proximal to the myocardial bridge. In two studies, this incidence was higher than 80%.[12,15] Curiously, these proximal lesions are frequently not detected by angiography, probably because the eventual lumen reduction due to the plaque is visually interpreted as a manifestation of the milking effect of myocardial bridging.

Placement of Doppler wires in the bridged segment has allowed identification of a peculiar flow pattern abnormality, present in approximately 90% of symptomatic patients, consisting of an abrupt early diastolic flow acceleration and rapid mid-diastolic deceleration followed by a mid- to late-diastolic plateau.[12,14,20,21]

The abrupt early diastolic flow acceleration has been termed the 'finger tip' phenomenon. The Doppler flow pattern in systole consists of reduced or even absent antegrade flow, and in some cases retrograde flow in late systole. Coronary flow reserve distal to the bridge, defined as the ratio of mean flow velocity achieved at peak hyperemia to mean resting flow velocity was shown to be abnormally reduced (<3) in several studies, ranging from 2.0 to 2.6.[13–17] Symptomatic patients with myocardial bridging frequently complain of exercise-induced angina. The invasive assessment exclusively performed at rest may leave undetected hemodynamic abnormalities present only during exercise or situations of increased inotropism, since the degree of phasic reduction in coronary diameter is dependent on extravascular compression and intramural tension. The importance of inotropic stimulation for the physiological assessment of myocardial bridging was demonstrated by Escaned et al, in a recent study that involved 12 symptomatic patients; all patients had abnormal non-invasive tests and/or electrocardiogram (ECG) changes that were suggestive of myocardial ischemia.[22] The authors measured fractional flow reserve (FFR) by the conventional method (using mean coronary pressure over the complete cardiac cycle) and diastolic FFR, calculated exclusively from diastolic pressures, to avoid the interference that the systolic overshoot occurring in myocardial bridging can have in conventional measurements of FFR.

Through a micromanometer-tipped guidewire, following intracoronary administration of 200 µg of nitroglycerin, baseline translesional pressure measurements were obtained during hyperemia induced by a 20 µg intracoronary adenosine bolus. A new set of pressure measurements was performed after an intravenous infusion of 5 µg/kg/min dobutamine was given for 5 min, followed by new measurements at progressive increases in dobutamine in 5 µg/kg/min doses, to a maximum dose of 20 µg/kg/min, or until the patient developed symptoms. At baseline, only one patient was found to have a hemodynamically significant myocardial bridging using diastolic FFR. During dobutamine inotropic challenge, five patients were shown to have significant reductions in diastolic FFR, and only one in conventional FFR. Then, there are patients with significant reduction in flow reserve detected by diastolic FFR, although it is not detected by conventional FFR. Curiously, the angiographic severity of myocardial bridging did not correlate with its functional relevance. The authors conclude that for patients with myocardial bridging studied using conventional FFR, a negative result, even after dobutamine challenge, does not preclude the possibility of a false negative. Many factors may influence the myocardial perfusion abnormality induced by myocardial bridging, including length, thickness, and location of the muscle bridge, presence of left ventricular hypertrophy, increased heart rate, coronary vasomotion, and enhanced platelet aggregation. In symptomatic patients, bridges tend to be longer (by QCA) and thicker at IVUS studies.[15] Patients with myocardial bridging and progressive left ventricular hypertrophy may present with myocardial ischaemia later in life, when the increase in wall tension aggravates the systolic compression of the coronary segment covered by the muscle band. Increases in heart rate by atrial pacing lead to magnification of the diastolic flow disturbances, as documented by Doppler flow measurements. Pharmacological vasodilators like nitroglycerin and sodium nitroprusside increase the coronary narrowing in patients with myocardial bridging, whereas vasoconstrictors like norepinephrine, phenylephrine, and ergonovine decrease it. Additionally vasospastic coronary constriction may be associated with myocardial bridging. Interestingly, at coronary angiography and at autopsy studies, atherosclerotic plaques are rarely found either at the level of intramural coronary arteries or in the distal segment of the bridge.[23]

The absence of atherosclerosis in the tunneled segment may be at least partially explained by both hemodynamic and constitutional factors. There is evidence that the intima in the tunneled segment could be protected by hemodynamic factors such as high shear stress, with consequent local production of nitric oxide (NO).[24] Additionally, the intima beneath the bridge does not contain the synthetic-type smooth muscle cells, that are known to proliferate during progression of atherosclerosis.[25,26] On the other hand, phasic compression of the tunneled coronary segment may cause trauma to the intima and damage to the endothelium, that could lead to acute coronary syndromes, due to platelet aggregation and vasospasm.[27-29]

Following the pioneer work of Noble et al[5] many clinical studies involving symptomatic patients with MB have been published.[5,7,12-17] In these series, 55–70% of all patients with greater than 50% systolic lumen narrowing of the LAD had typical angina, frequently of severe intensity. Rest angina is often reported among patients with atypical anginal symptoms. It is noteworthy that cases of unstable angina, acute myocardial infarction (MI), life-threatening cardiac arrhythmias, and even of sudden death have been atributted to myocardial bridging. When stress tests were performed, significant ischemic ST segment depression was detected in 28–67%, and stress-induced perfusion defects of the anterior wall or septum in 33–63% of the patients. These clinical and non-invasive signs of myocardial ischemia are comparable to those observed among patients with single-vessel coronary disease. Furthermore, as suggested by Bourassa et al, the long-term outcome of patients with myocardial bridging may be as favorable as that of patients with single-vessel coronary disease or even better, considering that little late disease progression is to be expected.[23]

Therapy

According to the pathophyisiological mechanisms that lead to myocardial ischemia, symptomatic patients with myocardial bridges may benefit from the three therapeutic modalities usually applied to patients with atherosclerotic coronary disease, namely medical therapy, percutaneous coronary intervention, and surgical myocardial revascularization. In addition, direct surgical myotomy may be indicated in highly selected patients. It is important to realize that the outcome of patients with myocardial bridges is benign, with an extremely low risk of serious cardiac events. Among 28 patients followed up for an average of 11 years, there was not a single case of MI.[7]

Asymptomatic patients should not be treated. Patients with symptoms and evidence of myocardial ischemia should initially be treated with optimal doses of beta-blockers, calcium-channel blockers in cases of contraindication to beta-blockers, and antiplatelet agents. Nitrates should be in general avoided, considering that they have been shown to increase the degree of systolic coronary narrowing and to provoke worsening of symptoms.[29] Additionally, during a 4-year follow-up of 185 patients with isolated myocardial bridges (in which there were three deaths and seven myocardial infarctions), the use of nitrates was shown to be significantly associated with a decrease in survival free of major cardiac events.[30] On the other hand, the risk of events was reduced among patients in use of aspirin.

Limitation of strenuous physical activity is recommended to avoid the unfavorable effects of tachycardia and strong inotropic stimulation.

In 15 symptomatic patients with myocardial bridges, anginal symptoms and ST changes triggered by rapid atrial pacing were abolished by the administration of esmolol, a short-acting beta-blocker, through reductions in systolic and diastolic vascular compression and in mid- to late-diastolic flow velocities within the bridged segment.[13]

At 1-year follow-up of a series of 12 patients with myocardial bridging, abnormal non-invasive tests and/or ECG changes suggestive of ischaemia, in which long-term treatment with beta-blockers was followed in all patients with hemodynamically relevant myocardial bridging, all patients remained asymptomatic and free of cardiac events.[31]

An apparently very small subset of patients may have symptoms refractory to treatment with beta-blockers, and should be further investigated by IVUS and coronary physiological studies with pressure and/or flow wires. Patients belonging to this subset may have hidden atherosclerotic plaques proximal to the bridged segment, detected by IVUS and missed by angiography. In the absence of proximal atherosclerotic plaques and of significant abnormalities in coronary flow dynamics, conservative treatment should be continued, percutaneous and/or surgical treatment being restricted to patients with positive results.

Before the current era of coronary stenting, surgical myotomy was an important treatment option for patients refractory to medical treatment, with good clinical results, although it was not infrequently associated with complications like severe arrythmias and even right ventricular perforation.[29]

In our view, surgical dissection of the overlying myocardium should nowadays be restricted to highly exceptional cases of extremely long intramyocardial segments not amenable to stenting or bypass grafting, in severely symptomatic patients with documented ischaemia refractory to treatment with beta-blockers.

Minimally invasive coronary artery bypass grafting (CABG) carries a low risk, and has been reported for myocardial bridging.[33] It may be the treatment of choice for patients with unsuccessful coronary stenting or in-stent restenosis. Additionally, internal mammary artery grafting might be indicated in patients with myocardial bridging and significant coronary disease in other vessels requiring coronary bypass surgery.

Coronary angioplasty with stenting was shown to be effective in abolishing phasic lumen compression, diastolic flow abnormalities, and anginal symptoms caused by myocardial bridges.[14,34] Haager et al reported successful coronary stenting in 11 myocardial bridge patients with repeat coronary angiography at 7 weeks and 6 months, as well as clinical follow-up at 2 years.[16] Stenting determined immediate normalization of systolic and diastolic flow abnormalities and cessation of systolic compression. At re-study, QCA showed a high in-stent restenosis rate of 46% (5 of 11 patients), although within the range commonly observed with bare-metal stents in lesions of 25 mm length in vessels of small diameter, as pointed out by the authors. Restenosis was treated in four patients: by repeat balloon angioplasty in two, and by coronary bypass surgery with an internal mammary artery graft to the LAD in two. In 2 years' follow-up, there were no cardiac events, and all remained asymptomatic.

Stenting of intramyocardial coronary segments or of lesions located immediately proximal to these segments may eventually be hazardous,[35–37] with reported cases of complications including coronary perforation and MI due to thrombus formation.

Problems may arise from inappropriate stent sizing, especially in long myocardial bridges, when a stent diameter adequate for the proximal reference segment may be oversized for the distal segment. Measurements of proximal and distal reference diameter, if possible by IVUS, are important for selection of balloon and stent sizes. Additionally, although it has not been our practice, we believe that inotropic challenge with dobutamine may be of great value in sizing the stent length, in order to avoid the hazardous consequences of incomplete coverage of the intramyocardial segment.

Accordingly, among the 12 patients studied by Escaned et al, dobutamine infusion determined a highly significant two-fold increase in stenosis length measured by QCA, from 12.40 ± 9.05 mm to 24.04 ± 9.17 mm.[22]

In summary, myocardial bridges, in addition to systolic coronary compression, may determine diastolic reductions in coronary diameter, diastolic flow abnormalities, reductions in coronary flow reserve, anginal symptoms, and myocardial ischaemia documented by non-invasive stress tests. Additionally, there is evidence that atherosclerotic plaques are not infrequently present in the coronary artery segment immediately proximal to the myocardial bridges.

However, long-term prognosis is excellent among symptomatic patients kept on medical therapy with beta-blockers, and for that reason percutaneous interventions are only indicated in cases of refractory symptoms and documented abnormal coronary flow dynamics. Special care should be taken in stent sizing, with meticulous measurement of reference diameters, and ideally with measurements of stenosis length during inotropic stimulation by dobutamine infusion.

CORONARY SPASM

Coronary spastic angina (variant angina) is classically characterized by spontaneous episodes of angina in association with ST segment elevation on the ECG.[38]

Spasm usually occurs in either normal or diseased vessels, at a single site or in more than one site, and also as a diffuse narrowing of long segments of the coronary tree.[39] It can usually be reversed by nitroglycerin or a calcium-channel blocker. In diseased vessels it is usually observed within 1 cm of an atherosclerotic plaque, whereas among cocaine users, spasm frequently occurs in the absence of angiographically documented coronary disease.[40]

Provocative tests in the catheterization laboratory (with either ergonovine, acetylcholine or hyperventilation) are indicated in patients with recurrent episodes of apparently ischemic chest pain at rest, in whom ECGs were not recorded during the anginal attacks, and the coronary angiogram revealed normal or only mildly abnormal coronary arteries. The test with ergonovine is the most sensitive and specific for provoking coronary spasm.[41,42] Coronary spasm induced by ergonovine use is rapidly reversible by nitroglycerin. Positivity of the test is defined as the induction of a spasm that triggers the patient's symptoms, and/or associated ST segment deviations. The recommended dose is 50–400 µg given intravenously, beginning with 50 µg, and repeating this dose at 5 minute intervals until a positive result or the maximum dose is reached.

Hyperventilation performed in the early morning can also be used as a provocative test for spastic angina and/or ST segment shifts, with moderate sensitivity and very high specificity for patients with angiographically documented spasm.[39,41,43] The sensitivity seems to be higher in patients with frequent episodes of angina than in patients with only sporadic symptoms.[41] Sensitivity can be enhanced if hyperventilation is followed by cold pressor testing during electrocardiographic and echocardiographic monitoring.[44]

Medical therapy

Pharmacological therapy with the administration of calcium-channel blockers (nifedipine, diltiazem, and verapamil) or nitrates should be complemented by cessation of smoking, use of statins, and modification of other risk factors, since spasm not infrequently occurs at the site, or in the vicinity, of atherosclerotic plaques. Calcium-channel blockers and nitrates are widely recognized to prevent coronary constriction. Propranolol and non-selective beta-blockers in general can exacerbate vasospasm, and are not recommended for patients with suspected spastic angina.[45] Aspirin should also be avoided, due to prostacyclin synthesis inhibition.[46]

Percutaneous coronary intervention

Among patients with variant angina, 5–30% continue to have recurrent episodes of angina in spite of full medical treatment with calcium-channel bockers and nitrates, with the risk of occurrence of MI and arrhythmic sudden death.[47–52]

Spastic angina can occur in patients with a wide spectrum of coronary anatomies, from angiographically normal coronary arteries to severe multivessel disease.[53] In about two-thirds of patients with variant angina, spasm occurs at the level of an atherosclerotic lesion.[54]

As a rule, coronary stenting should be contraindicated in patients with variant angina, and focal and minimal obstructive disease. In these cases multivessel coronary spasm is frequently observed.[55] On the other hand, stenting may be highly effective in cases of refractory medical treatment with vasospasm occurring in a segment with mild to moderate coronary disease. Gaspardone et al reported a series of nine patients with variant angina and persistent anginal attacks, despite aggressive medical treatment (up to 960 mg diltiazem or 100 mg nifedipine and nitrates) in whom coronary angiography demonstrated a segmental epicardial spasm induced by an ergonovine derivative.[56] In all patients, spasm was localized at the level of a mild to moderate atherosclerotic lesion; baseline reductions in coronary luminal diameter at the lesion site ranged from 36% to 65%. Stent placement was successful in all patients. Exercise thallium-201 myocardial scintigraphy and 48-h Holter monitoring were performed after 2 months, and coronary angiography was repeated after 6 months. Within 2 months, three patients developed recurrent episodes of angina at rest associated with ST segment elevation during Holter monitoring. During a mean follow-up of 10 months, six patients remained asymptomatic with Holter monitoring negative for transient episodes of silent myocardial ischemia. Repeat coronary angiography documented a patent stent in eight patients (89%). One patient had an asymptomatic intra-stent restenosis with lumen diameter narrowing of 54%. Intra-coronary administration of increasing doses of methylergometrine caused coronary spasm associated with ST segment ischemic changes and angina in the three patients presenting with ST segment elevation during anginal episodes at Holter monitoring. In two patients, coronary spasm occurred proximally to the previously implanted stent, and in the third patient, in whom the stent was placed in the right coronary artery, the spasm occurred in both the left anterior descending, and the circumflex coronary arteries. Thus, stent placement is an attractive therapeutic option for patients with vasospastic angina refractory to aggressive medical therapy, in whom the vasospasm occurs at the level of a mild to moderate atherosclerotic lesion. When severe organic stenosis is present, spasm occurs at the lesion site in a high proportion of patients, and there are several case reports of successful stenting for the treatment of medically refractory spastic angina and severe coronary stenosis.[57,58] However, multivessel spasm may occur even in patients with documented spasm at the site of a coronary lesion. In a recent study, 45 patients with coronary spastic angina and severe stenosis underwent spasm provocative testing with intracoronary acetylcholine, before and approximately 7 months after PCI (20 patients had angioplasty, and 25 patients had stenting), all free of restenosis.[59] Pre-intervention, spasm was induced at the site of severe stenosis in 30 patients, and at a different site in the stenotic vessel and/or in another vessel in the remaining 15 patients. Repeat provocative tests were performed in 43 of 45 patients. Spasm was induced at a different site in the dilated vessel and/or in another vessel in 33 (77%) of 43 patients. Multivessel spasm occurred in 62% of 45 patients on one or both provocations. Thus, in a high proportion of patients with variant angina and severe coronary obstruction, spasm continues to be induced by provocative tests after successful PCI in the absence of restenosis, usually at a site different from the initial stenosis. These findings indicate that patients with severe coronary narrowing, who present with signs and symptoms of variant angina, have a combination of atherosclerotic coronary disease and hyper-reactivity of coronary smooth muscle to constrictor stimuli.[54] For that reason it is suggested that therapy with calcium antagonists should be continued after coronary stenting. Patients with spastic angina and coronary arteries free of severe obstructive lesions have good prognosis, with overall 5-year survival greater than 95%.[52,60,61] The prognosis is poorer for patients with multivessel disease and severe coronary lesions,[61] and for patients who experience ventricular fibrillation during an episode of spasm. There are conflicting data regarding the role of calcium-channel blockers in survivors of cardiac arrest due to spasm-induced ventricular fibrillation. In one series, among seven patients with spasm-induced ventricular tachycardia or fibrillation, six patients remained free of symptoms for approximately 5 years on calcium-channel blockers.[62] Curiously, in a series of eight patients treated with calcium-channel blockers, ventricular arrhythmia recurred in all during a short follow up of 15 months.[63] The role of coronary stenting in survivors of spasm-induced ventricular fibrillation is still not known.

REFERENCES

1. Polacek P, Kralove H. Relation of myocardial bridges and loops on the coronary arteries to coronary occlusions. Am Heart J 1961; 61: 44–52.
2. Hansen BF. Myocardial covering on epicardial coronary arteries. Prevalence, localization and significance. Scand J Thorac Cardiovasc Surg 1982; 16: 151–5.
3. Ishii T, Hosoda Y, Osaka T, Imai T et al. The significance of myocardial bridge upon atherosclerosis in the left anterior descending coronary artery. J Pathol 1986; 148: 279–91.
4. Ferreira AG Jr, Trotter SE, Konig B Jr et al. Myocardial bridges: morphological and functional aspects. Br Heart J 1991; 66: 364–7.
5. Noble J, Bourassa MG, Petitclerc R, Dyrda I. Myocardial bridging and milking effect of the left anterior descending coronary artery: normal variant or obstruction? Am J Cardiol 1976; 37: 993–9.
6. Kramer JR, Kitazume H, Proudfit WL, Sones FM Jr. Clinical significance of isolated coronary bridges: benign and frequent condition involving the left anterior descending artery. Am Heart J 1982; 103: 283–8.
7. Juilliere Y, Berder V, Suty-Selton C et al. Isolated myocardial bridges with angiographic milking of the left anterior descending coronary artery: a long-term follow-up study. Am Heart J 1995; 129: 663–5.
8. Angelini P, Trivellato M, Donis J, Leachman RD. Myocardial bridges: a review. Prog Cardiovasc Dis 1983; 26: 75–88.
9. Alegria JR, Herrmann J, Holmes DR Jr, Lerman A, Rihal CS. Myocardial bridging. Eur Heart J 2005; 26: 1159–68.
10. Bourassa MG, Bernard P, Brevers G, Petitclerc R, Dyrda I. Systolic and early diastolic inflow obstruction in patients with muscular bridging of the left anterior descending artery. In: Bruschke AVG, van Herpen G, Vermeulen FEE, eds. Coronary Artery Disease Today. Princeton, NJ: Excerpta Medica, 1981: 380–94.
11. Navarro-Lopez F, Soler J, Magrina J et al. Systolic compression of coronary artery in hypertrophic cardiomyopathy. Int J Cardiol 1986; 12: 309–20.
12. Ge J, Erbel R, Rupprecht HJ et al. Comparison of intravascular ultrasound and angiography in the assessment of myocardial bridging. Circulation 1994; 89: 1725–32.
13. Schwarz ER, Klues HG, vom Dahl J et al. Functional characteristics of myocardial bridging. A combined angiographic and intracoronary Doppler flow study. Eur Heart J 1997; 18: 434–42.
14. Klues HG, Schwarz ER, vom Dahl J et al. Disturbed intracoronary hemodynamics in myocardial bridging: early normalization by intracoronary stent placement. Circulation 1997; 96: 2905–13.
15. Ge J, Jeremias A, Rupp A et al. New signs characteristic of myocardial bridging demonstrated by intracoronary ultrasound and Doppler. Eur Heart J 1999; 20: 1707–16.
16. Haager PK, Schwarz ER, vom Dahl J et al. Long term angiographic and clinical follow up in patients with stent implantation for symptomatic myocardial bridging. Heart 2000; 84: 403–8.
17. Schwarz ER, Klues HG, vom Dahl J et al. Functional, angiographic and intracoronary Doppler flow characteristics in symptomatic patients with myocardial bridging: effect of short-term intravenous beta-blocker medication. J Am Coll Cardiol 1996; 27: 1637–45.
18. Möhlenkamp S, Hort W, Ge J, Erbel R. Update on myocardial bridging. Circulation 2002; 106: 2616–22.
19. Alegria JR, Herrmann J, Holmes DR, Jr, Lerman A, Rihal CS. Myocardial bridging. Eur Heart J 2005; 26: 1159–8.
20. Sanchez V, Zamorano J. New approach to the diagnosis of myocardial bridging by intracoronary ultrasound and Doppler. Eur Heart J 1999; 20: 1687–8.
21. Kneale BJ, Stewart AJ, Coltart DJ. A case of myocardial bridging: evaluation using intracoronary ultrasound, Doppler flow measurement, and quantitative coronary angiography. Heart 1996; 76: 374–6.
22. Escaned J, Cortes J, Flores A et al. Importance of diastolic fractional flow reserve and dobutamine challenge in physiologic assessment of myocardial bridging. J Am Coll Cardiol 2003; 42: 226–33.

23. Bourassa MG, Butnaru A, Lesperance J, Tardif JC. Symptomatic myocardial bridges: overview of ischemic mechanisms and current diagnostic and treatment strategies. J Am Coll Cardiol 2003; 41: 351–9.
24. Masuda T, Ishikawa Y, Akasaka Y et al. The effect of myocardial bridging of the coronary artery on vasoactive agents and atherosclerosis localization. J Pathol 2001; 193: 408–14.
25. Ishii T, Asuwa N, Masuda S et al. Atherosclerosis suppression in the left anterior descending coronary artery by the presence of a myocardial bridge: an ultrastructural study. Mod Pathol 1991; 4: 424–31.
26. Campbell GR, Campbell JH. Smooth muscle phenotypic changes in arterial wall homeostasis: implications for the pathogenesis of atherosclerosis. Exp Mol Pathol 1985; 42: 139–62.
27. Ciampricotti R, el Gamal M. Vasospastic coronary occlusion associated with a myocardial bridge. Cathet Cardiovasc Diagn 1988; 14: 118–20.
28. Gertz SD, Uretsky G, Wajnberg RS, Navot N, Gotsman MS. Endothelial cell damage and thrombus formation after partial arterial constriction: relevance to the role of coronary artery spasm in the pathogenesis of myocardial infarction. Circulation 1981; 63: 476–86.
29. Maseri A, Chierchia S. Coronary artery spasm: demonstration, definition, diagnosis, and consequences. Prog Cardiovasc Dis 1982; 25: 169–92.
30. Iversen S, Hake U, Mayer E et al. Surgical treatment of myocardial bridging causing coronary artery obstruction. Scand J Thorac Cardiovasc Surg 1992; 26: 107–11.
31. Vaz VD, Feres F, Abizaid A, et al. Long-term prognosis of patients with isolated myocardial bridge. J Am Coll Cardiol 2006; 47 (suppl I): 187A [abstract].
32. Escaned J, Goicolea J, Alfonso F et al. Propensity and mechanisms of restenosis in different coronary stent designs: complementary value of the analysis of the luminal gain-loss relationship. J Am Coll Cardiol 1999; 34: 1490–7.
33. Pratt JW, Michler RE, Pala J, Brown DA. Minimally invasive coronary artery bypass grafting for myocardial muscle bridging. Heart Surg Forum 1999; 2: 250–3.
34. Prendergast BD, Kerr F, Starkey IR. Normalisation of abnormal coronary fractional flow reserve associated with myocardial bridging using an intracoronary stent. Heart 2000; 83: 705–7.
35. Hering D, Horstkotte D, Schwimmbeck P et al. [Acute myocardial infarct caused by a muscle bridge of the anterior interventricular ramus: complicated course with vascular perforation after stent implantation]. Z Kardiol 1997; 86: 630–8.
36. Agirbasli M, Hillegass WB Jr., Chapman GD, Brott BC. Stent procedure complicated by thrombus formation distal to the lesion within a muscle bridge. Cathet Cardiovasc Diagn 1998; 43: 73–6.
37. Antonellis IP, Patsilinakos SP, Pamboukas CA et al. Intracoronary stent placement proximal to a myocardial bridge: immediate and long-term results. Catheter Cardiovasc Interv 1999; 46: 363–7.
38. Prinzmetal M, Kennamer R, Merliss R, Wada T, Bor N. Angina pectoris. I. A variant form of angina pectoris; preliminary report. Am J Med 1959; 27: 375–88.
39. Okumura K, Yasue H, Matsuyama K et al. Diffuse disorder of coronary artery vasomotility in patients with coronary spastic angina. Hyperreactivity to the constrictor effects of acetylcholine and the dilator effects of nitroglycerin. J Am Coll Cardiol 1996; 27: 45–52.
40. Lange RA, Cigarroa RG, Yancy CW Jr et al. Cocaine-induced coronary-artery vasoconstriction. N Engl J Med 1989; 321: 1557–62.
41. Previtali M, Ardissino D, Barberis P et al. Hyperventilation and ergonovine tests in Prinzmetal's variant angina pectoris in men. Am J Cardiol 1989; 63: 17–20.
42. Hamilton KK, Pepine CJ. A renaissance of provocative testing for coronary spasm? J Am Coll Cardiol 2000; 35: 1857–9.
43. Nakao K, Ohgushi M, Yoshimura M et al. Hyperventilation as a specific test for diagnosis of coronary artery spasm. Am J Cardiol 1997; 80: 545–9.
44. Hirano Y, Ozasa Y, Yamamoto T et al. Hyperventilation and cold-pressor stress echocardiography for noninvasive diagnosis of coronary artery spasm. J Am Soc Echocardiogr 2001; 14: 626–33.

45. Robertson RM, Wood AJ, Vaughn WK, Robertson D. Exacerbation of vasotonic angina pectoris by propranolol. Circulation 1982; 65: 281–5.
46. Miwa K, Kambara H, Kawai C. Effect of aspirin in large doses on attacks of variant angina. Am Heart J 1983; 105: 351–5.
47. Freedman SB, Richmond DR, Alwyn M, Kelly DT. Late follow-up (41 to 102 months) of medically treated patients with coronary artery spasm and minor atherosclerotic coronary obstructions. Am J Cardiol 1986; 57: 1261–3.
48. Egashira K, Kikuchi Y, Sagara T, Sugihara M, Nakamura M. Long-term prognosis of vasospastic angina without significant atherosclerotic coronary artery disease. Jpn Heart J 1987; 28: 841–9.
49. Nakamura M, Takeshita A, Nose Y. Clinical characteristics associated with myocardial infarction, arrhythmias, and sudden death in patients with vasospastic angina. Circulation 1987; 75: 1110–16.
50. Veau P, Scholl JM, Benacerraf A et al. [Long-term prognosis of spastic angina with normal or irregular coronary arteries. Apropos of 48 cases]. Arch Mal Coeur Vaiss 1989; 82: 889–94.
51. Hannebicque G, Lablanche JM, Fourrier JL, Gommeaux A, Bertrand ME. [Long-term prognosis of coronary artery spasm]. Arch Mal Coeur Vaiss 1990; 83: 461–7.
52. Bory M, Pierron F, Panagides D et al. Coronary artery spasm in patients with normal or near normal coronary arteries. Long-term follow-up of 277 patients. Eur Heart J 1996; 17: 1015–21.
53. Maseri A, Severi S, Nes MD et al. 'Variant' angina: one aspect of a continuous spectrum of vasospastic myocardial ischemia. Pathogenetic mechanisms, estimated incidence and clinical and coronary arteriographic findings in 138 patients. Am J Cardiol 1978; 42: 1019–35.
54. Kaski JC, Crea F, Meran D et al. Local coronary supersensitivity to diverse vasoconstrictive stimuli in patients with variant angina. Circulation 1986; 74: 1255–65.
55. Okumura K, Yasue H, Horio Y et al. Multivessel coronary spasm in patients with variant angina: a study with intracoronary injection of acetylcholine. Circulation 1988; 77: 535–42.
56. Gaspardone A, Tomai F, Versaci F et al. Coronary artery stent placement in patients with variant angina refractory to medical treatment. Am J Cardiol 1999; 84: 96–8, A8.
57. Lopez JA, Angelini P, Leachman DR, Lufschanowski R. Gianturco–Roubin stent placement for variant angina refractory to medical treatment. Cathet Cardiovasc Diagn 1994; 33: 161–5.
58. Jeong MH, Park JC, Rhew JY et al. Successful management of intractable coronary spasm with a coronary stent. Jpn Circ J 2000; 64: 897–900.
59. Tanabe Y, Itoh E, Suzuki K et al. Limited role of coronary angioplasty and stenting in coronary spastic angina with organic stenosis. J Am Coll Cardiol 2002; 39: 1120–6.
60. Yasue H, Takizawa A, Nagao M et al. Long-term prognosis for patients with variant angina and influential factors. Circulation 1988; 78: 1–9.
61. Walling A, Waters DD, Miller DD et al. Long-term prognosis of patients with variant angina. Circulation 1987; 76: 990–7.
62. Chevalier P, Dacosta A, Defaye P et al. Arrhythmic cardiac arrest due to isolated coronary artery spasm: long-term outcome of seven resuscitated patients. J Am Coll Cardiol 1998; 31: 57–61.
63. Meisel SR, Mazur A, Chetboun I et al. Usefulness of implantable cardioverter-defibrillators in refractory variant angina pectoris complicated by ventricular fibrillation in patients with angiographically normal coronary arteries. Am J Cardiol 2002; 89: 1114–16.

25

Complications of drug-eluting stents: thrombosis and restenosis

J Eduardo Sousa and Luiz Alberto Mattos

Drug-eluting stent thrombosis • Drug-eluting stent restenosis • Incidence and predictors

DRUG-ELUTING STENT THROMBOSIS

Percutaneous coronary intervention (PCI) has evolved significantly since its introduction in 1977, by Grüentzig et al.[1] The balloon era demonstrated that the method was feasible and capable of effectively promoting myocardial revascularization, utilizing a non-surgical method. However, the balloon expansion was unpredictable in its intrinsic mode of action, and may promote some major complications as: spasm, coronary artery dissection, slow- or no-flow phenomena, coronary perforation, myocardial infarction (MI), a need for urgent coronary bypass surgery, and risk of death.[2]

Balloon-expandable stents were introduced in clinical practice in 1987. After a tortuous beginning, stents became the gold standard since 1995, when the pitfalls of early years were corrected, with optimal stent implantation, using high-pressure balloon expansion and adoption of a dual antiplatelet regimen (aspirin and ticlopidine or clopidogrel). Before this, the use of bare-metal stents suffered from the occurrence of subacute thrombosis, linked to under-expansion of stent struts, and also related to an uncorrected pharmacological regimen.[3]

Drug-eluting stents (DES) were introduced in 1999, and have been available for clinical practice since 2002.[4] From pioneer drug delivery programs using sirolimus and paclitaxel, many other pharmacological approaches were tested, and new agents will soon become available and effectively reduce the restenosis rates, with the concept of local drug delivery and blockage of cell cycle triggering.[5]

The understanding of the vascular biology of restenosis, coupled with the development of stents as local controlled delivery vehicles of therapeutic agents (polymer based) has generated the proof for the concept for the application of DES.[5]

DES avoids the disruption of central cellular processes inhibiting the downstream effects of injury-mediated growth factors and cytokines, allowing the blockage of the process of hyperplasia proliferative response that culminates with the narrowing of the lumen vessel size, with an excess of smooth muscle cell growth.[6]

The first generation of antiproliferative-coated stents, using sirolimus and paclitaxel, were able to effectively promote a drastic reduction in the restenosis rate (up to 70%) by intense inhibition of intimal hyperplasia, reflected by minimal late lumen loss indices, below 0.5 mm, measured by quantitative coronary angiography (QCA) analysis.[7,8]

From the First in Man (FIM) series, to large randomized controlled trials and to 'all comers' entry criteria registries, large amounts of data were soon gathered, but the specter of stent thrombosis, particularly in the long-term follow-up period, again returned, haunting the days of patients submitted to PCI, now with DES.[9–13]

Definitions

Stent thrombosis is defined in two different periods after a PCI:

- *acute* (<48 h) and *subacute,* when it occurs within the first 30 days
- *late,* from 30 days to long-term follow-up.

As DES promote delay in the endothelization process, creating a third subgroup has recently been accepted, so-called *very late stent thrombosis,* after one year post-DES implantation.[10]

Proof of a true DES thrombosis during the long-term follow-up period is not an easy task. Only angiographic documentation can really confirm that this complication has occurred in the target vessel already treated. However, without that, the association of natural progression of coronary heart disease plus the presence of multivascular coronary disease, or even mixed up cases treated with DES and bare-metal stents, may definitely create confounding variables that upset accurate evaluation of the rate of late occurrence of DES thrombosis.

Despite that, interventional cardiology has a long tradition of always being highly rigorous in its clinical evaluation, while accepting that patients previously submitted to DES implantation, and who suffered a clinically documented new MI (symptoms and electrocardiogram (ECG) Q wave confirmation), or sudden death, were probably exhibiting late DES thrombosis.

Incidence

In a systematic review from 2004, gathering large consecutive data from registries and randomized trials ($n = 22\,763$ patients), the incidence of late thrombosis (up to 1 year) with bare-metal stents was 1.2%, hence it is clear that it also occurs with this technology, when there is no antiproliferative drug delivery appliance.[14]

The first FIM series with DES did not document its occurrence. However, the patients included could be classified as being of low risk for clinical and angiographic profile, mainly because of the limitation of single DES stent usage in vessels up to 3.0 mm in size with lesions shorter than 20 mm in length.[4] As data were accumulated with daily practice registries, this scenario changed.[9–13]

The first meta-analysis encompassing the first large trials, with polymeric and non-polymeric DES compared with the bare-metal ones, was published in 2004 with results from 3646 patients.[15] The follow-up period analyzed was up to one year. The stent thrombosis rates were similar between DES and bare-metal stents (0.7% vs. 0.5%; P = not significant (NS), respectively), and also without significant difference between sirolimus or paclitaxel-eluting stents (0.6% vs. 0.7%; P = NS, respectively).

The warning signals initially came from anecdotal reports of consecutive series from interventional centers where there was extensive use of DES in a broad spectrum of clinical and angiographic percutaneous revascularization of coronary heart disease. All were complex cases; there were many diabetic patients, bifurcations, and overlapping stents, but the main link was the interruption of antiplatelet dual therapy or even just cessation of treatment with aspirin.[12,16]

The sirolimus-eluting controlled series did not report late catch-up thrombosis phenonema in its analysis.[17] However, the paclitaxel-eluting stents demonstrated a slight but worrying increase in the interim analysis from 1 to 2-year follow-up from the TAXUS IV trial (0.5% vs. 0%; $P = 0.77$, paclitaxel-eluting versus bare-metal stents).[18]

A more recent systematic review discussed 5030 patients from 10 randomized controlled trials (RCT) with a follow-up time ranging from 9 to 12 months. The late stent thrombosis rates were quite similar between DES and bare-metal stents, with six cases in each group (0.54% vs. 0.58%; $P = $ NS, respectively). The independent predictors were identified by multivariate analysis as stent length and more multiple stents.[19]

The Rapamycin-Eluting Stent Evaluated At Rotterdam Cardiology Hospital (RESEARCH) and Taxus Stent Evaluated At Rotterdam Cardiology Hospital (T-SEARCH) registries, from the Thoraxcenter, Rotterdam, analyzed the occurrence of stent thrombosis in real-practice DES cases. The acute rates were similar (1.5%, 1.6%, and 1.4%; $P = $ NS) between sirolimus-eluting (SES, $n = 1017$), paclitaxel-eluting ($n = 989$), and a historical matched cohort of bare-metal stents (PES, $n = 506$), respectively. The late incidence was 0.35% (0.3% for SES, and 0.5% for PES), with a follow-up of 1.5 years, demonstrating a high morbidity in these eight patients, all with Q wave MI, and with the occurrence of two deaths. In patients undergoing dual antiplatelet therapy this complication did not occur.[13]

More detailed analysis that allows better identification of late DES thrombosis from independent predictors in the complex population of angiographic patients (more than 80% with multivessel disease, 23% with bifurcations, and 17% with in-stent restenosis) comes from consecutive experience gathered together from two hospitals in Germany and Italy. The incidence of late stent thrombosis was 0.5% for SES and 0.8% for PES ($P = $ NS), as detected from angiographic evidence, Q wave MI occurrence, or death. The strongest independent predictors was discontinuation of antiplatelet therapy (odds ratio (OR) 89.78; 95% confidence interval (CI) 29.90–269.60)), plus renal failure, bifurcation lesion treatment, diabetes, and progressive increases of 1 mm in the stent length.[20]

The Washington Hospital Center interventional group reported experience in 2974 consecutive patients submitted to DES implantation. The acute incidence of thrombosis was 1%, but fortunately, the late rate was of 0.3% (8 cases). Independent multivariate analysis predictors were in-hospital renal failure, treatment of bifurcations, and in-stent restenosis, and also lack of clopidogrel continuation therapy.[21]

The incidence of late thrombosis did not differ between SES or PES use, as demonstrated by Kastrati meta-analysis with direct comparison of both stents (0.7% vs. 0.9%; $P = $ NS) in 3699 patients recruited in these head-to-head comparison trials.[22]

The Basel Stent Kosten Effektivitäts Trial (BASKET) trial late follow-up analysis (from 6 to 18 months) documented a significant increase in the occurrence of death (1.2% vs. 0%; $P = 0.09$) and MI (4.1% vs. 1.3% $P = 0.04$) after clopidogrel discontinuation, in patients who underwent DES compared to those with bare-metal stents. The rates of stent thrombosis doubled in this period comparing DES with bare-metal stents. The authors noted that for every 100 patients treated with a DES, 3.3 cases of cardiac death or MI are induced for a reduction of five cases of target lesion revascularization. However, some criticism arose because not all patients had angiographic documentation.[23] These results increased concern over the discontinuation of clopidogrel in high-risk cases submitted to DES. Further detailed analysis of large numbers is strongly warranted to confirm this.[22] Table 25.1 summarizes all these results.

Table 25.1 Summarized data on stent thrombosis rates in randomized trials and registries: comparison of drug-eluting with standard stents

Author	Number of patients	Method	Stent thrombosis (%)			Angiography performed
			0–360 days	30 days–1 year	1–2 years	
Babapulle[15]	5103	11 RCTs				Yes
All DES			0.7		–	
SES			0.6		–	
PES			0.7		–	
BMS			0.5		–	
Moreno19	5030	10 RCTs				Yes
All DES			0.58	0.23		
SES			0.57	0.11	–	
PES			0.73	0.42	–	
BMS			0.54	0.25	–	
SIRIUS[17]	1058	RCT				
SES			0.4	0.2	0.2	Yes
SES			0.6	0.4	0.4	All events
BMS			0.8	0.6	0	Yes
BMS			1.2	1.0	0.6	All events
TAXUS IV[18]	1314	RCT				Yes
PES			0.6%		0.5	
BMS			0.5		0	
RESEARCH and T-SEARCH[13]	1084	Registry				Yes
SES			0.4	0	–	
PES			1.4	0.34	–	
LAST[10]	2006	Registry				Yes
All DES				0.40	–	
SES			–	0.30	–	
PES			–	0.50	–	
Iakovou[20]	2229	Consecutive cohort				Yes + all events
SES			0.8	0.5	–	
PES			1.7	0.8	–	
Kuchulakanti[21]	2974	Consecutive cohort				Yes + autopsy
All DES			1.27	0.3	–	
Kastrati[22]	3669	6 RCTs				Yes
SES			0.92	–	–	
PES			1.10	–	–	
BASKET[23]	743	RCT				Yes + all events
All DES			2.6			
BMS			1.3			

BMS, bare-metal stent; DES, drug-eluting stent; PES, paclitaxel-eluting stent; RCT, randomized controlled trial; SES, sirolimus-eluting stent.

In conclusion, the evidence relating to DES thrombosis is as follows:

1. the incidence for DES and bare-metal stents is quite similar up to 9 months' follow-up and, depending on the profile of the patients treated, ranges from a mean of 0.3% to no more than 1.0%
2. the majority occurs in the first 30 days (acute and subacute phase)
3. late or very late stent thrombosis exists, but the incidence is less than 0.5%, ranging from 0.2% to less than 0.8%. There is no controlled series comparing the incidence of very late stent thrombosis between bare-metal and drug-eluting stents. Also, the profile of the patients enrolled in the recent series with DES, explores the treatment of patients with much higher risk in comparison with the ones treated with bare-metal stents, as left mains and bifurcations or even trifurcations
4. in order to avoid bias, angiographic documentation is essential for future relevance and judgement. Reports of only clinical events may not give a full assessment of late DES thrombosis
5. the morbidity after occurrence in the first 30 days is higher, with Q wave MI being diagnosed in 50–70% of cases and up to 45% mortality
6. discontinuation of dual antiplatelet therapy is the strongest independent predictor of thrombosis, from analysis of the period 1–24 months; stopping aspirin alone is also a strong predictor. Patients discontinuing that treatment had a 30% higher risk for stent thrombosis
7. the most common clinical and/or angiographic features are the presence of renal failure, treatment of bifurcations with two drug-eluting stents, in addition to overlapping stents for the treatment of long segments
8. there is no significant consistent difference in stent thrombosis rates between SES or PES
9. further controlled registries and trials with long-term follow-up are strongly recommended to clarify these issues.

Mechanisms of DES thrombosis

Drug-eluting stents were developed for delaying the endothelialization process after endothelial injury, requiring that dual antiplatelet therapy is maintained for at least 6 months and, in high-risk cases, for up to 1 year.[5]

Small series with angioscopy and a few post mortem analyses, mostly with SES implantation, demonstrated that only 13% of SES had complete coverage of the stent struts when compared to bare-metal ones. Portions of stents without any coverage of intimal hyperplasia presented with more thrombus attached. Late incomplete stent apposition has also led to controversy about the incidence of thrombosis, but in cases where this phenomenon is genuinely documented, by IVUS, late apposition may be a potentially good predictor for this adverse outcome.[23]

The second set of possible mechanisms is the same as for bare-metal stents: incomplete expansion, and/or significant residual stenosis after DES implantation, as demonstrated by Fugii K et al.[25] The incidence of acute and subacute thrombosis was higher in such cases. This includes treatment of bifurcations for example, where arterial branch points are foci of low shear and low flow velocity, predisposing for development of new atherosclerotic plaque, thrombus, and inflammation.[25]

Table 25.2   Potential causes for late drug-eluting stent thrombosis
• Cessation of dual antiplatelet therapy • Non-degradable polymers with residual drug • Incomplete endothelialization of stent struts • Stent malpositioning and incomplete stent expansion • Increased stent length • Stenting of bifurcations and overlapping segments

Finally allergic reactions to the non-degradable polymer used in the first generation of SES and PES, and even some small amount of residual drug trapped in the polymer from PES, might be the resource for inflammatory reaction and late thrombosis occurrence. The identification of these cases is very difficult and unpredictable. Only the new generation of DES with biodegradable polymer may limit the occurrence of this major and harmful side-effect.[26] Table 25.2 summarizes the potential causes of this phenomenon.

Treatment

The identification of stent thrombosis, regardless of the length of time since PCI, promotes the need for urgent percutaneous target vessel revascularization. The patient should receive the same rapid diagnosis and treatment as for cases of primary angioplasty in MI.

The 10 recommendations for treatment of DES thrombosis are:

1. restart dual antiplatelet therapy immediately. If clopidogrel was halted, introduce 600 mg oral as a bolus
2. despite of no definitive evidence of their use in this situation, glycoprotein IIb/IIIa inhibitors should be of mandatory use, with a preference for abciximab. The last systematic review for its use in primary PCI ($n = 3912$ patients) demonstrated a significant 29% reduction in mortality, and a 47% reduction in 30-day re-infarction rates[26]
3. bivalirudin might also be an option
4. proceed to rapid angiographic injection of the culprit vessel, recrossing it with the guidewire; give preference to prolonged balloon inflations (3–5 min) using a 1:1 matched relationship with the vessel size, if feasible
5. if there is serious concern about the angiographic result, IVUS should be mandatory, in order to identify incomplete expansion. If this is found, further expansion with a larger balloon should be performed, if it is feasible and safe. Massive calcification may not allow that so easily
6. after the use of a standard balloon, vessel patency is usually restored with achievement of epicardial Thrombolysis in Myocardial Infarction (TIMI) 3 flow. In case of a slow- or no-flow phenomena, the use of intracoronary adenosine will be necessary (30–50 µg). Some physicians use it as a routine, as prophylaxis to avoid thrombus formation
7. in the presence of slow-flow or no-flow that does not respond to adenosine, the other pharmacological measures should be started, until the last one, the use intracoronary epinephrine (50–200 µg)

8. the use of filter devices or mechanical aspiration of thrombus should be assessed on a case-by-case basis. If the expected stent length is longer than 25 mm, the vessel is large, or there is a clear large thrombus burden present, these methods might be indicated

9. the use of intracoronary abciximab or alteplase is also an option in the face of difficulties in restoring normal coronary flow with the routine measures

10. however, in an average of less than 5% of the cases of stent thrombosis (particularly those with late presentation and/or with longer delay for treatment), PCI will be not capable of restoring the antegrade coronary flow. The decision about these cases depends on the balance of the threat of myocardial, clinical, and hemodynamic instability. The decision to stop the procedure is always difficult but is acceptable if there is evidence of small branches with no symptoms at all (usually related to the presence of variable amount of previous fibrosis). Urgent coronary artery bypass surgery (CABG) is needed in less than 0.3% of PCI procedures, but might be necessary when there is a large amount of viable myocardium at risk, with no re-establishment of normal coronary flow. The reversal of all the antiplatelet agents already administered will be mandatory, and such cases must be viewed as a very high risk for elevated morbidity after CABG.

DRUG-ELUTING STENT RESTENOSIS

The restenosis rates after DES usage were dramatically reduced. However, according to the presence of diabetes and the angiographic profile from the vessel treated, the rates range from nearly zero to 15%.[27]

INCIDENCE AND PREDICTORS

Sirolimus-eluting stent

In SES, FIM registry and RAVEL (randomized comparison of a sirolimus-eluting stent with a standard stent for coronary revascularization) randomized trial data have demonstrated that it is feasible to obtain nearly 'zero' per cent restenosis, when the patients treated receive a single SES, with a vessel size greater than 2.80 mm and a lesion length that is less than 15 mm.[4] The sum of SIRIUS (sirolimus-eluting versus standard stents in patients with stenosis in a native coronary artery) series, called NEW SIRIUS demonstrated a rate of 5.1% segmental restenosis, with 3.1% in-stent restenosis. Some proximal edge effect occurred more frequently in SES.[28]

In the more complex RESEARCH registry, 441 lesions were treated with SES in 238 patients. Angiographic follow-up data were available for 70% of these. The incidence of SES restenosis was 7.9% (in-lesion), with 6.3% being located in-stent, 0.9% in the proximal, and 0.7% in the distal edge. Independent predictors were identified by multivariate analysis. In order of decreasing odds ratio, treatment of in-stent restenosis, ostial location lesions, diabetic patients, total stented length, and vessel reference size were identified. Again, the same variables already known in the bare-metal stent era re-appear, but fortunately, at a much lower rate (Figure 25.1).[29]

SIRIUS analyzed 31 patients with an in-stent restenosis pattern after SES implantation compared to bare-metal implantation. A focal pattern intimal hyperplasia was present in a majority of cases (87%) after Cypher stent implantation, compared to only 42% in the bare-metal stent group ($P < 0.001$). The majority (65%) was located in the proximal margin. A proliferative pattern was rare, only identified in two

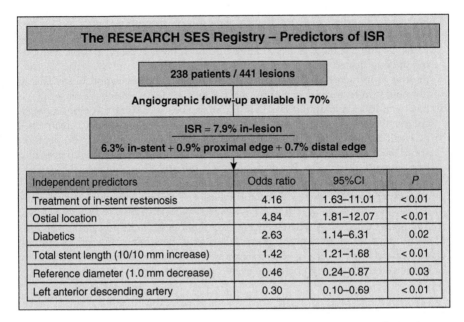

Figure 25.1 Inependent predictors (by multivariate analysis) of sirolimus-eluting in-stent restenosis according to RESEARCH registry analysis

patients. Diffuse restenosis was seen in the majority of the bare-metal stent group (65%), compared to no cases in the SES group ($P < 0.001$).[28]

Paclitaxel-eluting stent

As PES has less impact on late lumen loss index if compared to SES (0.34 mm vs. 0.15 mm; $P < 0.001$), a higher restenosis rate is to be expected in late angiographic follow-up of these cases. So, progressing to a more complex population of patients, from the TAXUS II to TAXUS IV trials, the restenosis rate increased from 5.1% to 12.4% respectively, with longer lesions and smaller vessels included in the last one. Fortunately, usually only half of cases discovered by angiographic investigation require further revascularization related to the presence of myocardial ischemia.[27,30]

The TAXUS IV angiographic subanalysis of 559 patients identified the in-stent restenosis pattern.[31] Focal restenosis was identified in the majority of cases (62%), but a little less than observed with SES. Certainly, the less powerful effect of paclitaxel than sirolimus on inhibiting intimal hyperplasia might explain that. When compared to bare-metal stent group, patients treated with PES had 50% less in-stent restenosis length (15.3 mm vs. 9.7 mm ; $P = 0.01$).[8]

The 12-month target lesion revascularization rates identified in the TAXUS IV series were bare stent use, lesion length, female sex, and no prior MI.[8]

Treatment

As DES implantation has become the current gold-standard technique. The issue of in-stent drug-eluting stent restenosis will become progressively more significant, although to a much lesser extent than for bare-metal stent technology.

The first report of treatment of DES restenosis described an overall recurrent restenosis rate of 43%, with a recurrent restenosis rate in *de novo* lesions of 18.2%. The risk was increased for patients with previous PCI, failed brachytherapy, early failure post-DES (less than 6 months), and post-SES restenosis treated only with balloon dilatation.[31]

A definitive recommendation for its treatment is still under discussion, whether with the same eluting stent, a different one, or with different doses.

The current recommendations from our own practice are as follows:

1. in face of a DES restenosis it is important to identify the possible mechanism of the failure: incomplete expansion, heavily calcified vessel, or DES failure related to strut fracture or polymer damage, or in the absence of that, the sole presence of intimal hyperplasia
2. the use of IVUS is highly recommended, if feasible, in order to clarify the possible mechanism of the failure
3. if there is incomplete expansion related to very fibrotic lesions or severe focal points of calcification, it is still acceptable to try balloon dilatation at least one more time, only. If there is another very early severe recurrence (less than 3 months of follow-up), surgical revascularization might be indicated, if the amount of myocardium at risk justifies the decision for this procedure
4. as the majority of the drug-eluting in-stent restenosis is focal, the initial approach is to use balloon dilatation
5. edge restenosis, mainly of the proximal edge, and a more diffuse pattern, will usually require implantation of another DES. Evidence for selecting one type of DES over another is scarce. The trend is toward SES selection in relation to its potency of inhibition of intimal hyperplasia, but this is still anecdotal. Our preference is for SES
6. refractory cases after a second DES implantation will require a definite solution, and, at present, surgical revascularization is considered necessary. Fortunately, this occurs in a very low number of patients. The final decision should be made on an individual, case-by-case and is a matter for discussion between the patient and interventionalist
7. refractory cases after a second DES implantation will require a definite solution, and, at present, surgical revascularization is considered necessary. Fortunately, this occurs in a very low number of patients
8. more data will be necessary to clarify this issue. However, as the restenosis rate has been decreased by 75% on average with DES, candidates for RCTs will be scarce.

REFERENCES

1. Grüentzig, AR, Senning A, Siegenthaler WE. Nonoperative dilatation of coronary-artery stenosis: percutaneous transluminal coronary angioplasty. N Engl J Med 1979; 301: 61–8.
2. Topol EJ, Serruys PW. Frontiers in interventional cardiology. [Editorial]. Circulation 1998; 98: 1802–20.
3. Colombo A, Hall P, Nakamura S et al. Intracoronary stenting without anticoagulation accomplished with intravascular ultrasound guidance. Circulation 1995; 91: 1676–88.
4. Sousa JE, Costa MA, Abizaid A et al. Lack of neointimal proliferation alter implantation of sirolimus-coated stents in human coronary arteries: a quantitative coronary angiography and three-dimensional intravascular ultrasound study. Circulation 2001; 103: 192–5.
5. Wessely R, Schomig A, Kastrati A. Sirolimus and paclitaxel on polymer-based drug-eluting stents: similar but different. J Am Coll Cardiol 2006; 37: 708–14.

6. Marx SO and Marks AR. The development of rapamycin and its application to stent restenosis. Circulation 2001; 104: 852–5.
7. Moses JW, Leon MB, Popma JJ et al. Sirolimus-eluting stents versus standard stents in patients with stenosis in a native coronary artery. N Engl J Med 2003; 349: 1315–23.
8. Stone GW, Ellis SG, Cox DA et al. A polymer-based, paclitaxel-eluting stent in patients with coronary artery disease. N Engl J Med 2004; 350: 221–31.
9. Ong ATL, van Domburg RT, Aoki J et al. Sirolimus-eluting stents remain superior to bare-metal stents at two years. Medium-term results from the Rapamycin-Eluting Stent Evaluated at Rotterdam Cardiology Hospital (RESEARCH) Registry. J Am Coll Cardiol 2006; 47: 1356–60.
10. Ong ATL, McFadden EP, Regar E et al. Late angiographic stent thrombosis (LAST) events with drug-eluting stents. J Am Coll Cardiol 2005; 45: 2088–92.
11. Ong AT, Hoye A, Aoki J et al. Thirty-day incidence and six-month clinical outcome of thrombotic stent occlusion following bare metal, sirolimus, or paclitaxel stent implantation. J Am Coll Cardiol 2005; 45: 947–53.
12. McFadden EP, Stabile E, Regar E et al. Late thrombosis in drug-eluting stents after discontinuation of antiplatelet therapy. Lancet 2004; 364: 1519–21.
13. Ong ATL, Serruys PW, Aoki J et al. The unrestricted use of paclitaxel-versus sirolimus-eluting stents for coronary artery disease in an unselected population. One-year results of the Taxus-Stent Evaluated at Rotterdam Cardiology Hospital (T-Search) Registry. J Am Coll Cardiol 2005; 45: 1135–41.
14. Cutlip DE, Baim DS, Ho KKL et al. Stent thrombosis in the modern era. A pooled analysis of multicenter coronary stent clinical trials. Circulation 2001; 103: 1967–71.
15. Babapulle MN, Joseph L, Bélisle P, Brophy JM, Eisenberg MJ. A hierarchical Bayesian meta-analysis of randomized clinical trials of drug-eluting stents. Lancet 2004; 364: 583–91.
16. Rodriguez AE, Mieres J, Fernandez-Pereira C et al. Coronary stent thrombosis in current drug-eluting stent era: insights from ERACI III trial. J Am Coll Cardiol 2006; 47: 205–7.
17. Weisz G, Leon MB, Holmes DR et al. Two-year outcomes after sirolimus eluting stent implantation. Results from the Sirolimus-Eluting Stent in de Novo Native Coronary Lesions (SIRIUS) Trial. J Am Coll Cardiol 2006; 47: 1350–5.
18. Stone GW. TAXUS IV: 2 year follow-up. Presented at the Transcatheter Cardiovascular Therapeutics, Washington DC, USA, 17 October 2005.
19. Moreno R, Fernandez C, Hernandez R et al. Drug-eluting stent thrombosis. Results from a pooled analysis including 10 randomized studies. J Am Coll Cardiol 2005; 45: 954–9.
20. Iakovou I, Schimidt T, Bonizzoni E et al. Incidence, predictors, and outcome of thrombosis after succesful implantation of drug-eluting stents. JAMA 2005; 293: 2126–30.
21. Kuchulakanti PK, Chu WW, Torguson R et al. Correlates and long-term outcomes of angiographically proven stent thrombosis with sirolimus- and paclitaxel-eluting stents. Circulation 2006; 113: 1108–13.
22. Pfisterer ME. Basel Stent Kosten Effektivitats Trial (BASKET). Presented at the American College of Cardiology 55th Annual Scientific Sessions, Atlanta GA, USA, 14 March 2006.
23. Kotani J, Awata M, Nanto S et al. Incomplete neointimal coverage of sirolimus-eluting stents: angioscopic findings. J Am Coll Cardiol 2006; 16: 2108–11.
24. Fugii K, Carlier S, Mintz G et al. Stent underexpansion and residual reference segment stenosis are related to stent thrombosis after sirolimus-eluting stent implantation. J Am Coll Cardiol 2005; 45: 995–8.
25. Nebeker JR, Virmani R, Bennett CL et al. Hypersensitivity cases associated with drug-eluting coronary stents. A review of available cases from the Research on Adverse Events and Reports (RADAR) Project. J Am Coll Cardiol 2006; 47: 175–81.
26. De Luca G, Suryapranata H, Stone GW et al. Abciximab as adjunctive therapy to reperfusion in acute ST-segment elevation myocardial infarction. A meta-analysis of randomized trials. JAMA 2005; 293: 1759–65.
27. Dawkins KD, Grube E, Guagliumi G, Banning AP et al. Clinical efficacy of polymer-based paclitaxel-eluting stents in the treatment of complex, long coronary artery lesions from a multicenter, randomized trial. Circulation 2005; 112: 3306–13.

28. Schluter M, Schofer J. The SIRIUS, E-SIRIUS, and C-SIRIUS trials. In: Serruys PW, Gershlick AH, eds. Handbook of Drug-Eluting Stents. London: Taylor and Francis; 2005: 121–32.
29. Lemos PA, Hoye A, Goedhart D et al. Clinical, angiographic, and procedural predictors of angiographic restenosis alter sirolimus-eluting stent implantation in complex patients. An evaluation from the rapamycin-eluting stent evaluated at Rotterdam Cardiology Hospital (RESEARCH) study. Circulation 2004; 109: 1366–70.
30. Colombo A, Drzewiecki J, Banning A et al. Randomized study to assess the effectiveness of slow- and moderate-release polymer-based paclitaxel-eluting stent for coronary artery lesions. Circulation 2003; 108: 788–94.
31. Lemos PA, van Mieghem CAG, Arampatzis CA et al. Post-sirolimus-eluting stent restenosis treated with repeat percutaneous intervention late angiographic and clinical outcomes. Circulation 2004; 109: 2500–2.

26

Coronary interventions in patients with antiplatelet therapy resistance

Dominick J Angiolillo and Marco A Costa

The degree and duration of platelet inhibition using glycoprotein IIb/IIIa receptor antagonists during percutaneous coronary intervention: clinical implications • Resistance to oral antiplatelet agents: aspirin, clopidogrel, or both • Management of patients with antiplatelet drug resistance undergoing percutaneous coronary intervention • Future directions • Conclusions

Platelets play a key role in the pathophysiology of thrombosis after plaque rupture.[1] Plaque rupture may occur spontaneously, as in patients with acute coronary syndromes (ACS), or may be iatrogenically induced, as in patients undergoing percutaneous coronary interventions (PCI). Antiplatelet therapy is therefore a cornerstone of treatment in these scenarios. Three classes of platelet-inhibiting drugs, aspirin, thienopyridines, and platelet glycoprotein (GP) IIb/IIIa inhibitors are most commonly used for the prevention and treatment of ischemic complications associated with plaque rupture. Given the pivotal role of platelets on the adverse events associated with plaque rupture, all these antiplatelet agents have proved to be clinically effective. Nevertheless, despite their efficacy, patients on these medications may continue to suffer from ischemic complications. This may be, at least in part, attributed to the fact that responsiveness to antiplatelet agents is not uniform in all patients. In particular, there is a growing degree of evidence showing that suboptimal responsiveness or 'resistance' to antiplatelet medications may contribute to adverse outcomes. Although the mechanisms of antiplatelet drug resistance remain to be established, there is increasing data to suggest that monitoring and tailoring antiplatelet therapy in the individual patient may help optimize clinical outcomes. In the present chapter we describe the impact of individual response variability to antiplatelet agents on clinical outcomes in patients undergoing PCI, and current and future directions for the treatment of patients with suboptimal responsiveness to antiplatelet agents.

THE DEGREE AND DURATION OF PLATELET INHIBITION USING GLYCOPROTEIN IIB/IIIA RECEPTOR ANTAGONISTS DURING PERCUTANEOUS CORONARY INTERVENTION: CLINICAL IMPLICATIONS

The initial evidence underscoring the importance of the degree of platelet inhibition on clinical events in patients undergoing PCI comes from pivotal GP IIb/IIIa receptor antagonist studies. The goal with abciximab treatment for PCI is to achieve and sustain a threshold of receptor blockade $\geq 80\%$.[2] In the Evaluation of IIb/IIIa platelet receptor antagonist 7E3 in Preventing Ischemic Complications (EPIC) study, patients receiving only a bolus of abciximab appeared to be fully protected from the need for urgent repeated interventions for a 4–6 h period, during which time it was likely that GP IIb/IIIa receptor blockade was $\geq 80\%$.[3] In contrast, patients in the placebo group showed no protection in the first 4–6 h, and patients receiving the bolus and 12-h infusion were protected for nearly the entire time of the infusion. Therefore, the EPIC study was the first to demonstrate the relevance of the degree of platelet blockade on outcomes, where the best outcomes were observed in patients with sustained platelet inhibtion.

Although standard dosing of GP IIb/IIIa receptor antagonists achieve $\geq 80\%$ platelet inhibition in most patients, interindividual variations in receptor blockade may occur even with this potent platelet inhibitor, and some patients may even have suboptimal platelet inhibition.[2] Variations in platelet count, density of GP IIb/IIIa receptors, intrinsic platelet functional competence, plasma levels of platelet cofactors, and other unknown factors may affect the functional response to given plasma levels of a GP IIb/IIIa antagonist, and thus lead to interindividual variation in responsiveness. The clinical impact of individual response variability was assessed in the GOLD study.[4] In this study, the level of platelet inhibition as measured by a point-of-care assay was shown to be an independent predictor for the risk of major adverse cardiac events in a cohort of 500 patients undergoing a PCI with the planned use of a GP IIb/IIIa inhibitor. In particular, one-quarter of all patients did not achieve $\geq 95\%$ inhibition 10 min after the bolus of abciximab, and experienced a significantly higher incidence of major adverse cardiac events (14.4% vs. 6.4%, $P = 0.006$). Patients whose platelet function was $< 70\%$ inhibited at 8 h after the start of therapy also had a higher event rate (25% vs. 8.1%, $P = 0.009$). By multivariate analysis, platelet function inhibition $\geq 95\%$ at 10 min after the start of therapy was associated with a significant decrease in the incidence of a major adverse cardiac events (odds ratio (OR) 0.46; 95% confidence interval (CI) 0.22–0.96; $P = 0.04$).

A clinical benefit of tirofiban, a non-peptidyl tyrosine derivative that produces a dose-dependent inhibition of GP IIb/IIIa-mediated platelet aggregation, has been documented in patients with unstable angina undergoing PCI. In the PRISM-PLUS (Platelet Receptor Inhibition in Ischemic Syndrome Management in Patients Limited by Unstable Signs and Symptoms) trial, the composite endpoint of death, myocardial infarction (MI), or refractory ischemia was significantly reduced in the heparin/ tirofiban group compared to the heparin alone group (10.0% vs. 15.7%; $P = 0.01$).[5] However, in the TARGET (Do Tirofiban and ReoPro Give Similar Efficacy Trial) study, in which abciximab was compared with tirofiban (used at the same dose as in PRISM-PLUS) in patients undergoing urgent and elective coronary revascularization, tirofiban offered lower protection from major ischemic events than abciximab.[6] There was a hypothesis that these results were attributed to the inadequate loading dose of tirofiban, leading to insufficient platelet inhibition during coronary intervention. When different antiplatelet regimens were compared in the COMPARE (Randomized COMparison of platelet inhibition with abciximab, tiRofiban and eptifibatide during percutaneous coronary intervention in acute coronary syndromes) trial, platelet aggregation at 15 and 30 min after drug administration was significantly less inhibited with tirofiban than after either abciximab, or eptifibatide.[7] On the other hand, increasing the bolus of tirofiban from 10 to 25 µg/kg has been proven to be safe and effective in the ADVANCE (additive value of tirofiban administered with the high-dose bolus in the prevention of ischemic complications during high-risk coronary angioplasty) trial.[8] Overall, these findings highlight the importance of achieving specific therapeutic targets when using antiplatelet medication. Dose adjustments, according to individuals' platelet function profile, measured by dedicated assays may be useful to reach therapeutic goals, reducing suboptimal responders, and improving the efficacy of antiplatelet treatment.

RESISTANCE TO ORAL ANTIPLATELET AGENTS: ASPIRIN, CLOPIDOGREL, OR BOTH

Aspirin resistance

Clinical trials have shown the efficacy of aspirin in both the primary and secondary prevention of MI, stroke, and cardiovascular death. The Antithrombotic Trialists' Collaboration found an approximately 25% reduction in stroke, MI, or cardiovascular death.[9] The ISIS-2 (Second International Study of Infarct Survival) trial demonstrated that acute aspirin use reduced mortality by 23% in acute ST elevation myocardial infarction (STEMI).[10] Aspirin was shown to be equally efficacious as thrombolytic therapy while having an additive benefit when used in conjunction with streptokinase. The antithrombotic effect of aspirin is mediated by the irreversible acetylation of platelet cyclooxygenase 1 (COX 1), and the subsequent inhibition of thromboxane A_2 synthesis, a potent agonist of platelet aggregation.[11] However, the antiplatelet effects of aspirin are not uniform in all patients, and its inhibition of platelet function is subject to interindividual and intra-individual variability.[12] This has led to the concept of aspirin 'resistance' or 'non-responsiveness', which refers to the subset of patients taking aspirin who do not have adequate inhibition of COX 1 as measured by platelet function assays or urinary 11-dehydrothromboxane B_2 levels.[13]

Interindividual variable response to aspirin is multifactorial, and can be attributed to clinical, cellular, and genetic factors.[14] In its broadest sense, the term 'resistance' refers to the continued occurrence of ischemic events despite adequate antiplatelet therapy and compliance.[13] There is emerging evidence showing the association between aspirin resistance and risk of major adverse cardiovascular events. However, currently there is no standard assay to measure platelet function, and methods range from the use of urinary 11-dehydrothromboxane B_2 levels to light transmittance aggregometry.[13] For this reason the incidence of aspirin non-responsiveness varies according to the assay chosen, and has been reported to range from 5% to 60%.[13,14] The lack of a standard definition of resistance, as well as the lack of a standard diagnostic modality has hampered the field in identifying and treating this clinical entity.

Using a variety of definitions of aspirin resistance, five studies in patients with coronary, peripheral, and/or cerebrovascular disease have reported 1.8–10-fold increased risk of thrombotic events.[15-19] The point-of-care determination of aspirin non-responsiveness appears to have important clinical implications in the PCI setting, with a significant increased risk of periprocedural MI in aspirin non-responsive compared to aspirin-sensitive patients.[20] This was evaluated by Chen et al in 151 patients pretreated with 300 mg of clopidogrel >12 h prior to PCI, and 75 mg the morning of the PCI.[20] Twenty-nine patients (19.2%) were found to be aspirin resistant. The incidence of any creatine kinase-MB (CK-MB) elevation was 51.7% versus 24.6% in the aspirin-resistant and aspirin-sensitive groups, respectively ($P = 0.006$). Notably, this occurred despite clopidogrel pretreatment. Elevation of troponin I (TnI) occurred in 65.5% of aspirin-resistant patients and 38.5% of aspirin-sensitive patients ($P = 0.012$). Variables associated with CK-MB elevation by univariate analysis were aspirin resistance ($P = 0.006$), bifurcation lesion ($P = 0.035$), B2/C lesion ($P = 0.029$), and number of stents used ($P = 0.04$). Multivariate analysis revealed aspirin resistance (OR 2.9; 95%

CI 1.2–6.9; $P = 0.015$) and bifurcation lesion (OR 2.8; 95% CI 1.3–6.0; $P = 0.007$) to be independent predictors of CK-MB elevation after PCI.

Clopidogrel resistance

Clopidogrel, a thienopyridine derivative similar to ticlopidine, is an inhibitor of platelet aggregation induced by ADP.[21] Abundant data from a number of studies have proven that clopidogrel is not only safer and more tolerable than ticlopidine, but also at least as efficacious following coronary stenting.[22] In addition, compared to ticlopidine, clopidogrel has the enormous advantage of being able to be administered as a loading dose, allowing antiplatelet effects to be achieved within hours following administration.[23] This has important clinical implications considering that stent thrombosis most commonly occurs within the first 24–48 h following PCI. Pooled data suggest similar rates of stent thrombosis and lower rates of major adverse cardiac events with clopidogrel, with a clear advantage for clopidogrel regarding undesired adverse events.[24] In addition, long-term dual antiplatelet therapy with clopidogrel and aspirin is more effective than aspirin alone in preventing major cardiovascular events in patients with ACS, including those treated with PCI.[25-27]

Treatment with clopidogrel is associated with a broad variability in antiplatelet effects.[28-31] This may be in part attributed to the levels of clopidogrel's active metabolite.[32] Clopidogrel in fact is an inactive prodrug, which requires oxidation by the hepatic cytochrome P450 3A4 (CYP3A4) to generate an active metabolite.[21] The active metabolite of clopidogrel inhibits platelet activation through an irreversible blockage of the platelet ADP $P2Y_{12}$ receptor. The $P2Y_{12}$ receptor inhibits adenylyl cyclase, and in turn decreases platelet cyclic adenosine monophosphate (cAMP) levels and cAMP-mediated phosphorylation of the vasodilator-stimulated phosphoprotein (VASP), critical for inhibition of GP IIb/IIIa receptor activation. Drugs which are substrates or inhibit CYP3A4 can potentially interfere with the conversion of clopidogrel into its active metabolite.[33]

Clopidogrel resistance, a concept related to aspirin resistance, has also been described.[34] Possible mechanistic explanations include increased platelet reactivity before clopidogrel dosing, drug–drug interactions inhibiting clopidogrel activation by CYP3A4, genetic polymorphisms, or defects in signaling pathways downstream from the receptor.[34] In a recent study, Lau and coworkers demonstrated that low baseline CYP3A4 activity, which decreases clopidogrel activation, is one mechanism for clopidogrel resistance, at least during the first days of treatment.[35] The metabolic activity of the CYP3A4 enzyme, which varies considerably among individuals, is under genetic control, and genetic polymorphisms of this enzyme have been shown to modulate individual responsiveness to clopidogrel.[36] Although a minor haplotype of the $P2Y_{12}$ receptor was found to be associated with increased platelet reactivity in non-medicated healthy volunteers,[37] these findings could not be duplicated by several authors studying patients with coronary artery disease treated with clopidogrel.[38,39] We recently demonstrated the lack of association between genetic polymorphisms of the GP IIb/IIIa and $P2Y_{12}$ receptors and platelet reactivity in patients on chronic clopidogrel therapy.[39] These findings are probably related to the fact that an active metabolite and not clopidogrel *per se*, is responsible for inhibition of the $P2Y_{12}$ receptor, suggesting therefore that an upstream target within clopidogrel's metabolic pathway has a more important modulating role of its downstream antiplatelet effects. Similarly to aspirin, clinical factors, such as compliance, increased body mass index, diabetes mellitus, in particular insulin-dependent diabetes mellitus, and acute coronary syndromes may all be implied in suboptimal responsiveness to clopidogrel therapy.[40–43]

The prevalence of clopidogrel non-response in patients is evaluated between 4% and 30% 24 h after administration.[34] The reported rates vary between studies because of the technique used to measure the extent of platelet aggregation and the presence of factors contributing to greater baseline platelet reactivity. Furthermore, the definition of non-responders is not standardized. The first study to hypothesize the clinical implications of clopidogrel responsiveness was reported by Muller et al, in which in a cohort of 105 patients undergoing PCI, two incidents of subacute stent thrombosis occurred and both patients were clopidogrel non-responders.[44] Barragan et al. carried out a prospective evaluation using a VASP assay, which is highly specific for the $P2Y_{12}$ pathway, in order to detect patients at high risk for subacute stent thrombosis, and patients experiencing subacute stent thrombosis had significantly enhanced platelet reactivity.[45] Recent data suggest that clopidogrel resistance is associated with increased risk of recurrent atherothrombotic events in patients with STEMI undergoing primary PCI. In a study from Matetzky et al, patients were stratified into four quartiles according to the percentage reduction of ADP-induced platelet aggregation.[46] Whereas 40% of patients in the first quartile sustained a recurrent cardiovascular event (STEMI, ACS, subacute stent thrombosis, and acute peripheral arterial occlusion) during 6-month follow-up, only one patient (6.7%) in the second quartile, and none in the third and fourth quartiles suffered a cardiovascular event ($P = 0.007$).

Combined aspirin and clopidogrel resistance

There are limited data on the simultaneous responses to both aspirin and clopidogrel. *In vitro* studies from our group have shown that patients with resistance to both aspirin and clopidogrel are characterized by markedly enhanced platelet function profiles.[47] Lev et al evaluated the response to clopidogrel among aspirin-resistant versus aspirin-sensitive patients undergoing elective PCI.[48] Patients ($n = 150$) treated with aspirin but not clopidogrel had blood samples drawn at baseline and 24 h after a 300 mg clopidogrel loading dose. Depending on the definition used, 9–15% were resistant to aspirin, and 24% to clopidogrel; ~50% of the aspirin-resistant patients were also resistant to clopidogrel. Overall, aspirin-resistant patients had lower response to clopidogrel than aspirin-sensitive patients. Elevation of CK-MB after stenting occurred more frequently in aspirin-resistant versus aspirin-sensitive patients (38.9% vs. 18.3%; $P = 0.04$) and in clopidogrel-resistant than clopidogrel-sensitive patients (32.4% vs. 17.3%; $P = 0.06$). Patients with dual drug resistance had higher incidence of CK-MB elevation than the respective sensitive patients (44.4% vs. 15.8%; $P = 0.05$).

MANAGEMENT OF PATIENTS WITH ANTIPLATELET DRUG RESISTANCE UNDERGOING PERCUTANEOUS CORONARY INTERVENTION

Aspirin and clopidogrel resistance are emerging clinical entities, with potentially severe consequences such as recurrent MI, stroke, or death. Given the clinical consequences of therapeutic failure, the problem thus becomes one of how a clinician can effectively treat resistance to antiplatelet agents. Unfortunately, the treatment for antiplatelet drug resistance is as yet undefined. An initial approach would be to correct the clinical factors that may cause resistance. Importantly, physicians must ensure proper patient compliance. Decreasing drug–drug interactions, and optimizing control of cholesterol and glucose levels can improve responsiveness to antiplatelet agents.

Management of aspirin resistance

Increasing the dose of aspirin has been suggested as a measure to overcome aspirin resistance. However, although it is possible that increased doses of aspirin may overcome aspirin resistance *in vitro* in an individual patient, currently, there is a lack of evidence demonstrating improvement in clinical outcomes through this strategy.[9] Importantly, data from clinical trials specify an increased risk of serious bleeding associated with high aspirin doses.[49,50] The CAPRIE (Clopidogrel versus Aspirin in Patients at Risk of Ischemic Events) study revealed modest, but significant, superiority of clopidogrel monotherapy over aspirin monotherapy.[51] Such benefit was increased in a high-risk subset of patients. Notably, aspirin resistance is more common in high-risk patients, such as patients with diabetes, diffuse atherosclerotic disease, or ACS, who are also those with a higher risk of developing future ischemic events.[14] Whether clopidogrel therapy is superior to aspirin in aspirin-resistant patients is currently unknown. The ASCET (ASpirin non-responsiveness and Clopidogrel Endpoint Trial) trial, currently ongoing in Scandinavia, will recruit stable patients with angiographically documented coronary artery disease to evaluate whether switching to clopidogrel will be superior to continued aspirin therapy in improving clinical outcomes among patients with aspirin resistance (measured using the PFA-100 system).

The ISAR-REACT (Intracoronary Stenting and Antithrombotic Regimen: Rapid Early Action for Coronary Treatment) trial has shown that abciximab did not reduce the incidence of ischemic complications in low-to-intermediate risk patients undergoing elective PCI after pretreatment with aspirin and a 600 mg clopidogrel loading dose.[52] Furthermore, those receiving aspirin and clopidogrel without abciximab were less likely than those receiving all three agents to have thrombocytopenia and to require transfusions. These data suggest that in patients at low-to-intermediate risk who undergo elective PCI after pretreatment with a high loading dose of clopidogrel, the use of a GP IIb/IIIa inhibitor, although more potent, is associated with no clinically measurable benefit within the first 30 days. In contrast, high-risk patients should receive triple antiplatelet therapy. Yet, the study by Chen et al suggests that aspirin and clopidogrel may be insufficient in aspirin non-responsive patients.[20] Therefore, this study in low- to medium-risk patients nearly identical to ISAR-REACT addresses an important gap area by further defining optimal antiplatelet treatments in up to 25% of patients undergoing PCI who are aspirin non-responsive, but currently treated with aspirin, clopidogrel, and heparin alone by the majority of interventional cardiologists. The ongoing Research Evaluation to Study Individuals who Show Thromboxane Or P2Y12 Receptor Resistance (RESISTOR) trial will investigate the use of clopidogrel in addition to aspirin prior to elective angioplasty. The trial will utilize a point-of-care assay (VerifyNow Rapid Platelet Function Analyzer) to identify patients as responders or non-responders, and then randomize patients to the intravenous GP IIb/IIIa inhibitor eptifibatide plus unfractionated heparin, or unfractionated heparin alone, and determine the impact on myonecrosis (CK-MB ≥ 2 times upper normal limit (UNL)) 24 h post-PCI.

Management of clopidogrel resistance

The CURE (Clopidogrel in Unstable angina to prevent Recurrent ischemic Events) and CREDO (Clopidogrel for the Reduction of Events During Observation) trials demonstrated the additive clinical benefit of clopidogrel to aspirin.[25-27] Such clinical benefit may be, at least in part, attributed to the presence of a considerable number of patients with suboptimal responsiveness to aspirin. Therefore, these patients may benefit from the addition of an antiplatelet agent which antagonizes one of the mechanisms contributing to the aspirin resistance phenomenon, which are increased exposure and/or sensitivity to ADP.[53] Nevertheless, *in vitro* studies have shown that in aspirin-resistant patients the addition of clopidogrel to aspirin does not overcome the aspirin resistance phenomenon, and these patients continue to have increased platelet reactivity.[54] Excessive formation of thrombin on the platelet surface may also contribute to the aspirin resistance phenomenon. It has been suggested that dipyridamole may be capable of overcoming increased prothrombinase complex formation and be in part able to compensate for aspirin resistance in patients with moderate carotid stenosis.[55] This phenomenon may explain the clinical advantages of combined therapy with aspirin and dipyridamole, known to reduce ischemic events in post-stroke patients as proven in clinical trials.[55] Overall, these findings support the presence of multifactorial mechanisms leading to individual response variability to antiplatelet agents.

Prospective clinical studies are also warranted to assess if the addition of clopidogrel to aspirin in aspirin-resistant patients will lead to improved clinical outcomes. Results from a substudy of the CHARISMA (Clopidogrel for High Atherothrombotic Risk and Ischemic Stabilization, Management, and Avoidance) trial, assessing whether clopidogrel added to aspirin attenuates the clinical risk associated with aspirin resistance (detected by measures of urinary 11-dehydro thromboxane B_2 levels) are pending.[56] Further, genetic analysis aimed to identify specific single nucleotide polymorphisms associated with antiplatelet drug responsiveness are currently ongoing, and will help to identify subjects who may benefit from specific drug regimens.

Several studies have focused on the impact of the dose of clopidogrel utilized in patients undergoing PCI, on drug responsiveness. Clopidogrel is currently the thienopyridine of choice used, in combination with aspirin, to prevent stent thrombosis. Clopidogrel is associated with higher platelet inhibition, lower adverse events after intervention, and a better safety profile as compared with ticlopidine.[22-24] Compared to ticlopidine, clopidogrel presents the advantage of being able to achieve rapid platelet inhibition which is achieved through the administration of a loading dose. A 300 mg loading dose of clopidogrel has been considered as the standard loading-dose regimen to be given in patients undergoing PCI. However, several functional studies have shown that a higher loading dose with 600 mg of clopidogrel causes an earlier and stronger inhibition of platelet function than does the 300 mg loading regimen.[29] A high-loading-dose regimen may prevent the reduction of platelet inhibition by concomitant use of statins metabolized by CYP3A4.[57] Furthermore, a high-loading-dose regimen of clopidogrel may reduce the rate of non-responders from ~30% after conventional dose to ~10% after a 600 mg loading dose.[29] The ARMYDA-2 (Antiplatelet therapy for Reduction of MYocardial Damage during Angioplasty) study showed the benefit of 600 mg of clopidogrel when compared with 300 mg of clopidogrel as pretreatment in reducing peri-procedural MI in patients undergoing PCI.[58] The utility of increasing the loading dose of clopidogrel to 900 mg has been recently evaluated in the ALBION (Assessment of the Best Loading Dose of Clopidogrel to Blunt Platelet Activation, Inflammation, and Ongoing Necrosis) trial and the ISAR-CHOICE (Stenting and Antithrombotic Regimen: Choose Between 3 High Oral Doses for Immediate Clopidogrel Effect) trials. Although a high-loading-dose regimen (600 and 900 mg) showed a greater and faster degree of platelet inhibition compared with a 300 mg loading dose of clopidogrel, the differences observed between a 600 and 900 mg loading-does-regimen were less remarkable.[59,60]

Recently, it was shown that administration of a 600 mg loading dose in patients already on chronic clopidogrel therapy results in an additional significant increase in inhibition of ADP-induced platelet aggregation, suggesting that the current recommended maintenance dose of clopidogrel may be insufficient in producing optimal platelet inhibition.[61] The currently used maintenance dose for chronic clopidogrel therapy (75 mg/day) was chosen because a degree of platelet inhibition is reached similar to that achieved with 500 mg ticlopidine per day. Therefore, it has been suggested that increasing the clopidogrel maintenance dose to 150 mg/day may improve individual responsiveness. Ongoing randomized studies are currently evaluating not only the impact of a high-clopidogrel maintenance regimen (150 mg) on individual responsiveness immediately after PCI, but also in clopidogrel low-responders already on chronic treatment. Specific emphasis is given to high risk patients (e.g. diabetes) more likely to have suboptimal responsiveness to standard drug regimens.

FUTURE DIRECTIONS

Beyond the use of aspirin and clopidogrel, with or without a GP IIb/IIIa receptor inhibitor, the options for medical therapy in patients with antiplatelet drug resistance remain limited. Novel $P2Y_{12}$ receptor antagonists with more potent antiplatelet effects are currently under clinical investigation. These novel molecules are all characterized by more potent antiplatelet effects, and therefore less likely to lead to resistance. Novel $P2Y_{12}$ receptor antagonists include prasugrel, AZD6140 and cangrelor. Prasugrel (CS-747) is a member of the thienopyridine class of oral platelet aggregation inhibitors. Like ticlopidine and clopidogrel, prasugrel (a third-generation thienopyridine) is a prodrug, and needs to be transformed in the liver into an active metabolite. The active metabolite of prasugrel, like the active metabolite of clopidogrel, leads to selective and irreversible blockade of the $P2Y_{12}$ receptor.[62] A single oral administration of prasugrel produces a dose-related inhibition of platelet aggregation in rats approximately 10- and 100-fold more potent than that of clopidogrel and ticlopidine, respectively. The anti-aggregatory effects of prasugrel are evident at 30 min and last until 72 h after dosing, indicating fast onset and long duration of action. The results of the JUMBO (Joint Utilization of Medications to Block Platelets Optimally) TIMI-26 phase II trial showed that prasugrel has safety profiles (significant, non-coronary artery bypass graft (CABG), bleeding through 30 days – the primary endpoint of the study) comparable to standard dose clopidogrel in patients ($n = 900$) undergoing PCI.[63] Clinical outcomes (secondary endpoint) in this trial were also similar with the use of either thienopyridine. The ongoing TRITON (Trial to Assess Improvement in Therapeutic Outcomes by Optimizing Platelet Inhibition With Prasugrel) TIMI-38 phase II trial will compare prasugrel and clopidogrel in over 13 000 patients with ACS undergoing PCI, with the primary endpoint of death, MI, and stroke at 12 months.

AZD6140 is a non-thienopyridine, and belongs to a new chemical class called cyclopentyl-triazolo-pyrimidine.[64] It is the first oral reversible ADP receptor antagonist. It does not require hepatic metabolism for its activity, and directly inhibits the $P2Y_{12}$ receptor. Platelet aggregation studies have shown that AZD6140 blocks platelet reactivity more consistently and completely than clopidogrel, with a lower degree of interindividual response variability. A phase II trial (DISPERSE II [Safety, Tolerability and Preliminary Efficacy of AZD6140, the First Oral Reversible ADP Receptor Antagonist, Compared with Clopidogrel in Patients with Non–ST Segment Elevation Acute Coronary Syndrome]) comparing AZD6140 to clopidogrel patients ($n = 990$) with ACS has recently finished enrolment. Results showed similar rates of bleeding in all groups (primary endpoint: total major/minor bleeding events at 4 weeks), and no significant difference in the composite endpoint of cardiovascular death, stroke, or recurrent ischemia.[65] A large-scale phase III clinical trial (PLATO [Study of Platelet Inhibition and Patient Outcomes]) will compare AZD6140 and clopidogrel in patients with ACS undergoing PCI with the primary endpoint of death, MI, and stroke at 12 months.

Cangrelor (also known as AR-C69931MX) is also a selective and competitive $P2Y_{12}$ antagonist, which is suitable for intravenous administration.[64] Cangrelor is an ATP analogue, with more potent antiplatelet activity than clopidogrel (90% inhibition of platelet aggregation at 1–4 µg/kg/min IV), and leads to selective inhibition of ADP-induced aggregation in a dose-dependent manner. Importantly, there is a rapid reversal of its dose-dependent effects. Reports proceeding from phase II clinical trials show that cangrelor in addition to tissue plasminogen activator (tPA) in patients with STEMI is associated with a greater degree of ST segment recovery in a dose-dependent manner.[66] Further, in patients undergoing PCI, cangrelor compares favorably with abciximab, both from a safety and clinical standpoint. A phase III trial with cangrelor (CHAMPION) is currently ongoing.

These novel ADP receptor antagonists may have advantages over currently available antiplatelet agents, which are probably related to the increased degree of platelet inhibition. Increased platelet reactivity, in fact, is an important predictor of ischemic events. However, increased platelet inhibition does not necessarily translate into better safety profiles, as more-potent antiplatelet agents may increase hemorrhagic risk. Results from phase III clinical trials will provide more definitive answers. Preclinical investigation of other ADP receptor antagonist such as INS-50589 (a dinucleotide intended for intravenous administration), and CT-50547 (a benzothiazolothiadiazine intended for oral administration) are also ongoing, and will further nurture this evolving field of research with the goal of identifying the optimal treatment of patients with atherothrombotic disease undergoing PCI.

Although, novel and more-potent P2Y12 receptor antagonists are being developed, it is likely that interindividual and intra-individual variability in responsiveness to antiplatelet agents will still persist. This is related to the multitude of stimuli to which to platelets continues to be exposed (Figure 26.1). In some individuals, alternative stimuli (i.e thrombin) may be particularly enhanced. This may explain why even with high loading doses of clopidogrel, although responsiveness may improve, a broad variability in platelet function profiles still persists.[29] Therefore, in line with this observation it is perhaps most correct not to characterize patients as simply resistant or sensitive to a medication, but to consider resistance/responsiveness as a continuous variable (Figure 26.2). In fact, as illustrated in Figure 26.2, a broad degree of responsiveness can be identified in a patient population equally treated, in which platelet reactivity may be markedly increased in some individuals (hyper-responders) and markedly reduced (hypo-responders) in others, enhancing their ischemic and hemorrhagic risk, respectively.

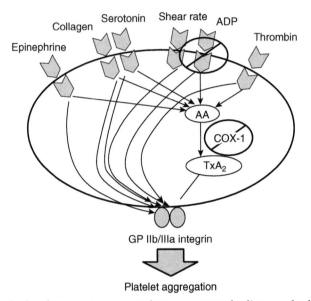

Figure 26.1 Platelets have numerous membrane receptors leading to platelet activation. Activation of the GP IIb/IIIa receptor represents the final common pathway leading to platelet aggregation. Even with inhibition of the cyclooxygenase 1 (COX-1) enzyme and ADP receptor with aspirin and clopidogrel, respectively, multiple other pathways remain unblocked. Therefore, variability in individual responsiveness to antiplatelet agents may depend on the presence of other pathways that lead to activation of the GP IIb/IIIa receptor. AA, arachidonic acid; TxA_2, thromboxane A_2.

In line with the contribution of not only cellular components (platelets) but also plasmatic components (thrombin) to thombotic events, Gurbel et al in the PREPARE-POST STENTING (Platelet reactivity in patients and recurrent events post-stenting) study investigated the relationship of high *ex vivo* platelet reactivity, rapid fibrin generation, and high thrombin-induced clot strength to post-discharge ischemic events in patients ($n = 192$) undergoing PCI.[67] Platelet reactivity to ADP by light transmittance aggregometry was measured. In addition, clot strength, a measure of thrombin-induced fibrin and platelet interactions, and the time to initial fibrin generation, a marker of thrombin activity, were measured by thrombelastography. The relationship of these measurements to ischemic event occurrence was prospectively examined over 6 months. Post-treatment ADP-induced aggregation ($63\pm12\%$ vs. $56\pm15\%$, $P = 0.02$) and clot strength were higher (74 ± 5 mm vs. 65 ± 4 mm, $P < 0.001$), and time to initial fibrin generation was shorter (4.3 ± 1.3 min vs. 5.9 ± 1.5 min, $P < 0.001$) in patients with events ($n = 38$). Cloth strength was most predictive of ischemic events. These findings may explain the occurrence of events despite treatment with COX 1 and P2Y12 inhibitors, suggesting the need to address thrombin inhibition during and after PCI.

CONCLUSIONS

Aspirin and clopidogrel resistance are emerging clinical entities. Although there is increasing evidence that monitoring and tailoring antiplatelet therapy in the individual patient may help optimize clinical outcomes, current clinical guidelines do not support routine screening for antiplatelet drug resistance. This is in part

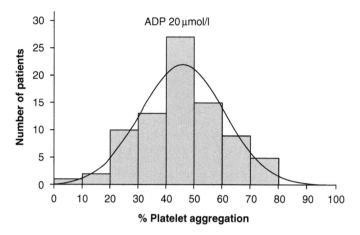

Figure 26.2   Platelet aggregation profile (20 μmol/l ADP-induced platelet aggregation using light transmittance aggregometry) in patients treated with aspirin (100 mg/day) plus clopidogrel (75 mg/day). Heterogeneous antiplatelet effects are observed in the overall patient population as depicted by the normal bell-shaped distribution of platelet aggregation. Patients with higher platelet aggregation (hyporesponsive) are at a higher risk of ischemic events, while those with lower platelet reactivity have an increased hemorrhagic (hyper-responsive) risk (data supplied by Angiolillo DJ et al, 2006).

because determination of the most appropriate screening test has not been established, and because of lack of clinical trials showing the impact on clinical outcomes of treatment modification in patients who are resistant to antiplatelet agents. Currently, many platelet function assays are expensive, time consuming, and not widely available. Therefore, rapid and accurate diagnosis of antiplatelet resistance also remains an issue. Widespread clinical application of antiplatelet resistance will require additional studies on larger populations that define antiplatelet resistance in a standardized manner using assays with consistency and reproducibility, that correlate the measurements with clinical outcomes, and that provide strategies for modifying antiplatelet regimens to improve outcome (e.g. increasing dose of antiplatelet agent, adding or substituting a second antiplatelet agent). Defining (a) the mechanisms leading to antiplatelet drug resistance; (b) the best diagnostic tool for its evaluation; and (c) therapeutic measures for its treatment will probably set the future basis for routine measurements of platelet function and a new era of individualized antithrombotic regimens similarly to that pursued to control other important prognostic variables such as blood pressure, cholesterol, and blood sugar levels.

REFERENCES

1. Fuster V, Stein B, Ambrose JA et al. Atherosclerotic plaque rupture and thrombosis. Evolving concepts. Circulation 1990; 82 (3 Suppl): II47–59.
2. Mascelli MA, Lance ET, Damaraju L et al. Pharmacodynamic profile of short-term abciximab treatment demonstrates prolonged platelet inhibition with gradual recovery from GP IIb/IIIa receptor blockade. Circulation 1998; 97: 1680–8.
3. Topol EJ, Califf RM, Weisman HF et al. Randomised trial of coronary intervention with antibody against platelet IIb/IIIa integrin for reduction of clinical restenosis: results at six months. The EPIC Investigators. Lancet 1994; 343: 881–6.

4. Steinhubl SR, Talley JD, Braden GA et al. Point-of-care measured platelet inhibition correlates with a reduced risk of an adverse cardiac event after percutaneous coronary intervention: results of the GOLD (AU-Assessing Ultegra) multicenter study. Circulation 2001; 103: 2572–8.

5. PRISM-PLUS Study Investigators. The platelet receptor inhibition in ischemic syndrome management in patients limited by unstable signs and symptoms. Inhibition of the platelet glycoprotein IIb/IIIa receptor with tirofiban in unstable angina and non-Q-wave myocardial infarction. N Engl J Med 1998; 338: 1488–97.

6. Topol EJ, Moliterno DJ, Herrmann HC et al. Do tirofiban and reopro give similar efficacy trial. Comparison of two platelet glycoprotein IIb/IIIa inhibitors, tirofiban and abciximab, for the prevention of ischemic events with percutaneous coronary revascularization. N Engl J Med 2001; 344: 1888–94.

7. Batchelor WB, Tolleson TR, Huang Y et al. Randomized COMparison of platelet inhibition with abciximab, tiRofiban and eptifibatide during percutaneous coronary intervention in acute coronary syndromes: the COMPARE trial. Comparison of measurements of platelet aggregation with aggrastat, reopro, and eptifibatide. Circulation 2002; 106: 1470–6.

8. Valgimigli M, Percoco G, Barbieri D et al. The additive value of tirofiban administered with the high-dose bolus in the prevention of ischemic complications during high-risk coronary angioplasty: the ADVANCE Trial. J Am Coll Cardiol 2004; 44: 14–19.

9. Antithrombotic Trialists' Collaboration. Collaborative meta-analysis of randomised trials of antiplatelet therapy for prevention of death, myocardial infarction, and stroke in high-risk patients. BMJ 2002; 324: 71–86.

10. ISIS-2 (Second International Study of Infarct Survival) Collaborative Group. Randomised trial of intravenous streptokinase, oral aspirin, both, or neither among 17 187 cases of suspected acute myocardial infarction: ISIS-2. Lancet 1988; 332: 349–60.

11. Patrono C, Garcia Rodriguez LA, Landolfi R et al. Low-dose aspirin for the prevention of atherothrombosis. N Engl J Med 2005; 353: 2373–83.

12. Rocca B, Patrono C. Determinants of the interindividual variability in response to antiplatelet drugs. J Thromb Haemost 2005; 3: 1597–602.

13. Patrono C. Aspirin resistance: definition, mechanisms and clinical read-outs. J Thromb Haemost 2003; 1: 1710–13.

14. Bhatt DL. Aspirin resistance: more than just a laboratory curiosity. J Am Coll Cardiol 2004; 43: 1127–9.

15. Eikelboom, JW, Hirsh J, Weitz JI et al. Aspirin resistant thromboxane biosynthesis and the risk of myocardial infarction, stroke, or cardiovascular death in patients at high risk for cardiovascular events. Circulation 2002; 105: 1650–5.

16. Gum PA, Kottke-Marchant K, Welsh PA et al. A prospective, blinded determination of the natural history of aspirin resistance among stable patients with cardiovascular disease. J Am Coll Cardiol 2003; 41: 961–5.

17. Mueller MR, Salat A, Stangl P et al. Variable platelet response to low-dose ASA and the risk of limb deterioration in patients submitted to peripheral arterial angioplasty. Thromb Haemost 1997; 78: 1003–7.

18. Grotemeyer KH, Scharafinski HW, Husstedt IW. Two-year follow-up of aspirin responder and aspirin non responder. A pilot-study including 180 post-stroke patients. Thromb Res 1993; 71: 397–403.

19. Grundmann K, Jaschonek K, Kleine B et al. Aspirin non-responder status in patients with recurrent cerebral ischemic attacks. J Neurol 2003; 250: 63–6.

20. Chen WH, Lee PY, Ng W et al. Aspirin resistance is associated with a high incidence of myonecrosis after non-urgent percutaneous coronary intervention despite clopidogrel pretreatment. J Am Coll Cardiol 2004; 43: 1122–6.

21. Savi P, Herbert JM. Clopidogrel and ticlopidine: P2Y12 adenosine diphosphate-receptor antagonists for the prevention of atherothrombosis. Semin Thromb Hemost 2005; 31: 174–83.

22. Bertrand ME, Rupprecht HJ, Urban P et al. Double-blind study of the safety of clopidogrel with and without a loading dose in combination with aspirin compared with ticlopidine in

combination with aspirin after coronary stenting: the clopidogrel aspirin stent international cooperative study (CLASSICS). Circulation 2000; 102: 624–9.

23. Cadroy Y, Bossavy JP, Thalamas C et al. Early potent antithrombotic effect with combined aspirin and a loading dose of clopidogrel on experimental arterial thrombogenesis in humans. Circulation 2000; 101: 2823–8.

24. Bhatt DL, Bertrand ME, Berger PB et al. Meta-analysis of randomized and registry comparisons of ticlopidine with clopidogrel after stenting. J Am Coll Cardiol 2002; 39: 9–14.

25. Yusuf S, Zhao F, Mehta SR et al; Clopidogrel in Unstable Angina to Prevent Recurrent Events Trial Investigators. Effects of clopidogrel in addition to aspirin in patients with acute coronary syndromes without ST-segment elevation. N Engl J Med 2001; 345: 494–502.

26. Mehta SR, Yusuf S, Peters RJ et al. Clopidogrel in Unstable angina to prevent Recurrent Events trial (CURE) Investigators. Effects of pretreatment with clopidogrel and aspirin followed by long-term therapy in patients undergoing percutaneous coronary intervention: the PCI-CURE study. Lancet 2001; 358: 527–33.

27. Steinhubl SR, Berger PB, Mann JT 3rd et al. CREDO Investigators. Clopidogrel for the Reduction of Events During Observation. Early and sustained dual oral antiplatelet therapy following percutaneous coronary intervention: a randomized controlled trial (CREDO). JAMA 2002; 288: 2411–20.

28. Angiolillo DJ, Fernandez-Ortiz A, Bernardo E et al. Identification of low responders to a 300 mg clopidogrel loading dose in patients undergoing coronary stenting. Thromb Res 2005; 115: 101–8.

29. Angiolillo DJ, Fernandez-Ortiz A, Bernardo E et al. High clopidogrel loading dose during coronary stenting: Effects on drug response and interindividual variability. Eur Heart J 2004; 25: 1903–10.

30. Gurbel PA, Bliden KP, Hiatt BL et al. Clopidogrel for coronary stenting: response variability, drug resistance, and the effect of pretreatment platelet reactivity. Circulation 2003; 107: 2908–13.

31. Serebruany VL, Steinhubl SR, Berger PB et al. Variability in platelet responsiveness to clopidogrel among 544 individuals. J Am Coll Cardiol. 2005; 45: 246–51.

32. Taubert D, Kastrati A, Harlfinger S et al. Pharmacokinetics of clopidogrel after administration of a high loading dose. Thromb Haemost 2004; 92: 311–16.

33. Lau WC, Waskell LA, Watkins PB et al. Atorvastatin reduces the ability of clopidogrel to inhibit platelet aggregation: a new drug–drug interaction. Circulation 2003; 107: 32–7.

34. Nguyen TA, Diodati JG, Pharand C. Resistance to clopidogrel: a review of the evidence. J Am Coll Cardiol 2005; 45: 1157–64.

35. Lau WC, Gurbel PA, Watkins PB et al. Contribution of hepatic cytochrome P450 3A4 metabolic activity to the phenomenon of clopidogrel resistance. Circulation 2004; 109: 166–71.

36. Angiolillo DJ, Fernandez-Ortiz A, Bernardo E et al. Contribution of gene sequence variations of the hepatic cytochrome P450 3A4 enzyme to variability in individual responsiveness to clopidogrel. Arterioscler Thromb Vasc Biol 2006; 26: 1895–900.

37. Fontana P, Dupont A, Gandrille S et al. Adenosine diphosphate-induced platelet aggregation is associated with P2Y12 gene sequence variations in healthy subjects. Circulation 2003; 108: 989–95.

38. von Beckerath N, von Beckerath O, Koch W et al. P2Y12 gene H2 haplotype is not associated with increased adenosine diphosphate-induced platelet aggregation after initiation of clopidogrel therapy with a high loading dose. Blood Coagul Fibrinolysis 2005; 16: 199–204.

39. Angiolillo DJ, Fernández-Ortiz A, Bernardo E et al. Lack of association between the P2Y$_{12}$ receptor gene polymorphism and platelet response to clopidogrel in patients with coronary artery disease. Thromb Res 2005; 116: 491–7.

40. Angiolillo DJ, Fernandez-Ortiz A, Bernardo E et al. Platelet function profiles in patients with type 2 diabetes and coronary artery disease on combined aspirin and clopidogrel treatment. Diabetes 2005; 54: 2430–5.

41. Soffer D, Moussa I, Harjai KJ et al. Impact of angina class on inhibition of platelet aggregation following clopidogrel loading in patients undergoing coronary intervention: do we need more aggressive dosing regimens in unstable angina? Catheter Cardiovasc Interv 2003; 59: 21–5.

42. Angiolillo DJ, Fernandez-Ortiz A, Bernardo E et al. Platelet aggregation according to body mass index in patients undergoing coronary stenting: should clopidogrel loading-dose be weight adjusted? J Invasive Cardiol 2004; 16: 169–74.
43. Angiolillo DJ, Bernardo E, Ramirez C et al. Insulin therapy is associated with platelet dysfunction in patients with type 2 diabetes mellitus on dual oral antiplatelet treatment. J Am Coll Cardiol 2006; 48: 298–304.
44. Muller I, Besta F, Schulz C et al. Prevalence of clopidogrel non-responders among patients with stable angina pectoris scheduled for elective coronary stent placement. Thromb Haemost 2003; 89: 783–7.
45. Barragan P, Bouvier JL, Roquebert PO et al. Resistance to thienopyridines: clinical detection of coronary stent thrombosis by monitoring of vasodilator-stimulated phosphoprotein phosphorylation. Catheter Cardiovasc Interv 2003; 59: 295–302.
46. Matetzky S, Shenkman B, Guetta V et al. Clopidogrel resistance is associated with increased risk of recurrent atherothrombotic events in patients with acute myocardial infarction. Circulation 2004; 109: 3171–5.
47. Bernardo E, Angiolillo DJ, Ramirez C et al. Prevalence of concomitant suboptimal responsiveness to aspirin and clopidogrel treatment in diabetic patients. J Am Coll Cardiol 2006; 47 (Suppl A): 364A.
48. Lev EI, Patel RT, Maresh KJ et al. Aspirin and clopidogrel drug response in patients undergoing percutaneous coronary intervention: the role of dual drug resistance. J Am Coll Cardiol 2006; 47: 27–33.
49. Topol EJ, Easton D, Harrington RA et al. Randomized, double-blind, placebo-controlled, international trial of the oral IIb/IIIa antagonist lotrafiban in coronary and cerebrovascular disease. Circulation 2003; 108: 399–406.
50. Peters RJG, Mehta SR, Fox KAA et al, for the Clopidogrel in Unstable angina to prevent Recurrent Events (CURE) Trial Investigators. Effects of aspirin dose when used alone or in combination with clopidogrel in patients with acute coronary syndromes: observations from the Clopidogrel in Unstable angina to prevent Recurrent Events (CURE) Study. Circulation 2003; 108: 1682–7.
51. CAPRIE Steering Committee. A randomised, blinded, trial of clopidogrel versus aspirin in patients at risk of ischaemic events (CAPRIE). Lancet 1996; 348: 1329–39.
52. Kastrati A, Mehilli J, Schuhlen H et al. A clinical trial of abciximab in elective percutaneous coronary intervention after pretreatment with clopidogrel. N Engl J Med 2004; 350: 232–8.
53. Valles J, Santos MT, Aznar J et al. Erythrocyte promotion of platelet reactivity decreases the effectiveness of aspirin as an antithrombotic therapeutic modality: the effect of low-dose aspirin is less than optimal in patients with vascular disease due to prothrombotic effects of erythrocytes on platelet reactivity. Circulation 1998; 97: 350–5.
54. Angiolillo DJ, Fernandez-Ortiz A, Bernardo E et al. Influence of aspirin resistance on platelet function profiles in patients on long-term aspirin and clopidogrel after percutaneous coronary intervention. Am J Cardiol 2006; 97: 38–43.
55. Serebruany V, Malinin A, Ziai W et al. Dipyridamole decreases protease-activated receptor and annexin-v binding on platelets of post stroke patients with aspirin nonresponsiveness. Cerebrovasc Dis 2006; 21: 98–105.
56. Bhatt DL, Fox KA, Hacke W et al; CHARISMA Investigators. Clopidogrel and aspirin versus aspirin alone for the prevention of atherothrombotic events. N Engl J Med 2006; 354: 1706–17.
57. Gorchakova O, von Beckerath N, Gawaz M et al. Antiplatelet effects of a 600 mg loading dose of clopidogrel are not attenuated in patients receiving atorvastatin or simvastatin for at least 4 weeks prior to coronary artery stenting. Eur Heart J 2004; 25: 1898–902.
58. Patti G, Colonna G, Pasceri V et al. Randomized trial of high loading dose of clopidogrel for reduction of periprocedural myocardial infarction in patients undergoing coronary intervention: results from the ARMYDA-2 (Antiplatelet therapy for Reduction of MYocardial Damage during Angioplasty) study. Circulation 2005; 111: 2099–106.
59. von Beckerath N, Taubert D, Pogatsa-Murray G et al. Absorption, metabolization, and antiplatelet effects of 300-, 600-, and 900-mg loading doses of clopidogrel: results of the

ISARCHOICE (Intracoronary Stenting and Antithrombotic Regimen: Choose Between 3 High Oral Doses for Immediate Clopidogrel Effect) Trial. Circulation 2005; 112: 2946–50.

60. Montalescot G. Assessment of the best loading dose of clopidogrel to blunt platelet activation, inflammation, and ongoing necrosis (ALBION) Study. In: EuroPCR. Paris, France: 2005.

61. Kastrati A, von Beckerath N, Joost A et al. Loading with 600 mg clopidogrel in patients with coronary artery disease with and without chronic clopidogrel therapy. Circulation 2004; 110: 1916–19.

62. Niitsu Y, Jakubowski JA, Sugidachi A et al. Pharmacology of CS-747 (prasugrel, LY640315), a novel, potent antiplatelet agent with in vivo P2Y12 receptor antagonist activity. Semin Thromb Hemost 2005; 31: 184–94.

63. Wiviott SD, Antman EM, Winters KJ et al; JUMBO-TIMI 26 Investigators. Randomized comparison of prasugrel (CS-747, LY640315), a novel thienopyridine P2Y12 antagonist, with clopidogrel in percutaneous coronary intervention: results of the Joint Utilization of Medications to Block Platelets Optimally (JUMBO)-TIMI 26 trial. Circulation 2005; 111: 3366–73.

64. van Giezen JJ, Humphries RG. Preclinical and clinical studies with selective reversible direct P2Y12 antagonists. Semin Thromb Hemost 2005; 31: 195–204.

65. Cannon C, Husted S, Storey R et al, for the DISPERSE 2 Investigators. The DISPERSE2 Trial: Safety, Tolerability and Preliminary Efficacy of AZD6140, the First Oral Reversible ADP Receptor Antagonist, Compared with Clopidogrel in Patients with Non-ST-Segment Elevation Acute Coronary Syndrome. In: American Heart Association Scientific Sessions, 2005, at Dallas, TX, USA, 2005.

66. Greenbaum AB, Grines CL, Bittl JA et al. Initial experience with an intravenous P2Y12 platelet receptor antagonist in patients undergoing percutaneous coronary intervention: results from a 2-part, phase II, multicenter, randomized, placebo- and active-controlled trial. Am Heart J 2006; 151: 689.e1–689.e10.

67. Gurbel PA, Bliden KP, Guyer K et al. Platelet reactivity in patients and recurrent events post-stenting: results of the PREPARE POST-STENTING Study. J Am Coll Cardiol 2005; 46: 1820–6.

Index